THE EDUCATION
OF AUDIOLOGISTS AND
SPEECH-LANGUAGE
PATHOLOGISTS

THE EDUCATION OF AUDIOLOGISTS AND SPEECH-LANGUAGE PATHOLOGISTS

Edited by
Judith A. Rassi and
Margaret D. McElroy

YORK PRESS   Timonium, Maryland

This book was manufactured in the United States of America. Typography by Brushwood Graphics, Inc., Baltimore, Maryland. Printing and binding by Maple-Vail Book Manufacturing Group, York, Pennsylvania. Cover design by Joseph Dieter, Jr.

ISBN 0-912752-30-0

Library of Congress Cataloging-In-Publication Data

Rassi, Judith A., 1939–
    The education of audiologists and speech-language pathologists /
Judith A. Rassi and Margaret D. McElroy.
        p.   cm.
    Includes bibliographical references and index.
    ISBN 0-912752-30-0
    1. Speech therapy—Study and teaching.   2. Audiology—Study and teaching.   I. McElroy, Margaret D.   II. Title.
    [DNLM: 1. Audiology—education.   2. Speech-Language Pathology—education.   3. Teaching—methods.   WV 18 R228e]
RC428.R37   1992
616.85′00711—dc20
DNLM/DLC
for Library of Congress   92-16758
                                                                                    CIP

Dedicated to
the Learners and Teachers of
Audiology and Speech-Language Pathology

Contents

SECTION V   Appendices

Foreword

> The world seldom notices who the teachers are; but civilization depends
> on what they do and what they say.
>
> —Anonymous

There is no doubt in my mind that this text, *The Education of Audiologists and Speech-Language Pathologists,* is long overdue. As professionals in audiology and speech-language pathology, we are involved in educational planning and in teaching activities at almost every point of our career cycle. We work most of the time as either teacher/clinician, teacher/supervisor, or teacher/faculty member. It is very hard in our profession to avoid any of these roles, individually or combined, or the impact of the educational activities produced by them.

Rassi and McElroy suggest that a change must occur in the routine education we have developed to foster teachers and teaching in communication sciences and disorders (CSD). They propose that we must " . . . inspire these instructors [CSD] to seek improvement in their teaching and to experiment with innovative strategies." Their advice is quite on-target because few of us working in higher education have been trained formally to teach in the classroom. There is the assumption that if one has a good grasp of the subject matter, one can teach a course about that subject. Rassi and McElroy challenge that assumption and raise serious questions about the quality of teaching in our educational programs.

The authors have done an excellent job of informing the reader about pedagogical and andragogical matters as they relate to CSD. The focus of the book is divided between academic education and clinical education in order to establish that a positive relationship exists between the two areas of learning and that whatever happens in the classroom will affect the activities in the clinic, and vice versa.

Teaching in one capacity or another involves everything we do along the professional continuum. It is time for professionals in CSD to take notice of the quality of our teachers for the sake of providing quality education to our students. We must showcase the important role of education and teaching, not only to the professionals in CSD, but also to our students, because today's student certainly will be tomorrow's teacher. For these reasons, the authors have emphasized the importance of maintaining quality in teaching and have described how best to implement quality teaching models that reflect societal changes. This direction is necessary in order to stimulate quality of thinking in our students because "civilization depends on what they do."

Charlena M. Seymour, Ph.D., CCC-SLP
Vice President for Quality of Service, 1990–1992
American Speech-Language-Hearing Association

Preface

The need for educational reform in this country, a topic of daily discussion in the mass media, is apparently pervasive. Charges of inadequacy, and worse, have been leveled at elementary, secondary, postsecondary, and higher education. One need only turn to *The Closing of the American Mind* (Bloom 1987) and *ProfScam* (Sykes 1988) to experience a painful glimpse into sweeping indictments of higher education. Regardless of the educational level at which the myriad problems occur, they do affect, either directly or indirectly, the preparation of audiologists and speech-language pathologists. While the quality of students entering graduate programs in communication sciences and disorders (CSD) is of specific concern to educators, an increasing number of professionals in the field—many of them practitioners—are questioning the quality of the educational programs themselves. Yet, as suggested by a survey of 192 instructors in programs accredited by the Educational Services Board (ESB) of the American Speech-Language-Hearing Association (ASHA), the instructors tend to think otherwise. They rate the quality of classroom teaching as very good to excellent in their own work settings and in other ESB programs, compared with mediocre to ordinary ratings for U.S. higher education as a whole (Rassi and McElroy 1988). Even so, as detailed in this book, there is an undercurrent of concern shared by speech-language-hearing professionals in diverse settings about numerous educational issues.

In considering whether education and teaching in our field—at undergraduate, graduate, or continuing education levels—ought to be explored to examine the present status and to upgrade quality, we realized the need for gathering and disseminating information that would lead to this end. Two sets of circumstances were compelling. Clinical supervision, or clinical teaching, had emerged as a viable area of research and study in the field, resulting in scholarly conferences, a growing body of literature, and burgeoning interest in applying sound educational principles to the clinical setting. But there was no corresponding attempt to look at classroom or laboratory teaching in the field of communication sciences and disorders. Likewise, we found, in comparable areas such as the allied health professions, medicine, nursing, social work, psychology, and psychiatry, as well as teacher education itself, many facets of teaching in a variety of settings and formats have been investigated—indeed, there are entire journals devoted to the subject. And, again, there has been no corresponding attempt to do this in our field.

The abundance of information produced by these sources contrasted strikingly with the void in CSD education; it also gave us a starting place. The data and experiences of those whose pursuits are similar to one's own can be quite beneficial, of course. In this case, we believe, the material provides a conceptual framework, a meaningful vocabulary, a fund of research ideas, and numerous applications that can be incorporated into CSD teaching.

It is our hope that this book will broaden the perspectives of classroom, laboratory, and clinical teachers in audiology and speech-language pathology and, in doing so, inspire these instructors to seek improvement in their teaching and to experiment with innovative strategies. The need for this (re)dedication was illustrated in another phase of the earlier mentioned survey (Rassi and McElroy 1988; McElroy and Rassi 1989). In a sample of some 175 classroom instructors from ESB programs, 73% indicated that, although they had some awareness or knowledge of 16 different teaching/learning factors, more than half of these factors were never applied in their teaching. This finding serves to corroborate a statement made by The Holmes Group (1986), a consortium of deans and other leaders in education from major research universities: "The case can be made, in fact, that the nation's troubles with student learning in schools are closely tied to popular and excessively simple conceptions of teaching" (p. 27). Indeed, the notion that educators in our field might view classroom teaching in its simplest terms will sound familiar to those supervisors in speech-language pathology and audiology who have, for so many years, struggled to convince their colleagues that clinical supervision is a substantive educational endeavor requiring planning and study.

Although a major emphasis is placed on teaching, other pertinent facets of education are addressed herein as well. The historical markers of CSD education as well as critical commentary and other observations appear throughout. We should note that occasional overlapping of information between chapters was necessary for the sake of clarity. And, to clarify our semantic choices: audiology and speech-language pathology are viewed as a single field or discipline, that is, communication sciences and disorders, but as representing two different professions—the order of the two terms alternates somewhat arbitrarily;

clinical supervision and clinical teaching are used interchangeably, as are patient and client; his/her is used consistently.

The purpose of this book, then, is to present distilled information from numerous sources and, at the same time, lead educators in our field to relevant literature that exists beyond the narrow confines of speech-language pathology and audiology. Enroute, we hope to persuade continuing-education planners, educational program administrators, curriculum planners, classroom and laboratory instructors, clinical supervisors, and student advisers that all areas of educational endeavor warrant scrutiny. Indeed, the futures of audiology and speech-language pathology depend on it.

Judith A. Rassi
Margaret D. McElroy

REFERENCES

Bloom, A. 1987. *The Closing of the American Mind.* New York: Simon and Schuster, Inc.

The Holmes Group. 1986. *Tomorrow's Teachers: A Report of The Holmes Group.* East Lansing, MI: Author.

McElroy, M. D., and Rassi, J. A. 1989. Instructors' perceptions of clinical teaching in ESB-accredited programs. In *Supervision: Innovations. A National Conference on Supervision,* ed. D. A. Shapiro. Cullowhee, NC: Western Carolina University.

Rassi, J. A., and McElroy, M. D. 1988, November. Classroom teaching in ESB-accredited programs: A survey of instructors. Miniseminar presented at the American Speech-Language-Hearing Association Convention, Boston.

Sykes, C. J. 1988. *ProfScam: Professors and the Demise of Higher Education.* Washington, DC: Regnery Gateway.

Acknowledgments

Writing and editing a book require the support and cooperation of many individuals, not only those whose names appear on the list of contributors. The sense of personal enrichment we gained from these associations goes well beyond the satisfaction derived from uncovering new information and seeing a book materialize. To these persons, we are indebted. In particular, we are grateful to Martha and Nicholas Bountress for helping us to launch this project; to Charlena Seymour for lending her endorsement and words to these pages; to Sandra Ulrich for her sage editorial advice; and to the staff of York Press.

Furthermore, respectively and respectfully:

I, Judith Rassi, thank David Zarefsky, Jeri Logemann, and Dean Garstecki of Northwestern University who showed their confidence in this venture by granting me a three-month leave to begin the work with my co-author. This administrative support has continued at Vanderbilt University where Fred Bess has generously given me words of encouragement along with the necessary time to complete the book. I also thank Sara Hoffman who graciously took on the task of manuscript reading and editing. A host of colleagues, friends, and family members has sustained me throughout, providing helpful advice and proper motivation. Thank you, all.

I, Margaret McElroy, know that the reality of this book would not have been possible for me without the administrative support of John Horner, Richard Talbott, and Robert Pate; the technological and moral support of Zahrl Schoeny; the unfailing patience and encouragement of family and friends; the kindness of Brenda Strawley and Annelle Hodges as readers; and the understanding of the graduate students in audiology at the University of Virginia. Particular acknowledgment is given to the late Dr. Helen Gunderson Burr for her specialness as my mentor, colleague, and friend.

Finally, we do want to thank those whose names appear on the list of contributors, that is, the chapter authors. Each an expert in the area of his/her chapter topic, has added authority, credibility, and dimension to this book.

Judith A. Rassi
Margaret D. McElroy

Contributors

Nicholas W. Bankson, Ph.D.
Professor and Chair
Department of
  Communication Disorders
Boston University
Boston, MA

John E. Bernthal, Ph.D.
Professor and Chair
Department of Special
  Education & Communication
  Disorders
University of Nebraska-
  Lincoln
Lincoln, NE

Glen L. Bull, Ph.D.
Associate Professor
Instructional Technology
  Program
Curry School of Education
University of Virginia
Charlottesville, VA

Paula S. Cochran, Ph.D.
Assistant Professor
Department of
  Communication Disorders
Northeast Missouri State
  University
Kirksville, MO

Ellen C. Fagan, M.S., Director
Continuing Education Division
American Speech-Language-
Hearing Association
Rockville, MD

Cynthia G. Fowler, Ph.D.
Audiology Section
Veterans Administration
  Medical Center
Long Beach, CA

Gloria D. Kellum, Ph.D., Director
Clinical Services
Department of Communicative
  Disorders
University of Mississippi
University, MS

Janet S. Leonards, Ph.D.
Educational Psychologist and
  Adjunct Faculty
University of Southern
  California
California State University
Long Beach, CA

Margaret D. McElroy, M.Ed., M.S.
Clinical Instructor of
  Audiology and
Coordinator of Audiology
  Services
Communication Disorders
  Program
University of Virginia
Charlottesville, VA

Judith A. Rassi, M.A.
Associate Professor and

Coordinator of Clinical
  Teaching
Division of Hearing and
  Speech Sciences
School of Medicine
Vanderbilt University
Nashville, TN

Robert L. Schum, Ph.D.
  Clinical Psychologist
  Department of Speech
    Pathology and Audiology
  Wendell Johnson Speech &
    Hearing Clinic
  University of Iowa
  Iowa City, IA

Charlena M. Seymour, Ph.D., Chair
  Department of
    Communication Disorders

University of Massachusetts-
  Amherst
Amherst, MA
Vice-President for Quality of
  Service
American Speech-Language-
  Hearing Association
Rockville, MD

Jo Williams, M.Aud., Director
  Audiology Branch
  American Speech-Language-
    Hearing Association
  Rockville, MD

Richard H. Wilson, Ph.D., Chief
  Audiology Section
  Veterans Administration
    Medical Center
  Long Beach, CA

SECTION I

Educational Framework

Chapter 1

Learning Teaching, Improving Teaching

Margaret D. McElroy and Judith A. Rassi

The preparation and training of teachers has long been a subject of debate in this country. While experts and would-be experts question the value of educational methods courses and other teacher-training efforts, charges of diminishing teaching quality are being leveled at educators from preschool through higher education. Should classroom instructors in higher education be trained in methods of teaching? Is the quality of teaching poorer now than it was twenty years ago? Have the publish-or-perish demands of academia discounted the value of quality teaching in the minds of those who do it? The questions are many, the answers few.

It is our belief that educational programs in speech-language pathology and audiology, and the teaching problems they reportedly have, represent a microcosm of the nation's attitudes toward, and shortcomings in, higher education. While a disproportionate number of students with poorer credentials than those of their predecessors may now be entering communication sciences and disorders (CSD) programs, this problem, too, belongs to higher education in general. Although we agree that every attempt should be made to recruit the brightest students into audiology and speech-language pathology, the odds are that not all of our students will ever represent the brightest available.

Given this probability then, CSD educators should expect to have students with a wide range of abilities. All need the best education possible. Those with less ability and/or with poorer educational backgrounds present special learning needs. Unlike their brighter and better-educated counterparts who can learn despite poor teaching, these individuals may find learning difficult. The challenge to educators in audiology and speech-language pathology, therefore, is to provide the best teaching possible.

This chapter discusses the means for learning and improving classroom teaching. It should be noted here that there is no comparable chapter in this book on the preparation of clinical teachers or supervisors. The reason is that the topic of supervisory training in this field has already been addressed in other writings (e.g., Rassi 1978; Anderson 1988; Casey, Smith, and Ulrich 1988; Anderson et al. 1989; Farmer and Farmer 1989) whereas classroom teaching has not been similarly examined.

TEACHER EDUCATION

The Carnegie Task Force on Teaching as a Profession (Weis et al. 1989) recommended in 1986 the creation of a National Board of Professional Teaching Standards (Carnegie Forum 1986). Among the board's objectives were establishing a new set of assessments for teaching; reaching concurrence on the knowledge base of teaching; and benefiting the curriculum for teacher education. Another body with similar aims, The Holmes Group (1986; Weis et al. 1989), endorsed the establishment of a professional school for teachers at the graduate level that is related to a research-based curriculum and a firm liberal arts education. A goal of this group is to develop the knowledge base of teaching in a curriculum that intensifies bonds with the university and raises the status of teaching. Both the Carnegie Task Force and The Holmes Group support advanced positions in teaching to attract and retain the best teachers.

Schools of Education

Schools of education and the teacher certification process are structured in accordance with state regulations (Gideonse 1989) and, thus, are subject to a certain amount of political scrutiny. Given the nation's problems, which have been directly or indirectly linked to the quality of education in general and the quality of teaching in particular, teacher-education programs are particularly vulnerable to criticism. In its deliberations on the need for change in teacher-education programs, The Holmes Group (1986), composed of deans from colleges of education and research-oriented schools, advised that the time required for preservice preparation be increased. Such an undertaking would require a professional teacher-preparation faculty. Indeed, all the proposals put forth by The Holmes Group would entail a major overhaul of schools of education.

It should be pointed out here that, whereas teacher education is the responsibility of teacher educators, the education of teachers is the responsibility of the entire college or university (Imig 1986). Thus, the leadership in a teacher education program must rely on its continuing working relationship with the institution's leadership.

Training College/University Teachers

More colleges and universities now offer teacher training, and in a greater variety of formats, than ever before. Indeed, the college/university teacher, heretofore left to his/her own devices, is being offered teaching assistance—albeit usually on an informal, voluntary basis—by those in teacher education at the teacher's own institution. Largely the result of students' complaints and their poor evaluations of instructors, along with an increasingly critical public, this concern for teaching quality has been addressed by university administrators who are being held accountable by their boards of trustees.

Not surprisingly, however, this concern seems to be taken less seriously at those universities where research continues to be the top priority and where, no matter what value is said to be placed on quality teaching, every faculty member knows that research productivity, more than teaching quality, is supported and rewarded. Stated differently, a productive researcher who happens not to be an effective teacher has the more secure position than does the nonproductive researcher whose teaching may be lauded. Achievement in both areas would be ideal, of course. But, faced with a choice of spending time on learning new teaching techniques and preparing for class, or on pursuing new research avenues, a university teacher/researcher is likely to opt for the latter.

Sykes (1988) asserts that "the neglect of teaching" (p. 61) can be detected when teachers:

- Merely regurgitate the textbook
- Rely on notes prepared when they were younger, more ambitious, and without tenure
- Dwell on their own specialties without bothering to translate the material from the arcane jargon of their specialty
- Turn their classes into rap sessions, a tactic that has the advantage of being both entertaining and educationally progressive
- Fail to prepare at all and treat their classes to an off-the-top-of-the-head ramble, leaping from topic to topic in what they think are dazzling intellectual trapeze acts but which are confusing, frustrating muddles for the students (p. 61)

Fortunately, this is not the case with every instructor. Many classroom teachers in colleges and universities are conscientious about their teaching and continually seek to improve it. And some of them seem to be in our field.

Teacher Preparation in CSD Programs. In a survey of CSD instructors on the topic of classroom teaching in ESB-accredited educational programs (Rassi and McElroy 1988; McElroy and Rassi 1989), 146, or 76%, of the 192 respondents indicated that they had had some kind of specific preparation for their roles as classroom instructors. They reported involvement in a variety of preparation activities, with most persons participating in more than one kind. In order of prevalence, their most frequent involvement was in: consulting with colleagues; serving as teaching assistants; taking educational methods courses; observing teacher models; student teaching; and studying independently.

An average five years prior to the survey marked the time of the group's most recent involvement in some kinds of teacher preparation or improvement activity. When their years of classroom instruction experience were compared with their most recent participation in improvement activities, over two-thirds of this group were found to have involved themselves in such activities during the second half of their teaching years. When asked how helpful this teacher training effort was for them, 49 subjects thought it was "very helpful but not essential," 42 indicated that it was "moderately helpful," 38 found it to be "essential to teacher role," 18 said it was "minimally helpful," and four found it to be "noncontributory" (McElroy and Rassi 1989, p. 108).

Of the 39 subjects who reported never having participated in any kind of classroom instructor preparation, most indicated that their reason for not doing so was the unavailability of appealing preparation opportunities. Importantly, only six of the untrained subjects considered additional preparation for classroom instructors in higher education to be unnecessary.

Some university schools or departments of education offering a program for the express purpose of training new college teachers or assisting untrained, experienced ones, have found a consultation format to be more workable than formal coursework. Studies have shown that student evaluations of teachers' effectiveness are higher in some cases following such consultation (Carroll 1977; Erickson and Erickson 1979). Where formal courses and workshops for college teachers are offered, improvement in teaching effectiveness also is demonstrated (Grasha 1978; Levinson-Rose and Menges 1981; Justice 1983). These courses frequently are offered through university faculty development centers or teacher support centers.

University Teacher Support Centers. Drawing from the representativeness of our own employer institutions, we present three examples of university teacher support centers. Northwestern University offers graduate students opportunities to increase their classroom experience through summer session programs. Department chairpersons and program directors are encouraged to identify graduate students who have distinguished scholastic records and have shown ability to work well with undergraduates in classroom settings. These individuals are then assigned summer school courses to teach. However, prior to the beginning of the summer session, each teacher-to-be must attend three of five seminars on instructional issues.

In Virginia, seven teacher-training research centers were established by the State Council of Higher Education (Richardson 1988). One of the centers, located at the University of Virginia, is developing a computer simulator of classroom teaching situations (Richardson 1988). Providing instantaneous feedback for teachers, the system and format have been found to increase the confidence of preservice teachers and allow them to compare their performances with a model of successful teaching.

At Vanderbilt University, the Center for Teaching (Staff 1990) offers a series of informal "brown bag seminars" for faculty and graduate teaching assistants. Many seminar speakers themselves have won teaching awards. One facet of the program is the videotaping of instructors' classroom teaching, which is then used for follow-up self-examination. General information about the craft of teaching is also provided through workshops, consultation, a newsletter, and a library. An orientation component of the program is required for foreign graduate teaching assistants (Wannamaker 1989). In operation since 1986, the program has been well received by faculty at all levels as well as by graduate assistants.

The Continuing Problem. Notwithstanding these kinds of fruitful efforts, it is important even now to note the concern, expressed in 1985, of the Association of American Colleges (1985) about "the failure of graduate schools to prepare holders of the doctorate degree for careers in teaching" (p. 29). The report points out that exposure to teaching is by chance and occurs only in the capacity of a teaching assistant with periodic supervision by senior faculty. During work toward the doctorate, students are seldom exposed to any of the components that compose "the art, the science, and the special responsibilities of teaching" (p. 29). A national survey of teaching assistants conducted by Diamond and Gray (1987) indicates varied expectations of teaching assistants and variation in their support systems. Although university teaching centers undoubtedly have helped to improve this situation, we are unaware of the numbers of graduate programs, inside or outside of CSD, that require that their doctoral students take advantage of the support that is available.

Preparation Modes

Subject Knowledge, Self-Study. Lowman (1984) considers intelligence and academic preparation germane to competent teaching. Eble (1988) stresses the need for teachers at the university level to be familiar with testing, grading, planning readings and assignments, and developing a course. He suggests these books for beginning teachers: *Teaching Tips: A Guidebook for the Beginning College Teacher* (McKeachie 1986); *Teaching and Learning in Higher Education* (Beard 1972); *Studies of College Teaching* (Ellner and Barnes 1983); *A Practical Handbook for College Teachers* (Fuhrmann and Grasha 1983); and *The Art and Craft of Teaching* (Gullette 1982).

Practice Teaching. Teacher preparation usually includes practice teaching and discussion groups composed of teaching assistants and other individuals interested in teaching who meet periodically during the semester (Eble 1988). In some institutions, practice teaching is supervised, whereas in others, it is carried out in collaboration with peers and faculty (Eble 1988). Supervision by a regular faculty member is mandatory in some programs.

The need for larger numbers of outstanding teachers to serve as models was noted by Eble in 1980. However, more recently, Eble (1988) pointed out that future teachers should focus on analytical examination of diverse teaching situations rather than concentrate on models taken from graduate school observations. Ericksen (1984) also stated that teaching models do not necessarily represent the real effects of teaching on a day-to-day basis. He pointed to the interaction between the teacher and learner as critical to teaching and to the manner in which the instructor affects the learner's "motivation and values, learning, memory, problem solving, and learning how to learn and to think independently" (p. 5).

Teaching Apprenticeship. As a variation on the practice teaching theme, Lowman (1984) suggests a teaching apprenticeship—an arrangement whereby an experienced instructor teaches a course, which is first observed by the graduate student who will teach it in a subsequent school term. During both the observation stage and the participation stage, the apprentice becomes involved in preparing the course, attending class, and meeting on a regular basis with the instructor.

Teaching Seminars. Another teacher preparation suggestion made by Lowman (1984) is that of a seminar in college teaching for graduate students before they begin teaching. It requires more organization than the apprentice model, but may be a more efficient use of faculty time (Lowman 1984). In this format, the graduate student can lead small group discussions, give lectures, and have firsthand experience in grading. Seminars in teaching give faculty and students the opportunity to work as colleagues (Eble 1988), sharing information about the various components of teaching.

Supervised Teaching. No matter what initial approach is used in teacher education, the instructor-to-be needs a strong support system in the person of a consultant or supervisor during the first semester or term in the classroom. This teaching consultation should include classroom observations with feedback sessions. Videotapes of the classroom also can be useful.

Experiential Bases. Ericksen (1970) points out that new instructors may favor specific teaching techniques based on previous observations of their teachers. Their personal images of good teaching are, in many cases, based on these experiences. Cantrell (1973) found that some instructors who relied upon their own student experiences in developing teaching techniques said they concentrated on their memories of bad teaching, then avoided repeating these mistakes. Other individuals interviewed by Cantrell reported that they adopted a specific "method" (Jason and Westberg 1982, p. 79) to avert possible problems.

In some institutions, department chairpersons, deans, or well-established professors may advise the beginning instructor on classroom conduct and administrative responsibilities related to the particular institution. However, in Jason and Westberg's study of teaching in medical schools in the United States (1982), it was found that such individuals may not be available or the faculty are unaware of the availability of such persons.

A simulation on lecturing described by Jason and Westberg (1982) addresses a new faculty member's desire to improve his/her lecturing technique in a medical school. The simulation was used to ascertain faculty members' concepts of effective and ineffective lecturing; the sources of information faculty members consider appropriate for assessing instructional problems; the resources and strategies the faculty suggest for improving lecturing; and the strategies these same faculty members use to help colleagues. Approaches used by faculty members were found to include: talking with the individual who wants assistance in improving his/her lectures; observing the individual's lecture; talking with students who are taking the individual's course; examining the individual's lecture notes; and offering suggestions to the individual about improving the lecture style. This study further revealed that most faculty members employed direct observation to analyze the problem at hand; most adopted the approach of talking with colleagues who were recognized as good lecturers; most seemed willing to assist colleagues in improving their lectures; and most seemed to respect videotaping and self-review as instructional strategies.

Developing Teaching Skills

Teaching skill, according to Eble (1988), is "not so much taught as it is nurtured into existence" (p. 206). The skills to be developed by teachers are many, of course. In the following paragraphs, some of the basic ones are discussed relative to teacher education.

Eble (1988) stresses the importance of creating a comfortable atmosphere in the classroom to augment good teaching. In the first class meeting, a teacher usually focuses on texts to be used, the course outline, requirements for the course, and other details. Also at this time, the teacher establishes the temperament of the class through questions, remarks, gestures, and even through the ways in which he/she looks at students and walks. Eble encourages teachers to be open and humorous when appropriate. He suggests two resources that address humor, "Humor and Enjoyment of College Teaching" by Jean Civikly (1986) and "Everything You Always Wanted to Know About Humor in the Classroom But Were Afraid to Ask" by Howard Pollio (1985/86).

How students and the instructor address each other also affects classroom atmosphere. Many teachers use an approach that is comfortable for them. However, a worthwhile professional skill is remembering students' names for which a seating chart may be helpful, especially for larger classes. Being available to students also is desirable. Ishler and Ishler (1980) emphasize the need for teachers to identify basic or technical skills within their own teaching styles. In so doing, teachers can expand their confidence and proficiency.

Some of the technical skills associated with teaching, and, therefore, to be instilled in new university classroom teachers, include the ability to: establish with students a rapport that is conducive to their involvement in the lesson at hand; teach a lesson from several different points of view; attain closure by blending major points of newly gained knowledge with past knowledge to give students a sense of achievement; use questions effectively; understand and respond to students' behavior in the classroom; find different ways to foster classroom interaction; give feedback to students; use rewards and penalties appropriately; and analyze and initiate teaching models (Allen and Ryan 1969).

Hudgins (1974) asserts that specific fundamentals should be applicable to the attainment and utilization of teaching skills. For example, in teaching concepts, Hudgins would have the teacher evaluate the students' preinstructional knowledge; explain the concept and provide distinct examples; blend negative examples with these illustrations, asking students to note if each example meets the criteria established for the concept; provide feedback to the students after each response; and then assess the students' learning of the concept (Gage 1978). To ensure that teachers can use these steps, teacher education should enable the teacher to learn the general model of the teaching skill, practice the skill in a self-contained setting, and practice the skill in the actual classroom (Gage 1978, p. 46).

The approaches used to help graduate assistants or prospective teachers in developing their own teaching methods continue to vary. Indeed, a number of studies have shown that student teachers demonstrate little change in their teaching methods from the beginning to the end of their student teaching assignments (Gage 1978). Furthermore, as noted by Sykes (1988), there are a number of problems associated with university teaching assistants. He describes these individuals as being largely responsible for undergraduate education while being underpaid, underprepared, and under-recognized for the responsibilities they assume. The result, he maintains, is a lack of education for some undergraduate students and a lack of personal contact between students and teachers.

TEACHER EFFECTIVENESS

Definitions and descriptions of teacher effectiveness vary considerably among educational researchers, hence different criteria are used in its measurement. Those indicators of effectiveness will be addressed here.

In describing distinguished-teaching award nominees, Lawrence (1982) said that a composite of characteristics cited most frequently includes "an inspirational instructor" who demonstrates concern for students, "an active scholar" who is esteemed by colleagues, and "an efficient, organized professional" who is available to students and associates (p. 9). Ericksen (1984) speaks of "good" teachers as having the ability to motivate students (p. 3). He believes that teaching should be described in terms of its effect on students, taking into account individual differences among students. Ericksen (1984) further recognizes the following indicators of good teaching, where the teacher: recognizes knowledge as having lasting value; directs students in comprehending the meaning of this knowledge; and develops and fosters the motivation to learn and retrieve. Csikszentmihalyi (1982) identifies the effective instructor as one who can bring out and sustain the students' intrinsic motivation to learn.

Lowman (1984) refers to an instructor identified with "superior college teaching" (p. 2) as being skillful in giving clear, knowledgeable lectures and conducting discussions, and skillful in interpersonal relations such that teacher-student relationships are a source of motivation to the students. Eble (1988) maintains that the interactions of teachers and students are "the center of all teaching and learning" (p. xvii). Effective instructors, according to Lowman (1984), exemplify joy in learning and foster the same in their students. Eble (1972), in agreeing with students that there should be relevance in teaching, says that effective teachers "always establish relevance in one way or another" (p. 82).

In his book, *Mastering the Techniques of Teaching*, Lowman (1984) presents a two-dimensional model of teaching effectiveness that connects a college teacher's skill in effecting intellectual stimulation and genuine rapport in learners to the quality of instruction. Dimension I, Intellectual Excitement, looks at the explicitness of a teacher's communication and its constructive effect on students. Dimension II, Interpersonal Rapport, comprises a sensitive interpersonal category in which certain psychological factors are examined. A Dimension II item, for example, is that of decreased motivation on the students' part if they believe the instructor disapproves of them. It is Lowman's opinion that teachers who are recognized for their classroom effectiveness are outstanding in one or both of these two dimensions. To be competent, according to Lowman, a teacher should be moderately skillful in each dimension.

In his study of college teachers who were identified as outstanding and effective on the basis of student performance, student attrition, description by academic deans as being "exemplary," and interviews with the teachers themselves, Guskey (1988) was unable to distinguish specific personality characteristics or background traits common to these individuals. The only experience shared by the majority of these 28 teachers was their teaching experience in either elementary schools or high schools prior to teaching at the college level. Most of these individuals had had some form of formal educational instruction and had obtained teaching certificates. Importantly, Guskey did find consistencies in these teachers' teaching behaviors. They devoted considerable time to planning and organizing their courses and activities, emphasizing student learning; they shared a positive regard for students' strengths, weaknesses, and interests; they encouraged and promoted student participation; and they used feedback and reinforcement as a motivational strategy.

Erickson and Erickson (1980) cite the following steps as necessary for an instructor to be effective: give introductions that excite interest and reflect organization; provide examples that clarify material; pose questions that stimulate and guide thinking; use a variety of materials and approaches; show respect and concern for students; devise valid and reliable examinations; and provide feedback that assists students in monitoring their own progress. In their study of teachers and teaching in U.S. medical schools, Jason and Westberg (1982) linked effective teaching to instructor flexibility, spontaneous reactions to unanticipated questions, and a readiness to act without having all relevant information at hand.

While teacher effectiveness was not defined in our study of classroom teaching in ESB-accredited CSD programs (Rassi and McElroy 1988; McElroy and Rassi 1989), all of the survey respondents were asked if they thought their effectiveness had changed since they first assumed the role of teacher. Ninety percent, or 172, of the respondents, indicated that it had improved. Over half attributed this improvement, at least partially, to their teaching experience. Other less frequently reported reasons for improved teaching effectiveness included student feedback, self-confidence, peer consultation, as well as study, self-evaluation, and continuing education. Of the 12 persons in this study who indicated that their teaching effectiveness had not improved since they began teaching, several listed reasons that included a lack of sufficient time to prepare for class and diminishing enthusiasm for teaching. Although conclusions about teaching quality cannot be based on reports of self-perceived effectiveness, these findings do suggest that instructors have an awareness, for whatever reasons, of their own change and growth in teaching proficiency.

Private Practice and Effective Teaching

Given the comparatively late arrival of audiologists and speech-language pathologists as health professionals in private practice, their linkup with education has happened only in more recent years. And, although some private practices have served as off-campus practicum sites, the actual part-time involvement of university educators in private practice has emerged more slowly. Moreover, those faculty members who do split their careers between private practice and the university do not necessarily mix the two.

Faculty members who engage in private professional practice maintain that this involvement enhances their classroom and clinical teaching and, in some instances, provides extra clinical practicum opportunities for their students. In addition, according to Cunningham et al. (1989), this involvement fosters professional autonomy, as experienced through participation in "the unification model" at the University of Louisville School of Medicine. Here, CSD students are given the opportunity to become familiar with the business elements of private practice and to benefit from faculty members' ongoing management of diagnostic techniques and treatment protocols in this setting. This particular model provides an opportunity for faculty members to supplement their teaching salaries, but it also directs a percentage of private practice income into the graduate program. Time spent in private practice by faculty members is limited by university policy. Reportedly, the arrangement has been beneficial to all parties involved (Cunningham and Windmill 1990).

Another reported benefit of classroom teachers' participation in private-practice endeavors is the first-hand information teachers can bring to the classroom regarding a specific kind of case seen in private practice (Parsons and Felton 1987). Shames (1961), summarizing the reasons that faculty members should engage in private practice, stated that it provides expanded and enhanced services for the client, a means for obtaining new teaching materials, models for evolving professional ideals, and a stimulus for research. Ryan and Barger-Lux (1985) found that medical faculty members at Creighton University increased their publications and research as the result of involvement in private practice. Role modeling of superior practice was found by Munroe et al. (1987) to be related to faculty involvement in private practice.

Awards for Teaching Excellence

Awards given for excellence in teaching by institutions, organizations, and corporations reflect recognition of the value of effective teaching. As the move to improve education in this country continues, the number of these awards is likely to increase. Nominations for such awards typically are generated by present or former students, but also may come from colleagues, parents of students, or the public.

University classroom teachers in CSD are eligible for teaching awards in their own institutions and, in fact, a number have won such awards. In at least one instance, a clinical supervisor has been the recipient. Another teaching award, this one specifically available to audiology educators, was the Beltone Distinguished Teaching Award in Audiology, offered by Beltone Electronics Corporation from 1982 through 1988.

The importance of teaching awards should not be underestimated. They give quality teaching the visibility it needs and accomplished teachers the recognition they deserve. Awards also symbolize the value of teaching and, we would hope, are seen by teachers as a prize worth striving for. If our field had more teaching awards available, offered substantial monetary grants tied to CSD-based educational research, and publicized these efforts, both the value and quality of teaching might be upgraded. As is already being practiced by the Council of Supervisors in Speech-Language Pathology and Audiology through its annual Supervisor of the Year Award, other professional organizations might also consider recognizing teaching excellence through awards.

EVALUATION OF CLASSROOM TEACHING

A majority of educational researchers seems to agree that no single teacher evaluation can assess a teacher's effectiveness completely (Page and Loeper 1978). Teachers, according to Ericksen (1984), want the evaluation process to reflect the uniqueness of their interactions with students as well as specific elements of the course content. Different kinds of measures are needed to examine the various parameters involved in teaching. The weight given to evaluations by students, by peers, or by administrators may vary depending on the purpose of the evaluation.

An evaluation system should be broad based to avoid penalizing an instructor for a teaching approach that might differ from the tradition of the department or institution. Also, an evaluation should separate the features of a specific course from the person who teaches the course. By their nature, some courses are more interesting than others, and some teachers have the capacity to make a dreary course interesting (Ericksen 1984). Regardless of the type of teaching evaluation, it can be an effective means for the improvement of teaching if constructed well and taken seriously.

Evaluation by Students

Although many institutions use student feedback to evaluate teaching, students typically do not have the knowledge or ability to observe many of the factors related to teaching that can be addressed in an evaluation conducted by a teacher's peer or administrator. However, student evaluations do give information to teachers about matters students consider to be important. Indeed, student evaluations can be factors in teachers' salary increases and promotions. As discussed later in this section, they can also effect change in teachers and teaching. Professionally prepared evaluation questionnaires have been found to provide essentially stable results (Overall and Marsh 1982).

McKeachie (1986) indicates that student evaluations of teaching are important because such ratings influence the teaching "climate." He states that both students and teachers must have confidence in the methods used to evaluate teaching. Centra (1979) advocates conciseness in student evaluation forms, and recommends that they be designed for completion in 10 to 15 minutes.

Student evaluations take different forms, including written appraisals, rating scales, and interviews (Braskamp, Brandenburg, and Ory 1984). Because interviews with individual students and groups of students, often conducted by a faculty peer or staff member, tend to be time consuming, this form of evaluation is used less often than other forms. With few exceptions, student evaluations respect anonymity.

A majority of institutions use some form of objective course evaluation. Information from these evaluations can benefit students as well as teachers (Guskey 1988). Instructors can gain information regarding their effectiveness in the classroom. Both general and specific information can be gleaned from such evaluations, thus signaling to teachers the areas of instruction that need improvement. In order for the evaluation process to be as effective as possible, the instructor should receive feedback promptly. This ensures better recall on the part of the teacher and expedites changes in instructional approach or technique.

Coleman and Thompson (1987) reported an evaluation process involving student evaluations of classroom and clinical teaching faculty in nursing, although different evaluation criteria were used for the two settings. In a study of the relationship between nursing students' evaluations of teaching effectiveness and the contact time between students and teachers, Dawson (1986) found that nursing students' impressions of teachers in the clinical environment seemed to affect their feelings about the same teachers in the classroom. In other words, the set of ratings a teacher received in the clinical setting became a predictor of that teacher's classroom teaching effectiveness. Thus, it was concluded, students may be influenced by the amount of interaction time they have with teachers. The possible relationship between students' perceptions of clinical and classroom teaching effectiveness merits study in our field.

Studies of student ratings indicate that second to the instructor's ability to make clear presentations of material, students regard the relationships between teacher and student as most important (Abbott and Perkins 1978; Reardon and Waters 1979). According to Eble (1972), such findings contrast with the notion held by some faculty members that students give too much weight to an instructor's personal attributes in their ratings of teaching effectiveness. Teachers who may be considered demanding or trying are just as likely to receive outstanding evaluations by students as are teachers not identified with these traits (Lowman 1984). Similarly, students' ratings of teachers do not reflect negatively on work assignments given to students (Frey 1978; Abrami et al. 1980; Howard and Maxwell 1980; Peterson and Cooper 1980). On the whole, student ratings seem to mirror the extent to which a teacher is able to make clear presentations of material and nourish constructive relationships with students (Lowman 1984).

In our study of classroom teaching in ESB-accredited programs (Rassi and McElroy 1988), survey participants indicated that their courses and/or course instruction were evaluated. Of the 185 respondents who answered this question, 106 reported that students, only, did the evaluating. Nearly 78% of the instructors evaluated, including those who were evaluated by individuals other than students, considered the evaluations to be valuable. The respondents who found value in course evaluations cited different reasons for this opinion. The two reasons reported most frequently were that evaluations reveal areas of strengths and weaknesses and that evaluations provide necessary feedback. A number of subjects also reported that evaluations contain suggestions for improvement and reveal student perceptions. Although 26 subjects saw no value to course evaluations, 18 of those instituted changes recommended in these evaluations. Moreover, all 15 subjects who were equivocal about the value of course evaluations indicated that they would follow through with recommended changes.

The above findings apparently are not uncommon. Eble (1972) states that subjective evidence indicates teachers "are changed for the better by student ratings" (p. 69). The assumption here is that their teaching probably improves as well. Specific instructional or other course changes may occur as a result of student comments. Through evaluation by students, for example, teachers can learn about the effectiveness of textbooks, media, testing format, and lectures, or about the physical state of the classroom and other similar factors. For the most part, student evaluations seem to have a positive impression on the majority of teachers who have participated in the evaluation process. At the very least, student ratings exert pressure on faculty members to maintain minimum levels of teaching competence.

Evaluation by Peers

Although student evaluations of teaching are worthwhile and even mandatory in many universities, they do have some basic problems and can be viewed as incomplete if considered alone (Brannigan and Burson 1983; Knox and Morgan 1985). Cohen and McKeachie (1980) point out that only faculty have the qualifications to look at dimensions of teaching other than classroom performance, for example, the teacher's knowledge base, course content selection and organization, use of resource materials, and instructional methods. Thus, peer evaluations provide a different frame of reference than do student evaluations. Often conducted by a review committee, peer evaluations can focus on research and service as well as teaching, but they are carried out relatively infrequently, depending on university or departmental policy.

Although possibly the oldest form of teacher evaluation, peer evaluation is sometimes controversial. Centra (1975) found peer evaluation outcomes to be generous compared to those contributed by students. Still, these same evaluations were criticized because of the limited time available for classroom appraisal observations, the varied views held by faculty members regarding effective teaching methods, and a distrust among faculty members in evaluative roles. On the other hand, peer evaluations can yield explicit, helpful suggestions for improved teaching techniques, and they can reinforce self-respect and encourage cooperation among educators (Hulsmeyer and Bowling 1986).

Hulsmeyer and Bowling (1986) developed a peer evaluation tool for assessing classroom teaching in nursing education. Their evaluation form contains items in the following observation categories: the teacher's level of knowledge and capability in transmitting this knowledge; the teacher's teaching methodology; the teacher's zeal for teaching and interactions with students; and the teacher's interest in, and intent to refine, teaching. Faculty members reported benefits from the identification of strengths as well as weaknesses, from the promotion of teaching effectiveness, and from unprecedented collaboration among colleagues.

In the peer evaluation process for both clinical and classroom teaching described by Harwood and Olson (1988), faculty members can negotiate with the dean to use a peer evaluation format. Should the faculty member choose this format, he/she submits a list of names of potential peer evaluators to the dean who, in turn, has the option of designating one or all of the selected individuals to serve in this role. The instructor then makes arrangements with the individual(s) chosen to conduct the evaluation, which is to be based on classroom observations, and also provides the evaluator(s) with the tools selected for this process. The use of evaluative tools is optional. The completed evaluation is given to the dean, and a copy to the evaluated faculty member.

A peer evaluation approach specifically designed to examine course materials, content, and form is presently being encouraged at the University of Virginia and at other institutions of higher learning. Elsewhere, Rabada-Rice and Scott (1986) have used a tool for evaluating effective team teaching. Its twofold purpose is to study in a comprehensive way the individual contributions to a team approach and to gather information that can be used to promote individual professional growth. Thus, the instrument design is based on behaviors that meet team-teaching requirements while also providing a standard for distinguishing individual strengths and weaknesses.

Self-Evaluation

Self-appraisal is another means of evaluating teaching. Through informal conversations with colleagues and students, through workshops, in-service presentations, professional publications, and through self-observation and self-monitoring, classroom instructors can gain information useful for making changes in their courses and teaching methods. Student achievement also should be taken into account in evaluating teaching (Eble 1972).

In evaluating their own teaching, instructors may use a scaled form or a written format to facilitate teachers' observations of their teaching methods. Viewing videotapes also can be a component of this process (Centra 1975). Eble (1972) considers the self-evaluation to be a useful source of information and the impetus for one to improve his/her own teaching skills.

A direct way to gauge reactions to one's teaching is to observe students' classroom behavior (McKeachie 1986). As discussed in other chapters, instructors should encourage student participation in class discussions for teaching-learning purposes. In addition, for the purpose of teacher self-evaluation, such participation can reveal students' understanding or misunderstanding of information and enable the teacher to correct misconceptions. More blatant indications that students are bored or not understanding what the instructor is saying are evident through students' yawns, whispers, or blank stares. Another means for obtaining feedback about one's teaching is through individual conferences with students. The problem of one student might represent others' problems. For larger classes, McKeachie (1986) suggests that the instructor meet with a class representative to discuss various aspects of the course.

Self-Assessment Questionnaires. Some universities and colleges employ questionnaires to obtain information about faculty members' evaluations of their own teaching. In other academic settings, an instructor may devise his/her own questionnaire with general questions to students concerning presentation of content.

Another form of self-evaluation is an individual contract plan (ICP) such as that used at the Medical College of Georgia's School of Allied Health Sciences (Mitcham and Vericella 1985). This format enables faculty members to devise a plan in which they specify their activities to be accomplished during the year ahead, the manner in which they will accomplish the activities, the amount of time they will give to the activities, the criteria to be used in evaluating their efforts, and the way in which the effectiveness of their performance will be measured. The completed plan is discussed between the faculty member and chairperson. When an understanding is reached, the plan is executed, then reviewed each quarter and modified as necessary. It is evaluated on an annual basis. Bortz (1986) offers an entire system for planning, organizing, documenting, and rewarding faculty activity, including teaching.

Personality Tests. Personality tests are available for individuals seeking improvement in their university or college teaching. One of the more frequently used tests for this purpose has been the Myers-Briggs Type Indicator (MBTI) (Myers and Briggs 1967), which is based on Jung's concept that behavior is related to "observable and measurable differences in mental functioning" (Claxton and Ralston 1978, p. 26). According to Jung (Roberts 1977), two ways of perceiving are through sensing and intuition, and two ways of judging are thinking and feeling. Depending on individual preferences for each, there also are personal inclinations towards extroversion or introversion. Hence, the four scales of the MBTI are: Extroversion-Introversion; Sensation-Intuition; Thinking-Feeling; and Judging-Perceiving. Test findings reflect an individual's approach to his/her environment in these domains.

Results of studies conducted with the MBTI have yielded information that is useful for those interested in improving college level teaching. Roberts (1977) found, for example, that sensing and judging individuals demonstrate a preference for an organized approach to learning, one that allows them to use their senses. Intuitive and perceptive individuals, on the other hand, prefer less structure and have a greater interest in writing and verbalizing. Through administration of the test to themselves as well as to students, course instructors can, thus, become sensitive to the differences in personality types and their relation to learning and teaching approaches.

Student Achievement Measures. A summative evaluation, which involves testing students at the end of a course, can be used to assess course effectiveness, based on the assumption that if the students have the information being assessed, they will apply the information. When used for this purpose the test is ungraded. In using this student achievement approach, the instructor must have a listing of course objectives. The results are subjected to these analyses: ascertaining the degree to which the course attained its objectives; and ascertaining the success of this course compared to that of other courses with the same objectives (Westmeyer 1988).

A variation of the above course evaluation method involves use of a formative evaluation that is administered to students while the course is in progress. By monitoring student progress in the midst of the instructional process, the effectiveness of teaching can be determined (Westmeyer 1988). A midterm examination can be used as a formative evaluation, for instance, if its results are used by the instructor to reorganize the second part of the course, to consider remedial procedures for students who have not demonstrated proficiency, or to monitor progress toward goals to be evaluated at a later time. In addition, the instructor can, at this juncture, gather information on how students' attitudes may be affected by a particular teaching activity, whether or not they are enjoying the course, the relevance of the course content to their interests, and other learning matters (Kozma, Belle, and Williams 1978).

Combined Evaluation

Boland and Sims (1988) describe a comprehensive tool for evaluation of faculty that can be used by students, peers, administrators, and also by those evaluated. The 80 items included in this evaluation are taken from a pool of items appropriate to each evaluator's knowledge of the individual to be evaluated. In other words, the evaluator does not assess the instructor in areas in which the evaluator has no knowledge. The instrument design incorporates performance expectations and, when used in combination with a computer software program, has the potential for yielding a broad range of data. Although this tool was designed for nursing school faculty, the multi-evaluation concept could easily be adapted to educational programs in other disciplines.

Teacher Evaluation and Job Satisfaction

It is reasonable to assume that a teacher might be more receptive to being evaluated if it were known that evaluation results can have a positive effect on teaching. In fact, effective teaching can reflect job satisfaction and vice versa. Without opportunities for faculty members to be productive, to grow, and to be satisfied, evaluations serve no purpose (Bobbitt 1985). It is crucial that institutions provide teachers with the impetus to improve their instructional methods and the means to do so.

As previously mentioned, although many institutions do provide teaching improvement opportunities, there still may be administrative preoccupation with research and less emphasis on teaching (Jason and Westberg 1982). This seems to be the case in universities containing ESB-accredited CSD programs where a survey sample of classroom instructors (Rassi and McElroy 1988) indicated that their university administrators perceive research as being more important than classroom teaching. Both areas need to be supported in order to provide a sense of satisfaction for teachers.

Satisfaction is identified with personal gratification (Clark and Lewis 1988). In studies conducted by Clark and Corcoran (1983, 1985, 1986), faculty found satisfaction in working with students and ideas, in the flexibility of arranging their work schedules, in relationships with colleagues, and in their teaching experiences. However, findings of a survey of 5000 faculty conducted by the Carnegie Foundation (1985), when compared with previous studies, revealed a decline in faculty satisfaction. Moreover, 40% of the respondents reported decreased enthusiasm about their careers.

In another part of our study on classroom teaching in ESB-accredited programs (Rassi and McElroy 1988; McElroy and Rassi 1989), we examined respondents' personal enjoyment and professional satisfaction derived from various work activities. On linear scales where minimal enjoyment and satisfaction were represented by 1.0 and maximal satisfaction and enjoyment by 5.0, the survey participants' mean group ratings for classroom teaching were 4.0 on both dimensions, ranking higher than clinical supervision, research, clinical and educational program administration, and student advising. Only the work activity, "other," earned a rating close to that for classroom teaching in personal enjoyment, and matched classroom teaching in professional satisfaction. Respondents named such activities in the "other" category as professional committee work, outside consulting, and private practice endeavors. The personal enjoyment derived from classroom teaching was attributed by respondents to three main factors: interactions with students; student feedback and responsiveness; and helping students to learn, grow, and develop. The primary attribution factors for professional satisfaction in classroom teaching were similarly student oriented.

Changing Teacher Behavior

There are a number of ways to approach changes in teacher behavior. One such method, microteaching (also discussed in Chapter 11 relative to clinical teaching), is based on the premise that teaching can be organized into specific skills that can be explored, illustrated, performed, and then reviewed with accompanying feedback (Ishler and Ishler 1980). Microteaching focuses on the technical skills identified by Allen and Ryan (1969), which were mentioned earlier in this chapter. The teacher directs his/her attention to one skill at a time. After receiving an explanation of the specific skill, the teacher views a film or videotape that demonstrates the particular skill, then incorporates this skill into teaching a lesson of five or ten minutes (Ishler and Ishler 1980; Gage 1978). The session is videotaped for review or is analyzed directly, with feedback coming from teacher-consultants and students. Teaching sessions are continued with the same or different groups of "learners" until the teacher masters this specific skill. The microteaching approach enables teacher trainees to be active in the training period as observers, analysts, learners, and leaders (Ishler and Ishler 1980). It also allows a teacher to focus on one particular aspect of teaching at a time (Gage 1978).

The minicourse has evolved as another means of changing teaching behavior. It is composed of packets of materials, self-administered tests, and films for use with videotapes and with pupils (Gage 1978). In this approach, the teacher becomes familiar with a set of skills explained in the teacher's handbook; looks at a film depicting these skills; teaches a lesson to practice these skills; and then self-evaluates the lesson. Next, the teacher follows the microteaching plan by teaching the lesson with three or four students outside the regular classroom, followed by teaching a full class of students in the regular classroom. The entire minicourse format takes approximately one hour a day for 16 days. Observers determine the teacher's teaching skills prior to involvement in a minicourse, and again after it has been completed (Gage 1978).

Other approaches to improving teaching behaviors are those used in teacher development programs, as discussed in the following section. In addition, the already-mentioned teacher evaluations by students and peers can lead to changes in teacher behaviors.

FACULTY DEVELOPMENT

Instructional development refers to "the instructional situation rather than faculty competence," whereas faculty development is "a comprehensive term that covers a wide range of activities ultimately designed to improve student learning . . . and describes a purposeful attempt to help faculty members improve their competence as teachers and scholars" (Eble and McKeachie 1985, p. 11). Gaff (1975) explains:

> Faculty development focuses on faculty members and seeks to promote their individual growth and development. Because the instructional role is a major part of the faculty members' professional lives, most programs help them to explore their attitudes about teaching and learning, acquire more knowledge about educational matters, develop additional skills, enhance their sensitivities, improve their relationships with students and colleagues, and consider the teaching role in relation to other responsibilities (p. 8).

In earlier years, faculty development programs focused on research and scholarship because achievement in these areas led to advancement in academic rank and brought prestige to the institution (Guskey 1988). The function of these development programs expanded in the late 1960s and early 1970s, when more attention was given to assisting new faculty members and experienced professors in increasing their teaching effectiveness. As suggested before, student evaluations called attention to the need for faculty development, and the pressure to find more effective methods to evaluate teaching were strong (Eble and McKeachie 1985).

Various reviews and evaluations of effective staff development programs (Levinson-Rose and Menges 1981; Ging and Blackburn 1986) revealed four general characteristics in common (Guskey 1988): (1) a balance of administrators and faculty members involved in program planning; (2) a requirement that the change process be gradual and have strong administrative support; (3) the practice of giving faculty members feedback on the results of their efforts to incorporate change into their teaching; and (4) the continuation of support and the follow-up activity provided for faculty members who seek to improve their instructional methods. The opportunity to consult with colleagues about ideas concerning perspectives and strategies and to search for solutions to problems is very helpful to many college instructors (Joyce and Showers 1980). Moreover, the collaborative learning associated with colleague consultation can enable faculty members to develop similar skills in their students (Copeland and Jamgochian 1985). Even so, says Boice (1986), there may be a need for so-called "field developers," that is, chairpersons or middle-aged faculty who can succeed in encouraging reluctant faculty members to participate in a development progam.

Faculty development programs have the potential to help instructors in different ways: achieving professional growth; developing additional teaching skills; gaining a better understanding of, and improving interpersonal relationships with, students; increasing understanding of the effect of a specific discipline's organizational structure on student learning; developing greater intrinsic motivation for teaching; and learning from one's own teaching experience as well as from colleagues (Eble and McKeachie 1985). Depending on the availability of funding, institutions of higher learning may have faculty exchange programs, grants, and awards in addition to other opportunities for faculty development.

Many faculty development programs are available through universities and colleges; some may be offered during the regular academic year, others in the summer. Such programs usually offer individual instructional consultation similar to that described in conjunction with university teacher support centers. In an initial conference, the instructor and consultant(s) discuss the instructor's general and specific areas of concern regarding classroom preparation or presentation. Then, following direct observation of the instructor's teaching or review of a videotaped version, and/or small-group discussion with the instructor's students, the consultant gives feedback to the instructor.

Jason and Westberg, in 1982, cited the inattentiveness of medical practitioner-teachers to the need for competence in teaching. Of the development activities for new faculty being initiated at that time by some institutions, Jason and Westberg felt that workshops and short courses were among the more appropriate for individuals in the health care professions because of the limited time commitment to teaching. Furthermore, these investigators reasoned, strategies that incorporated practice and critique of new skills appealed to this group. Among the approaches they found to be most applicable were: trigger tapes or brief videotaped parts or file clips of events or topics that allowed the participants to practice managing the specific situation presented; master teachers whose strategies could be emulated; and a log of teaching experiences. Basic science medical school faculty, Jason and Westberg (1982) found, favored a faculty development program that included workshops on lecturing, evaluation of instructional effectiveness, and making optimal use of instructional technology.

Sabbaticals traditionally have been used to give an instructor the time and opportunity to pursue his/her own professional development. The attractive feature of a sabbatical is that the individual can plan the activities. However, this needs to be done carefully because even planned activities can take more time than anticipated (Carmack

1987). A less positive aspect of the sabbatical is that fewer institutions than in the past are awarding this kind of leave, and a number of individuals may not be able to afford them because of the possibility of reduced income (Clark and Lewis 1988).

Conferences, workshops, and convention presentations outside the university are obvious sources for professional development (Brittingham 1986). However, if information on teaching is not available within an instructor's own discipline, it becomes necessary to attend such sessions offered by other professional associations. Such an effort is not likely to be pursued by many individuals unless the presentations are given at nearby locations.

CONCLUSION

Educational research indicates that preparation for the teaching role can help to improve teaching in higher education. More than ever before, instructors have available and accessible resources to make this happen. With improved teaching comes improved learning, a need that apparently exists in CSD educational programs. Sustained individual effort on the part of each instructor is necessary to cultivate and maintain teaching skills.

REFERENCES

Abbott, R. D., and Perkins, D. 1978. Development and construct validation of a set of student rating-of-instruction items. *Educational and Psychological Measurement* 38:1069–1075.

Abrami, P. C., et al. 1980. Do teacher standards for assigning grades affect student evaluations of instructors? *Journal of Educational Psychology* 72:107–18.

Allen, D. W., and Ryan, K. 1969. *MicroTeaching*. Reading, MA: Addison-Wesley.

Anderson, J. L. 1988. *The Supervisory Process in Speech-Language Pathology and Audiology*. Austin, TX: Pro-Ed.

Anderson, J. L., Brasseur, J. A., Casey, P. L., Hunt-Thompson, J., Laccinole, M. D., McCrea, E., Rassi, J. A., Smith, K. J., and Ulrich, S. R. 1989. Preparation models for the supervisory process in speech-language pathology and audiology. *Asha* 31(3):97–106.

Association of American Colleges. 1985. Integrity in the college curriculum. *Chronicle of Higher Education* 2:12–13.

Beard, R. M. 1972. *Teaching and Learning in Higher Education*. Harmondsworth, England: Penguin.

Bobbitt, K. C. 1985. Systematic faculty evaluation: A growing critical concern. *Journal of Nursing Education* 24(2):86–88.

Boice, R. 1986. Faculty development via field programs for middle-aged, disillusioned faculty. *Research in Higher Education* 25:115–35.

Boland, D. L., and Sims, S. L. 1988. A comprehensive approach to faculty evaluation. *Journal of Nursing Education* 27(8):354–58.

Bortz, R. F. 1986. *Recognizing Faculty Contribution.* Carbondale, IL: Training Systems Designers.

Brannigan, C. N., and Burson, J. Z. 1983. Revamping the peer review process. *Journal of Nursing Education* 22(7):287–89.

Braskamp, L. A., Brandenburg, D. C., and Ory, J. C. 1984. *Evaluating Teaching Effectiveness.* Beverly Hills, CA: Sage Publications.

Brittingham, B. 1986. Faculty development in teacher education: An agenda. *Journal of Teacher Education* 37(5):2–5.

Cantrell, T. 1973. How do medical staff learn to teach? *Lancet* 2:734.

Carmack, B. J. 1987. Faculty sabbatical. *Nurse Educator* 12(5):29–32.

Carnegie Forum on Education and the Economy. 1986. *A Nation Prepared: Teachers for the 21st Century.* New York: Carnegie Forum.

Carnegie Foundation for the Advancement of Teaching. 1985. The faculty: Deeply troubled. *Change* 17:31–34.

Carroll, J. G. 1977. Assessing the effectiveness of a training program for the university teaching assistant. *Teaching of Psychology* 4:135–38.

Casey, P. L., Smith, K. J., and Ulrich, S. R. 1988. *Self-Supervision: A Career Tool for Audiologists and Speech-Language Pathologists.* Rockville, MD: National Student Speech Language Hearing Association.

Centra, J. A. 1975. Colleagues as raters of classroom instruction. *Journal of Higher Education* 46(1):327–37.

Centra, J. A. 1979. *Determining Faculty Effectiveness.* San Francisco: Jossey-Bass.

Civikly, J. M. 1986. Humor and the enjoyment of college teaching. In *New Directions for Teaching: Communicating in College Classrooms* (no. 26), ed. J. M. Civikly. San Francisco: Jossey-Bass.

Clark, S., and Corcoran, M. 1983. Professional socialization and faculty career vitality. Paper presented at the annual meeting of the American Educational Research Association, Montreal.

Clark, S., and Corcoran, M. 1985. Individual and organizational contributions to faculty vitality: An institutional case study. In *Faculty Vitality and Institutional Productivity: Critical Perspectives for Higher Education*, eds. S. M. Clark and D. R. Lewis. New York: Teachers College Press.

Clark, S., and Corcoran, M. 1986. Perspectives on the professional socialization of women faculty: A case of accumulative disadvantage? *Journal of Higher Education* 57:20–43.

Clark, S. M., and Lewis, D. R. 1988. Faculty vitality: Context, concerns, and prospects. In *Higher Education: Handbook of Theory and Research, Vol 2*, ed. J. C. Smart. New York: Agathon Press, Inc.

Claxton, C. S., and Ralston, Y. 1978. *Learning Styles: Their Impact on Teaching and Administration.* AAHE-ERIC/Higher Education Research Report No. 10. Washington, DC: Association for Higher Education.

Cohen, P. A., and McKeachie, W. J. 1980. The role of colleagues in the evaluation of college teaching. *Improving College and University Teaching* 8(4):147–54.

Coleman, E. A., and Thompson, P. J. 1987. Faculty evaluation: The process and the tool. *Nurse Educator* 12(4):27–32.

Copeland, W. D., and Jamgochian, R. 1985. Colleague training and peer review. *Journal of Teacher Education* 36(2):18–21.

Csikszentmihalyi, M. 1982. Intrinsic motivation and effective teaching: A flow analysis. In *Motivating Professors to Teach Effectively*, ed. J. L. Bess. San Francisco: Jossey-Bass.

Cunningham, D. R., and Windmill, I. M. 1990. Faculty private practice: Implications for the future of audiology. *Audiology Today* 2(6):18–21.

Cunningham, D. R., Baker, B. M., Steckol, K. F., and Windmill, I. M. 1989. The unification model. Ten years of faculty private practice. *Asha* 31(9):87–89.

Dawson, N. 1986. Hours of contact and their relationship to students' evaluations of teaching effectiveness. *Journal of Nursing Education* 25(6):236–39.

Diamond, R. M., and Gray, P. J. 1987. *A National Study of Teaching Assistants*. Syracuse, NY: Center for Instructional Development, Syracuse University.

Eble, K. E. 1972. *Professors as Teachers*. San Francisco: Jossey-Bass.

Eble, K. E. 1980. Future considerations and additional resources. In *Improving Teaching Styles*, ed. K. E. Eble. San Francisco: Jossey-Bass.

Eble, K. E. 1988. *The Craft of Teaching* (2nd ed.). San Francisco: Jossey-Bass.

Eble, K. E., and McKeachie, W. 1985. *Improving Undergraduate Education through Faculty Development*. San Francisco: Jossey-Bass.

Ellner, C. L., and Barnes, C. P. 1983. *Studies of College Teaching*. Lexington, MA: D. C. Heath.

Ericksen, S. C. 1970. Earning and learning by the hour. In *Effective College Teaching*, ed. W. H. Morris. Washington, DC: American Association for Higher Education.

Ericksen, S. C. 1984. *The Essence of Good Teaching*. San Francisco: Jossey-Bass.

Erickson, B. L., and Erickson, G. R. 1980. Working with faculty teaching behaviors. In *New Directions for Teaching and Learning: Improving Teaching Styles* (no. 1), ed. K. E. Eble. San Francisco: Jossey-Bass.

Erickson, G. R., and Erickson, B. L. 1979. Improving college teaching: An evaluation of a teaching consultation procedure. *Journal of Higher Education* 50: 670–83.

Farmer, S. S., and Farmer, J. L. (eds.). 1989. *Supervision in Communication Disorders*. Columbus, OH: Merrill Publishing Company.

Frey, P. W. 1978. A two-dimensional analysis of student ratings of instruction. *Research in Higher Education* 9:69–91.

Fuhrmann, B., and Grasha, A. 1983. *A Practical Handbook for College Teaching*. Boston: Little, Brown and Company.

Gaff, J. G. 1975. *Toward Faculty Renewal: Advances in Faculty Instructional and Organizational Development*. San Francisco: Jossey-Bass.

Gage, N. L. 1978. *The Scientific Basis of the Art of Teaching*. New York: Teachers College Press, Columbia University.

Gideonse, H. D. 1989. The Holmes Group proposals: Critical reactions and prospects. In *Crisis in Teaching. Perspectives on Reforms*, ed. L. Weis, P. G. Altbach, G. P. Kelly, H. G. Petrie, and S. Slaughter. Albany: State University of New York Press.

Ging, T. J., and Blackburn, R. T. 1986. Individual and contextual correlates of faculty adoption on an innovation. Paper presented at the annual meeting of the American Educational Research Association, San Francisco.

Grasha, A. F. 1978. The teaching of teaching: A seminar on college teaching. *Teaching of Psychology* 5:21–23.

Gullette, M. M. (ed.). 1982. *The Art and Craft of Teaching*. Cambridge, MA: Harvard Danforth Center for Teaching and Learning, Harvard University.

Guskey, T. R. 1988. *Improving Student Learning in College Classrooms*. Springfield, IL: Charles C Thomas Publisher.

Harwood, C. H., and Olson, J. 1988. Peer evaluation: A component of faculty performance appraisal. *Journal of Nursing Education* 27(8):377–79.

The Holmes Group. 1986. *Tomorrow's Teachers: A Report of The Holmes Group*. East Lansing, MI: Author.

Howard, G. S., and Maxwell, S. E. 1980. Correlation between student satisfaction and grades: A case of mistaken causation. *Journal of Educational Psychology* 72:810–20.

Hudgins, B. B. 1974. *Self-Contained Training Materials for Teacher Education: A Derivation from Research on the Learning of Complex Skills.* Bloomington, IN: National Center for the Development of Training Materials in Teacher Education, Indiana University.

Hulsmeyer, B. S., and Bowling, A. K. 1986. Evaluating colleagues' classroom teaching effectiveness. *Nurse Educator* 11(5):19–23.

Imig, D. G. 1986. The greater challenge. *Phi Delta Kappan* 68:33.

Ishler, R. E., and Ishler, M. F. 1980. Developing desirable teaching behaviors. In *Improving Teaching Styles,* ed. K. E. Eble. San Francisco: Jossey-Bass.

Jason, H., and Westberg, J. 1982. *Teachers and Teaching in U. S. Medical Schools.* Norwalk, CT: Appleton-Century-Crofts.

Joyce, R. B., and Showers, B. 1980. Improving inservice training: The messages of research. *Educational Leadership* 37:379–85.

Justice, E. 1983. Evidence for the effectiveness of graduate teacher training. Paper presented at the 28th annual meeting of the Southeastern Psychological Association, Atlanta.

Knox, J. E., and Morgan, J. 1985. Important clinical teaching behaviors as perceived by university nursing faculty, students and graduates. *Journal of Advanced Nursing* 10(1):25–30.

Kozma, R. B., Belle, L. W., and Williams, G. W. 1978. *Instructional Techniques in Higher Education.* Englewood Cliffs, NJ: Educational Technology Publications, Inc.

Lawrence, J. H. 1982. *Descriptions of Exemplary Teachers—An Explanatory Study of Awards.* Ann Arbor, MI: Center for Research on Learning and Teaching, University of Michigan.

Levinson-Rose, J., and Menges, R. J. 1981. Improving college teaching: A critical review of the research. *Review of Educational Research* 51:403–34.

Lowman, J. 1984. *Mastering the Techniques of Teaching.* San Francisco: Jossey-Bass.

McElroy, M. D., and Rassi, J. A. 1989. Instructors' perceptions of clinical teaching in ESB-accredited programs. In *Supervision: Innovations. A National Conference on Supervision,* ed. D. A. Shapiro. Cullowhee, NC: Western Carolina University.

McKeachie, W. J. 1986. *Teaching Tips: A Guidebook for the Beginning College Teacher* (8th ed.). Lexington, MA: D. C. Heath.

Mitcham, M. D., and Vericella, B. J. 1985. The use of individualized contract plans as a method of performance evaluation for allied health faculty. *Journal of Allied Health* 14(4):351–62.

Munroe, D. J., Sullivan, T. J., Lee, E. J., and Sarter, B. 1987. Establishing an environment for faculty practice: The primary affiliation. *Journal of Nursing Education* 26(7):297–99.

Myers, I. B., and Briggs, K. C. 1967. *The Myers-Briggs Type Indicator.* Princeton, NJ: Educational Testing Service.

Overall, J. J., and Marsh, H. W. 1982. Students' evaluations of teaching: An update. *Bulletin of the American Association for Higher Education* 35(4):9–12.

Page, S., and Loeper, J. 1978. Peer review of the nurse educator: The process and development of a format. *Journal of Nursing Education* 17(9):21–29.

Parsons, M. A., and Felton, G. 1987. Practice: A sanctioned faculty role. *Journal of Nursing Education* 26(3):123–25.

Peterson, C., and Cooper, S. 1980. Teacher evaluation by graded and ungraded students. *Journal of Educational Psychology* 72:682–85.

Pollio, H. R. 1985, Fall/1986, Winter. Everything you always wanted to know about humor in the classroom but were afraid to ask (with apologies to

Woody Allen et al.). *Teaching-Learning Issues* 57. Knoxville, TN: Learning Research Center, University of Tennessee.

Rabada-Rice, F., and Scott, R. S. 1986. A peer evaluation for measuring team teaching effectiveness. *Journal of Nursing Education* 25(6):255–58.

Rassi, J. A. 1978. *Supervision in Audiology*. Baltimore: University Park Press.

Rassi, J. A., and McElroy, M. D. 1988, November. Classroom teaching in ESB-accredited programs: A survey of instructors. Miniseminar presented at the annual convention of the American Speech-Language-Hearing Association, Boston.

Reardon, M., and Waters, L. K. 1979. Leniency and halo in student ratings of college instructors: A comparison of three ratings procedures with implications for scale validity. *Educational and Psychological Measurement* 79:159–62.

Richardson, J. 1988, June 19. Teaching revolution under way. *The Daily Progress*, F1, 2.

Roberts, D. Y. 1977. Personalized learning processes. *Revista/Review Inter-Americana* 7:139–43.

Ryan, S. A., and Barger-Lux, M. J. 1985. Faculty expertise in practice: A school succeeding. *Nursing & Health Care* 6:75–78.

Shames, G. H. 1961. Private practice in speech pathology in addition to full-time service on a university faculty. *Asha* 3:211–13.

Staff. 1990. On campus. *Vanderbilt Magazine* Spring:2.

Sykes, C. J. 1988. *ProfScam: Professors and the Demise of Higher Education*. Washington, DC: Regnery Gateway.

Wannamaker, A. 1989, August 13. U. Va. undergrads rip teaching assistants. *The Daily Progress*, B1, 2.

Weis, L., Altbach, P. G., Kelly, G. P., Petrie, H. G., and Slaughter, S. (eds). 1989. *Crisis in Teaching. Perspectives on Reforms*. Albany, NY: State University of New York Press.

Westmeyer, P. 1988. *Effective Teaching in Adult and Higher Education*. Springfield, IL: Charles C Thomas Publisher.

Chapter 2

Learning and Teaching

Margaret D. McElroy and Judith A. Rassi

In order to plan teaching and carry it out effectively, classroom, laboratory, and clinical instructors need to understand learning and the ways in which teaching and learning interact. This understanding is just as important for instructors in higher or continuing education as it is for those who teach at elementary and secondary levels.

THE LEARNING PROCESS

Learning is "a relatively permanent change in behavior which occurs as a result of experience," according to Tarpy (1975, p. 4). In their definition of learning, Douglas, Hosokawa, and Lawler (1988) equate learning with "the acquisition of knowledge leading to a process of behavior change" (p. 44). Gagne (1974) views learning as a process permitting people (and animals) to alter their behavior in an instantaneous way, usually not requiring the same change in every new circumstance. Learning is thus inferred by a change in an individual's performance.

Typically, the learning process entails interaction with the peripheral environment and occurs over the life of an individual (Douglas, Hosokawa, and Lawler 1988). Learning theories take into account the manner in which individuals are influenced by their environment (Craig 1976). Learning involves discerning "the personal meanings and relationships of ideas to existing knowledge, skills, and past experiences" (Douglas, Hosokawa, Lawler 1988, p. 46).

The broader viewpoint of learning encompasses the concept of learning as a lifelong process. From this perspective, education is continuous throughout the life cycle, changing in purpose and structure to meet individuals' needs at various phases of their maturation (Darkenwald and Merriam 1982). In viewing learning as a lifelong process, one becomes aware that education is influenced indeed by society, culture, and the environment. As change occurs in any of these sectors, it also must occur in education to enable individuals to make adjustments in their professional preparedness. Chapters 15 and 16 address lifelong learning in greater detail.

Developmental Factors

Development is a successive schedule of changes taking place in an anticipated pattern and resulting from "an interaction between biological and environmental factors" (Salkind 1985, p. 2).

Chronology. In infancy and early childhood, it is well known that specific skills may not be learned until related growth and maturation have occurred. Although maturation cannot be hastened, learning can take place with adequate stimulation and incentive (Fincher 1985). The effect of education, regardless of level, relates to the learner's developmental state at the time (Chickering 1969; Feldman and Newcomb 1976).

Adolescence is considered to be, approximately, the teen years, although the end of adolescence is variable. Kuhlen (1952) is among those who suggest that the end of this period is related to the individual's adjustment rather than to age. Adolescence is the time span affected by what precedes it and what is to occur as the individual progresses from dependence to independence (Breslin 1974). Higher education, according to Feldman and Newcomb (1976), enables adolescents to become adults.

Adult Learners. As interest in educational pursuits for adults has heightened, the study of behavioral changes in the adult years has increased. Teachers need to be aware of the characteristics of adult learners before adopting instructional methods.

Knowles (1980) originated the term *andragogy* to differentiate between the process of assisting adults in their learning and the more familiar approach used in teaching children, or pedagogy. Andragogy is based on these four main suppositions about adults as learners: (1) adults view themselves as self-directing and reliable; (2) adults have masses of experience that can serve as a promising resource for their own learning as well as the learning of others; (3) adults are motivated to learn to the degree that they discern timely relevance to their life activities; and (4) adults center their interests less on abstract hypotheses and more on problem solving. The concept of andragogy encompasses a number of learning theories and concepts, including reinforcement, individual differences, and self-evaluation (Mast and Van Atta 1986).

Adult learners have individualized learning styles that have evolved through the years; some learn more readily through interactive approaches, whereas others may be more responsive to reflective strategies (Mast and Van Atta 1986). Quickness in learning and quickness in retention may characterize some adult learners; slowness in learning but more permanent retention may describe others. Adults tend to be at ease with their individual learning styles and are not eager to adopt other styles (Warren 1974). Being anxious about making mistakes in the presence of peers or younger students and being hesitant to change their approach to tasks are concerns of many adult learners. In addition, adult learners often must exercise caution to ensure that their self-concept and sense of competence, solidly based on previous experiences of their lives, do not decrease in the new learning situation.

Adults tend to learn best in nonintimidating settings in which they are perceived as individuals (Douglas, Hosokawa, Lawler 1988). Adults are interested in learning that is useful to them. They are attracted to the application of knowledge and tend to react positively to a problem-based approach. Adults prefer information about their progress in contrast to being evaluated formally (Douglas, Hosokawa, and Lawler 1988).

Seaman and Fellenz (1989) report that adults utilize "an independent or individual mode" (p. 25) for learning as opposed to group-learning approaches. Tough (1978a, 1978b) and his colleagues found that most adult learning endeavors are self-initiated, meaning that the learner and instructor, at times, are one and the same. Nevertheless, even in self-directed learning, Mast and Van Atta (1986) point out, the instructor's position is significant. Self-directed learning implies a lesser role for the instructor, but, in reality, the instructor is vital as a resource, reinforcer, and supporter of the learning process (Cooper 1983).

Learners in communication disorders have various reasons for returning to a higher education program or for becoming involved in continuing education outside the university. Some may want to renew certification or update their knowledge or clinical base. Others may be entering the specialization area for the first time or taking courses simply for the joy of learning. These individuals may be older than the average student and require more time and effort to become self-directed.

Psychosocial Development. The relationship between students' behavior and their development of skills with personal and professional correlates (Coles 1970; Erikson 1968, 1982) should be of interest to educators as well as to practitioners in communication disorders. In Erickson's eight-stage theory of psychosocial development from infancy to old age, for example, a primary task must be managed successfully at each stage to secure the individual's success in future undertakings. These stages, in order, are: (1) trust and mistrust; (2) autonomy and shame/doubt; (3) initiative and guilt; (4) industry and inferiority; (5) identity and role confusion; (6) intimacy and isolation; (7) generativity and stagnation; and (8) ego integrity and despair. There must be a propitious balance between the two dissimilar segments of each task in order to obtain a successful outcome (Erikson 1963).

In accordance with this theory, then, an individual would not: be self-reliant or autonomous until having a feeling of trust; show initiative until having a feeling of freedom to decide what to do; be industrious until having a feeling of trust in his/her own instincts; have an identity until having a feeling of involvement and gratification in applying him/herself to learning; have knowledge of intimacy until having a feeling of who he/she is and how he/she is accepted; experience honesty, expressed as a feeling of attainment and completeness, until having a feeling of creating and fostering. Erikson's psychosocial theory, which already has proved to be applicable in the clinical and academic components of nursing education (Wallhead 1986), has the same potential for education in other health care professions, including audiology and speech-language pathology.

Perceptual Development.   Perception, a psychological phenomenon, is the individual's means of maintaining contact with the environment through the use of his/her senses (Campbell and Bickhard 1986; Kemp and Smellie 1989). Vision, hearing, and touch are the main senses involved. The senses gather information for the nervous system where the impressions are altered into electrical impulses that initiate additional electrical and chemical events in the brain. The end product is an internal knowledge of an entity or incident. Perception foreruns communication (Kemp and Smellie 1989).

Perception is a component of cognition; it takes meaningful information from a peripheral or external response (Craig 1976). The process involved in perception is the basis for a child's intelligence or cognition as he/she grows. Perception serves as the basis for more involved elements of cognitive development, including eye-hand coordination. Individual differences are prevalent in perception. People perceive stimuli from their own advantage in terms of scope, merits, learning, and moral principles (Craig 1976).

Infancy and early childhood make up the period in which most changes occur in perceptual development. As an individual's attention expands, he/she becomes more aware of the significance of smaller clues. According to Gibson (1969), an appreciable amount of perceptual learning and development is related to differentiating among or attending to the unique elements of an entity or object. The specificity and abundance of meaning associated with perceptions increase in individual ways even through adulthood. As people age, their perceptions become more evident as mirrors of their experiences (Craig 1976).

The effect of individual differences in perception is evident throughout educational endeavors, but especially so in one-to-one clinical teaching.

Attitude Development.   An attitude is "an acquired internal state that influences the choice of personal action towards some class of things, persons, or events" (Gagne 1974, p. 66). Attitudes are representative of a definite category of learning effects. Those attitudes affecting the social realm may be learned in the home or in social interactions. They may involve thoughtfulness, cooperation, and tolerance for social differences. Another class of attitudes relates to preferences an individual might have for specific activities or events. Attitudes can be likened to values when viewed as learned capabilities. Values, however, are regarded as being more general, whereas attitudes are directed toward specific choices (Gagne 1974). Moreover, attitudes may have positive or negative influences.

Emotional Development. The matter of shared dependency of emotional and intellectual growth was pointed out by Perry (1970), especially regarding effects of students' emotions on the intellectual ability to be productive. Realizing the strength and breadth of cognitive skills is largely dependent on one's emotional development. Teachers' rapport with students can nourish emotional development in the classroom (Katz and Henry 1988).

Personality Development and Self-Concept. A majority of theorists believe that basic personality is established by the age of eight years. At this time, the child's self-concept, having begun to form at an earlier age (Craig 1976), becomes more evident and the child is able to clarify his/her individuality. Between the ages of eight and ten years, the self-concept is shaped and evolves into the nucleus of the child's personality (Breslin 1974). The self-concept is considered a vital personal possession; it serves as the heart of one's personality (Breslin 1974). People need to know themselves as well as possible because their behavior will be based on their perception of themselves.

There is a reciprocal relationship between self-concept and socialization; one assists the other in the individual's development. Although children do not emulate all individuals in their environment, they can be affected by their own preference for certain models. These attitudes and ideals can be influential in molding their self-concept (Craig 1976).

Self-concept is believed to be directly related to learning, as evidenced by the better learners who utilize self-reference. These individuals may be more discriminating about their selection of material; they may even discount variant data (Pervin 1984) and concentrate more on information similar to that associated with previous experience (Rogers, Rogers, and Kuiper 1979). Thus, students' self-concepts can have a great impact on the manner in which they function in a classroom, laboratory, or clinical learning situation. In certain instances, teachers need to make a concerted effort to help students improve and expand their self-concepts.

Cognitive Development. Changes in cognitive development accompany changes in one's physical and physiological maturation from childhood through adolescence (Breslin 1974). Cognitive development involves changes in the manner in which a person interprets and delineates problems. According to Piaget's (1970, 1972) theory of cognitive development (Lorton and Lorton 1984), definitive stages are evident. Each level is dependent upon the preceding level and occurs at progressive and sequential stages. Despite an age-related sequence, individuals do not reach each stage at the same time. Progression from sensorimotor actions established in infancy to concrete thinking and then to abstract reasoning is dependent on variables of age, maturation, experience, and intelligence (Breslin 1974).

The levels or stages are composed of "concrete operational thinking and formal operational thinking" (Fuhrmann and Grasha 1983, p. 265). Individuals are inclined to use specific procedures or concrete operations from the age of seven to eleven years, thus preferring the actual, the genuine, and the present. In addition, they lean toward utilization of rules for problem solving and toward logical reasoning. Formal operational thinking comes into play after the age of eleven when reasoning ability encompasses time beyond the present. These thinkers look at possibilities beyond the concrete; they utilize the hypotheticodeductive approach; and they are able to use abstract thinking (Fuhrmann and Grasha 1983). Because not everyone fully attains this formal operational thinking stage, it follows that those who eventually become college students might benefit from a classroom environment that nurtures formal operational thinking skills used in "applying, analyzing, synthesizing, and evaluating information" (Fuhrmann and Grasha 1983, pp. 266–267).

Memory. As a component of cognition, memory cannot be separated readily from the process of learning. There is an interrelatedness of intelligence, problem-solving ability, personality, and memory with learning potential, especially in older individuals (Hayslip and Kennelly 1985). Whereas learning concerns the manner in which information is acquired, memory pertains to the manner in which information is stored and its later retrieval (Ellis 1972; Botwinick 1967, 1973, 1978). In operation, memory involves the components influencing performance in the learning process itself and in the retention period (Ellis 1972). Cognitive theorists agree that the vital component of memory is information processing.

In the views of Melton (1963) and Waugh and Norman (1965), sensory register, short-term memory, and long-term memory make up "three interconnected memory systems" (Fuhrmann and Grasha 1983, p. 56). The sensory register or sensory memory is believed to be a preparatory part of short-term memory. Involved with short auditory or visual tracking of the information presented for learning, it deteriorates fast. A limited amount of information derived from the sensory register, then, is stored in short-term memory for a brief time. Short-term memory can be increased through repetition or categorization of information.

Information based on a meaningful code is taken from short-term memory and converted into long-term memory. Use of labeling and mental imagery helps to make information meaningful. For this reason, concrete concepts are easier to retain than abstract concepts (Bower 1970). Information relegated to long-term memory can be retained indefinitely. The inability to remember is not a result of memory loss but rather the inability to retrieve information (Fuhrmann and Grasha 1983).

Given that repetition of information is helpful to short-term memory, such a device is useful in teaching students. Instructors who stress major points of a presentation two or three times give students more opportunity to commit the information to memory. Having students ask questions or asking them to paraphrase what has been said are other methods that assist in processing information. Just as short-term memory capacity can be broadened as a result of categorizing information, long-term memory can be expanded by the meaningfulness of information (Fuhrmann and Grasha 1983).

Information-Processing Theory. The importance of short-term and long-term memory in learners' information processing has been emphasized by other researchers, among them Anderson and Bower (1973). As already suggested, information processing is that part of the thinking process by which individuals discern, systematize, and remember the large quantity of information acquired on a daily basis (Norman 1976). In other words, information processing looks at memory in terms of " 'the flow of information' through the person, from its initial encoding, to storage, and finally to retrieval" (Ellis 1972, p. 111). Information processing stresses differentiation between storage and retrieval, as demonstrated in computer programs (Ellis 1972; Sahakian 1976). In fact, through the use of computer programming or simulation, theorists have offered explanations of the way in which the human central nervous system can solve problems and form concepts as part of the elaborate cognitive process (Sahakian 1976).

Information processing presumes active learning, thereby emphasizing intrinsic motivation (discussed later in this chapter) that teachers can foster through the incorporation of critical thinking and problem solving in their courses. Memory is also an important element. The teacher's facilitative role in this regard is significant. Allowing students to participate in course design; offering ways for them to organize content; and using mental imagery in teaching are just a few examples of how teachers can encourage processing of information in the classroom (Fuhrmann and Grasha 1983).

Kemp and Smellie (1989), in reference to the information-processing theory, say that instruction should focus on directing the mind to new stimuli (the selection process) and on stimulation of encoding (converting stimuli into a summary system for memory). To attain these objectives, theorists of information processing recommend that attention be focused on:

Use of advanced organizers, such as examples and analogies that relate information to be learned to already learned knowledge

Development of instruction-based aids, such as synonyms for difficult words, questions placed in a text, summaries, and review questions that can serve as cues

Use of learner-generated cues, such as key words, rhymes, acronyms, and images for encoding and building associations that are helpful for information recall and pattern recognition. (Kemp and Smellie 1989, p. 17)

These techniques are also important in planning instructional media for classroom use.

Transfer of Learning. Transfer of learning has to do with ways in which new learning is influenced by earlier learning (Ellis 1972). It is based on those abilities and attitudes that are helpful to an individual in new situations. Thus, a person benefits from having an awareness of the reason a happening might occur and from considering his/her attitude regarding an unfamiliar happening. Another positive aspect of the transfer of learning is the individual's ability to consider possible options prior to solving a problem. One is more apt to solve a problem successfully if logic can be employed in approaching the problem. Self-image is part of the transfer process in that the individual who has a relatively good self-image will attempt to solve a problem without having a definite solution. Even if a solution is unworkable, a different option can emerge by relating the failure to previous learning (Lapp et al. 1975).

In evaluating the transfer of learning, one contrasts the learning of one task with two or more consecutive tasks. The learning of one task can enhance or conflict with the learning of another task, thereby resulting in either a positive or negative transfer. Or, the learning of one task may influence the performance of tasks learned earlier or those to be learned later. The direction of learning effect may be from an earlier task to a later task, or in the opposite direction (Catania 1979).

Other Contributing Factors

Attribution Theory. Although Atkinson (1964) and Rotter (1966) are recognized for their attribution theories, Weiner's (1979, 1985, 1986) attribution theory is examined here because of its focus on decisions made by individuals in distinct task-based situations (Stipek 1988). In addition, this theory appears to have practical application in the classroom and other learning environments.

Attribution theorists postulate that individuals intuitively seek insight into the reasons for happenings, especially when the result is unanticipated or significant (Stipek 1988). For example, a student is likely to search for an explanation as to why his/her test performance was better or poorer than expected. Attribution learning theory has as its foundation the cognitive processes of "meaningfulness, understanding, and organizational abilities" (Kemp and Smellie 1989, p. 18), which are fundamental to human behavior (Weiner 1980, 1986; Kemp and Smellie 1989). Attribution refers to the supposition made by an individual concerning the causes that effect an occurrence or a specific result (Kemp and Smellie 1989). The discernment of cause that contributes to achievement is termed causal attribution. In achievement situations, typical causal attributions point to ability ("I did well because I'm smart"; "I did poorly because I'm dumb") and effort ("I did/did not study") (Weiner 1986). Weiner (1979, 1985, 1986) maintains that, where achievement is concerned, the dimensions of the attributions are more important than the explicit attributions themselves. Effort and ability, as used in the example, differ meaningfully in their implications for behavior, according to Weiner, in that effort is controllable and variable, whereas ability is typically viewed as uncontrollable and fairly stable. (Stipek 1988). Attribution theorists use a causal scale to look at the ways in which individuals explain specific causes. It is the "individual's own interpretation that influences the individual's behavior in an achievement situation" (Stipek 1988, p. 82).

In their study of the antecedents and consequences of certain attributions, researchers have found value in knowing if the objective of an attribution is to improve students' motivation in academic situations. Indeed, some causal attributions may be more conducive than others to the stimulation of constructive, achievement-related behavior. It is, therefore, important for an instructor to be aware of the circumstances attending productive attributions by students (Stipek 1988). Moreover, Weiner contends, teachers can, through manipulation of the classroom environment, alter or modify students' causal attributions (Stipek 1988). If, for example, a teacher provides information about all class members' test performance, this can influence an individual student's impression about the cause of his/her own achievement. If all students obtain a low grade on a test, an external, uncontrollable attribution (e.g., task too difficult) might be made. But if only one student receives a low test grade, that student is apt to ascribe his/her performance to an internal, controllable attribution (e.g., too little study time). In the latter scenario, the result can be motivating and positive. For this reason, effort attributions are believed to be beneficial to learning (Stipek 1988). Ability attributions, on the other hand, may be counterproductive.

Self-Actualization. Self-actualization, a component of human motivation promoted by humanists such as Maslow (1954), also appears in his classic hierarchy of needs. In Maslow's view, self-actualization refers to one's desire for self-fulfillment or for attaining what one is capable of attaining. He identifies the following 15 basic personality traits of self-actualized individuals:

1. They detect the spurious, the fake, and the disinterest in personality and judge people correctly and efficiently.
2. They accept themselves and their own nature without chagrin or complaint.
3. They are spontaneous in their inner life, thoughts, impulses, etc. Their behavior is marked by simplicity and naturalness.
4. They are strongly focused on problems outside themselves; they are problem centered rather than ego centered.
5. They can be solitary without harm to themselves and without discomfort. They positively like solitude and privacy to a definitely greater degree than the average person.
6. They are independent of the physical and social environment.
7. They have a capacity to appreciate again and again, freshly and naively, the basic goods of life.
8. They have mystic experiences.
9. They have for human beings in general a deep feeling of identification, sympathy, and affection.
10. They have deeper and more profound interpersonal relations than any other adults.
11. They are democratic people in the deepest possible sense. They can be and are friendly with anyone of suitable character regardless of class, education, political belief, race, or color.
12. They are strongly ethical.
13. They are humorous but not in a hostile manner.
14. They have a special kind of creativeness or originality or incentiveness.
15. They maintain a certain inner detachment from the culture in which they are immersed. (pp. 153–174)

The core of Maslow's philosophy is that education should foster self-actualization by assisting individuals to become "the best." Furthermore, he says, educators should focus on promoting intrinsic, not extrinsic, learning. In other words, their teaching should be in the direction of "learning to be a human being in general, and, second, learning to be *this* particular human being" (Maslow 1976, pp. 120–121). Similarly, Rogers (1983), who has made a significant contribution to the humanistic realm of education, stresses experiential learning as a necessary expression of self-actualization (Darkenwald and Merriam 1982). Known for his research in human nature, Allport looks at the adult as a self-actualizing learner (Schultz 1977). He believes that people's self-awareness, beliefs, and interests in other people should be promoted in educational situations (Darkenwald and Merriam 1982).

Creativity. Creativity, another factor contributing to the learning process, has been defined by Torrance (1978) as:

> . . . a process of becoming sensitive to or aware of problems, deficiencies, and gaps in knowledge for which there is no learned solution; bringing together existing information from the memory storage or external resources; defining the difficulty or identifying the missing elements; searching for solutions, making guesses producing alternatives to solve the problem; testing and retesting these alternatives; perfecting them and finally communicating the result (p. 146).

Children who have been reared in an environment characterized by creativity and stimulation tend to be the most creative (Breslin 1974). According to Breslin (1974), the creative individual is identified with several of the following traits:

1. A tendency to talk fluently with a flow of ideas and speed in relating ideas that appear unrelated.
2. A tendency to have flexibility and adaptability in compliant settings and restlessness and impatience in rigid situations.
3. A tendency for thinking to digress and be creative rather than be concentrated and amiable.
4. A good memory and associational thinking helpful in viewing much that is familiar in supposedly unfamiliar circumstances.
5. A tendency to demonstrate humor and playful attitudes in a number of situations.
6. A reputation for foolish or flighty ideas.
7. Work that is characterized by some ideas that are considered different.
8. Display of a good opinion of self.
9. A willingness to acknowledge sentiments and emotions. (Bernard 1972, p. 207)

Usually, a creative individual is not the outstanding student in the average class and may not have the highest intelligence. A creative person may possess information that he/she can apply to inventive and original tasks but not to problems found in an intelligence test.

Motivation. Ericksen (1984) regards motivation as being "prerequisite for learning" (p. 86). An individual who is motivated to learn tends to learn more readily than an individual who is not motivated. Self-motivation or intrinsic motivation is a highly desired trait in the learning process (Breslin 1974).

Students' classroom behavior can be positively or negatively affected by intrinsic motivation. In particular, intrinsic motivation is augmented in situations where students are permitted to select the tasks (Stipek 1988). A challenge for teachers is to devise tasks and learning conditions that enhance intrinsic motivation.

Grolnick and Ryan (1984) suggest that intrinsically motivated students may acquire better conceptual knowledge of a subject than students whose recompense is external. This may be related to Nicholls' (1979, 1983) contention that these persons are more focused on an activity. Furthermore, intrinsically motivated activities are sources of greater gratification than are extrinsically motivated activities, according to Csikszentmihalyi (1975). Thus, the report by Heimstra (1976) that adult learners are highly motivated to learn should be encouraging to instructors in higher education and especially to those in continuing education.

In understanding all that occurs in the classroom, a teacher must be cognizant of the importance of motivation. Teachers' attitudes can have a forceful effect on students' motivation. An atmosphere characterized by enthusiasm and interest in the subject material on the teacher's part is conducive to fostering motivation in students (Ericksen 1984). Encouragement by the teacher, signified by a nod of the head or verbal reinforcement, can nurture motivation. To maintain motivation, the teacher needs to present problems that students are capable of solving. In children motivation is cultivated as a result of parents' encouragement to perform well and their establishing goals that are attainable (McKeachie 1986).

Other links in the connection between learning and motivation are those of curiosity and competence, both intrinsic motives. Unanticipated questions appear to be the most effective in piquing curiosity.

The preparation of instructional materials provides an opportunity for the promotion of "successful motivation" (Keller 1983, p. 18). Keller specifies four required conditions and the strategies to implement them:

1. Interest—arousing and sustaining the learner's curiosity and attention. *Strategies:* Use of novel, surprising, incongruous, or uncertain events in instruction. Give people the opportunity to learn more about things they already know about or believe in, but also give them moderate doses of the unfamiliar and unexpected.

2. Relevance—relating the instruction to how a learner can satisfy personal needs or a highly desired goal. *Strategies:* Use concrete language, examples, and concepts that are related to the learner's experience and values. Provide opportunities to achieve standards of excellence under conditions of moderate risk.
3. Expectancy (confidence)—perceiving the likelihood of success in learning and the extent to which success is under learner control. *Strategies:* Increase expectancy for success by increasing experience with success or by using attributional feedback and other devices to help learners connect success to personal effort and ability.
4. Satisfaction—combining extrinsic rewards and intrinsic motivation to influence the accomplishment of the instructional goal and provide further motivation to continue pursuing similar goals. *Strategies:* Use task-endogenous rather than task-exogenous rewards. Use verbal praise and informative feedback rather than threats, surveillance, or external performance evaluation. (Kemp and Smellie 1989, p. 18)

McKeachie (1986) stresses the importance of the teacher's role in stimulating motivation, and points out that teachers' eagerness and ideals are sources of motivation in learning. Some related strategies are discussed in Chapter 5.

Theories of Learning

No single theory of learning can delineate all factors involved in teaching and learning. The majority of learning theories were promoted to explain behaviors demonstrated in the laboratory and clinic. Only later were attempts made to relate theoretical precepts to educational settings. Therefore, although some components are applicable to the educational environment, others do not fit. Likewise, because people learn in different ways, it is not possible to group learning theories under one heading. For the most part, theories of learning can be categorized under the headings of cognition, behaviorism, or humanism, but even within these groups, there is variability (Fuhrmann and Grasha 1983). Composed of different elements, all three approaches to learning are in accordance with the idea that the learning process involves "thinking, language, decision making, and problem solving" (Joyce and Weil 1980, p. 44). Having already looked at cognition, particularly in its developmental manifestations, we examine the remaining two theories, behaviorism and humanism, in the following paragraphs.

Behaviorism. Well-known proponents of behaviorism include Watson (1924) and Skinner (1968, 1971). This learning theory emphasizes environmental stimuli as the basis for discerning and managing behavior. It stresses individuals' observable behavior (Lorton and Lorton 1984). When this theory was proposed by Watson, it was believed that behaviors were controlled by direct responses (Sahakian 1976); external stimuli were necessary to initiate action. Skinner, on the other hand, looked at the role of the organism as more active and, in fact, capable of influencing its surroundings. He advocated the use of rewards or penalties, that is, operant conditioning, as a means of controlling behavior. Behaviorists see students' previous and current environments as influencing behavior (Mathis and McGaghie 1974). Positive reinforcement in the form of rewards in a classroom motivates students. Contracts between teacher and students are a means of establishing positive reinforcement. The student engages in specific activities helpful in earning a particular grade. To assist students in gaining information, a structured setting for learning is arranged. Another way to encourage students' acquisition of information is to use self-pacing to allow for individual differences in the learning process. Behaviorists emphasize mastery of information through established criteria or the learning of particular skills. The importance of providing immediate feedback to students concerning their learning of content is also stressed (Fuhrmann and Grasha 1983).

Humanism. Humanistic education views the student as a person and combines "cognitive learning and affective experience" (Rich 1988, p. 7). From this perspective, the teacher is interested in students' personal growth—not their acquisition of knowledge—and assists them in the learning process (Fuhrmann and Grasha 1983; Rich 1988). Humanism stresses an individual's value as a human being (Axelrod 1970). It is the humanists' belief that more emphasis should be given to the affective segment of education and an integration of the affective domain and cognitive learning. Emotions, values, attitudes, and feelings are components of the affective domain (Rich 1988).

In teaching, humanism centers on the quality of the relationship of teacher and student. From a humanistic perspective, the teacher becomes a facilitator of learning through active interactions with students. The concept of facilitator is credited to Rogers (1969). The facilitator has the responsibility of fostering a genuine relationship with the learner. Through an atmosphere of understanding and assurance, the facilitator encourages students' genuineness (Mathis and McGaghie 1974; Darkenwald and Merriam 1982). No judgments are made and students are not coerced.

From the humanistic viewpoint, motivation for learning is based, at least partially, on self-actualization that prompts individuals to pursue new experiences (Fuhrmann and Grasha 1983). Rogers (1969) contends that self-actualization is prominent in the classroom, particularly in regard to learning course content. In Maslow's hierarchy, needs for personal growth and needs related to deficiencies were identified as sources of motivation (1954). These proponents' views on motivation have obvious meaning for the classroom. Through encouragement from facilitators, students can perform activities that will help them to attain their potential and/or to realize their self-actualization (Fuhrmann and Grasha 1983).

Student Learning Styles

Learning styles vary from student to student. To become more cognizant of their students' learning styles, one approach used by teachers is to ask students to spend about ten minutes writing about what they have learned in a specific course and how they have learned it. This reflection can give valuable information to the students and teacher, and, at the same time, serve as a means for improving learning and incentive (Katz and Henry 1988). Another approach used to gain information about student learning is a teacher review of students' notes taken in conjunction with a specific course.

Student learning style refers to "the manner in which an individual perceives and processes information in learning situations" (Foley 1983, pp. 244–45) and takes into account personality traits. These traits are composed of students' attitudes and ideals about learning, the ways in which they think, and the manners in which they prefer information to be presented. Learning-style models have been developed as a means of grouping particular dimensions of personality (Fuhrmann and Grasha 1983) and of cognition. Some are presented in this chapter, others in Chapter 9.

Cognitive Models

Field Independence and Dependence. Particular attention has been given to the study of cognitive styles, especially those involving field independence and dependence, which make up a research area initiated in the 1950s. These two styles are concerned with the way people process information. Those persons who prefer field independence depend on internal stimuli to process information; those who favor field dependence lean toward external clues. The former rely less on others in making decisions than do the latter. Thus, students who are field independent prefer little structure and guidance in the learning process, whereas those who are field dependent tend to prefer instructional approaches involving discussion and small groups (Witkin, Goodenough, and Oltman 1977).

Field independence is represented by analytical and logical thinking, and field dependence by global or universal thinking. Field-independent persons are, therefore, noted for their observations of distinct traits (Fincher 1985) and their ability to concentrate and focus on specifics, carry out activities in an organized manner, and think logically and critically. In addition, they are able to discern differences among homologous experiences (Schmeck 1988). Field-dependent individuals, on the other hand, view people, occurrences, and places more as a nebulous composite (Fincher 1985). Persons in this category exhibit intuitive thinking, random attention, and a lack of organization for detail. They have a tendency to be more impulsive and look more at similarities than differences (Schmeck 1988). In other words, field-dependent individuals tend to be "heavily influenced by the surrounding field," and, conversely, those who are field independent "are relatively uninfluenced by the surrounding field" (Claxton and Ralston 1978, p. 11).

Witkin (1976), Witkin et al. (1977), and others involved in research on field independence and field dependence stress that criteria to determine which of these two modes of perception is optimal are lacking. Nonetheless, Cross (1976), Witkin (1976), and Tyler (1978) are among those researchers who emphasize the importance of field independence and dependence in education. Witkin speculates that tests emanating from research on cognitive styles may supplant intelligence tests. In particular, he considers field independence germane to the judgments and preferences of college students in choosing their profession. According to Tyler (1978), teachers who prefer field dependence may favor group discussion and projects as an instructional approach. Learners who are field dependent may demonstrate a preference for social reinforcement in their studying, and also may have a particular interest in professions related to human services. Learners in both groups tend to be people-oriented, acceptive of others' opinions, and responsive to influence (Cross 1971).

Garity (1985) reported on the application of Witkin's field-independent and field-dependent learning styles to teaching and learning in the nursing profession. Two groups representing these styles were compared on a number of factors, including interpersonal orientation and group behavior. Garity found that field-dependent people demonstrate a more interpersonal orientation and show their feelings, compared with those who are more field-independent. Mezoff's (1979) observations of human-relations training groups revealed that people identified as field-independent were active participants, took leadership roles, and were at ease in trying their ideas in the group situation. Conversely, the field-dependent individuals exhibited a more passive role, confining themselves to the status of spectator, and could be swayed to change their opinions as a result of peer pressure. Although differences in these two learning styles have been found in a number of studies, neither style is favored over the other. A specific style may be more suited for specific circumstances.

Two related investigations center on learning preferences in allied health professions (Rezler and French 1975; Rezler and Rezmovic 1981). Most of the subjects favored only "concrete and teacher-structured learning conditions and situations" (Garity 1985, p. 13). Similar findings were revealed in testing administered by Garity (1985) to graduate students in nursing who were employed for the first time. Even so, Garity points out the need for different learning styles in different learning situations.

In another study of learning style in the nursing field cited by Garity (1985), findings suggested that nursing students are more successful in their coursework, more proficient collaborators in the teaching-learning mode, and more accommodating in handling learning projects as a result of knowledge about their own learning styles. Lange (1972) found that fewer nursing students failed or withdrew from specific courses when they were matched in learning styles with their instructors. The traits associated with field independence and field dependence would seem to have as much relevance and application to teachers and learners in communication disorders as they do in nursing education. This topic is explored further in Chapter 9.

Cognitive Mapping. This specific approach looks at evaluating the cognitive elements of learning styles. It is directed toward the processes that individuals tend to use in acquiring information, in thinking, in making decisions, and in becoming concerned for themselves, other people, and objects in their environment (Hill and Nunney 1972; Hill 1976; Fuhrmann and Grasha 1983). In Hill's Cognitive Style Mapping Inventory, these four general divisions are dissected into 27 cognitive traits. Students reply to 244 descriptive statements (e.g., "I hear the daily news on the radio"). Ratings are obtained on the 27 traits. Students' learning styles are "mapped" based on these elements, and instructional approaches and courses are designed to be compatible with these styles of learning (Claxton and Ralston 1978; Fuhrmann and Grasha 1983). In a study conducted by Sims and Ehrhardt (1978), positive experiences were reported by both students and teachers as a result of mapping. Students believed the maps were beneficial in providing information about the way in which they learned. They used this information in selecting courses and deciding study approaches. Teachers reported mapping to be helpful in comprehending student learning practices. Moreover, it assisted teachers in changing their instructional methods.

Another cognitive learning model, the Kolb model (1976), and two learning models based on social interaction, the Fuhrmann-Jacobs model (1980) and the Grasha-Riechmann model (1974), are discussed in Chapter 9.

TEACHING STYLES

Each teaching method an instructor uses is chosen in an effort to create an environment to facilitate learning (Sanders and McCutcheon 1986). Eble (1980) likens style in college teaching to "teaching excellence" (p. 1). He cites studies conducted by Yamamoto and Dizney (1966) and Wilson and his colleagues (1975) in which the influence of teaching modes and student preferences on student achievement was demonstrated. Other studies, such as the one by Tennyson, Boutwell, and Frey (1978), have found that students show "an overwhelming preference for a professor who sees himself, and is seen, as a teacher rather than researcher, administrator, or socialite" (p. 196). Eble's concept of a good teaching style is one that requires a lifetime process. Accordingly, styles rather than style should be considered, as no one style need be effective in all instructional settings. Many styles can be effective (Sheffield 1974).

While it is recognized that faculty development programs in higher education assist teachers in improving their teaching skills, Eble (1980) feels that such programs should address personality and character development at the same time they are focusing on improvement in instructional approaches. Eble says "developing an exemplary teaching style is to be achieved by painstaking and loving and artful attention to the particulars of what one does—both as a person and teacher" (p. 5).

Mann et al. (1970) identified six roles teachers play in the classroom. These teaching styles—some are discussed from a different perspective in Chapter 5—are mandated by the needs of the class. They result in teacher behavior associated with roles that, in turn, are related to the teaching method used:

The teacher as *expert* conveys information, tending toward intellectual preparation of classes, being comfortable with presenting material and responding to questions. Students may be afraid of seeming stupid.

The teacher as *formal authority* establishes objectives and methods for obtaining objectives, identifying plans and criteria for assessment of student performance. This role tends to cause dependency in students; students may be afraid of failing.

The teacher as *socializing agent* attempts to define goals and a vocational course for students following the course of study, attempting to assist students in readying for the profession. The teacher serves as a guide. Students should define their interests; they may be afraid of rejection by the profession.

The teacher as *facilitator* attempts to foster development and productivity in students' own terms, trying to be responsive to student needs. Students' self-discovery may expand, but they may be afraid of not having a distinct and workable individuality.

The teacher as *ego ideal* wants to convey the excitement and merit of intellectual inquiry in a specific area of study. Teacher serves as a model for students to follow after entering the field. Although students like having a model, they may fear boredom.

Teacher as *person* wishes to communicate that teachers are people who possess human needs and skills. The teacher fosters openness and eagerness in students. On the whole, students value the teacher's wish to be a person and to know them as more than a student. Students fear being ignored or treated as a product. (Mann et al. 1970; Fuhrmann and Grasha 1983; McKeachie 1986)

Familiarity with student learning and teacher styles is important to being more effective in the classroom. Cross (1976) offers the following comments regarding the use of cognitive models:

People will probably be . . . more productive if they are studying . . . via a method compatible with their style.

No one method should be regarded as a panacea for all students in all subjects.

We need to be knowledgeable in devising . . . strategies to teach [the subjects all students must learn].

Educators need to be aware of the cognitive styles of students in order to provide the appropriate kinds of reinforcement.

The learning program [should not be] biased in favor of a particular cognitive style.

More attention needs to be given to the potential of cognitive style for educational and vocational guidance.

Relatively greater attention should be given to [building] on the strengths of individuals.

Educators should remain flexible and experimental in their use of the concept [of learning style]. (Cross 1976, pp. 130–33)

Elaborating on Cross' ideas, Fuhrmann and Grasha (1983) suggest that student learning styles be matched with teaching approaches. They point out that benefits might result from considering instructional methods compatible with the class profile, or from taking individual student learning styles and giving these students corresponding assignments. Conversely, mismatching teaching and learning styles might foster growth in another learning style. Using either approach—that is, matching or mismatching the two styles—might force teachers to change their teaching style, thus expanding their repertoire.

Awareness of teacher and student styles is helpful also in understanding why some teacher/student relationships are better than others (Fuhrmann and Grasha 1983). Personalities are also an important factor in teaching and learning styles. Assessment of teachers' and students' personalities by means of such tests as the Myers-Briggs Type Indicator (MBTI) (Myers and Briggs 1967) can, in many cases, increase teachers' sensitivity to the differences and similarities among personality types and their relation to learning and instructional approaches (Roberts 1977).

Regardless of information about student/teacher learning styles presented in this chapter and elsewhere in this book, an instructor's own ideas about choosing teaching methods are just as viable as the ones addressed in this chapter. There is no formula concerning the best approach. The important point is that personalities should be taken into account.

TEACHING-LEARNING MODELS

Research findings emphasize the importance of facilitating the interaction between teaching and learning styles (Fincher 1985). Eble (1980) argues that teaching and learning cannot be separated. Douglas, Hosokawa, and Lawler (1988) state that " . . . good teachers work hard to understand and apply the principles of the teaching and learning process" (p. 2).

Aptitude-Treatment-Interaction Models

In an effort to determine the instructional approaches that might be best for specific people, studies of aptitude-treatment-interaction (ATI) have been conducted. Interactions between conventional teaching methods and aptitude differences, such as tension, intelligence, cognitive style, and personality traits, were analyzed. Included in these studies were lectures, classroom media, and the Personalized System of Instruction (Cronbach and Snow 1977), which is discussed below. Results indicate the interaction differences are more statistical than "actual" in that the differences were observed among individuals within a large population of students. According to Snow and Peterson (1980), however, the results have value because they lend support to those who advocate the need for making teaching approaches compatible with student learning styles. Tobias (1982), in looking at aptitude-treatment-interaction, emphasized the importance of the manner in which students use their time and thinking during study as opposed to the instructional method and time devoted to study.

Teachers and students give credence to aptitude tests as measures of intelligence, although such tests are not the sole indicators of performance. As already discussed, there are other factors that contribute to one's learning, including motivation. And, besides intelligence and motivation, "background preparation and personal characteristics" (Ericksen 1984, p. 86) are elements essential to learning. Just as an individual's preparation for college varies, so, too, do individuals' attitudes. Some may be positive and some may be negative. Both preparation and attitudes are important to classroom learning, a point underscored in Chapter 5. The classroom teaching environment is affected by the range of differences in personal attributes, such as interests, expectations, and ideals, each of which allows students to respond to information the teacher says and the way it is said (Ericksen 1984).

Ericksen (1984) stresses that the learner's process of comprehension is just as important to learning as is the presentation of information. Because people differ in their selection, encoding, remembering, and understanding of information, the Personalized System of Instruction (PSI) has been found useful in helping instructors adjust instruction to the individual student and promote independence in learning. There are three features related to PSI that offer special support for learning by the individual student: (1) students do not move to the next unit until they have mastered the previous unit; (2) the self-pacing aspect of PSI allows the student to regulate his/her learning rate; and (3) immediate feedback about performance fosters positive attitudes on the student's part and serves as a support in attaining goals (Ericksen 1984).

Behavioral Models

As explained in the discussion on behavioral theory, this idea regards development as a learning activity that progresses in accordance with particular learning tenets or precepts. The primary incentive for growth and development, based on the behavioral model, is in the environment. Although there may be variability in the significance of the environment, depending on the specific theory within this model, the organism is considered reactive (Salkind 1985).

Practically all behavioral theories regard behavior as an activity of environmental effects. In situations where the behavior's effects are positive, the activity is apt to continue; in circumstances where behavioral results are negative, the activity may alter or cease. According to the behavioral model, principles of learning and the effect of environment are foremost in the developmental process. Conditioning and semblance enable individuals to learn suitable behaviors and make adjustments. In fact, it is possible for behaviors to be modified into their fundamental components (Salkind 1985).

It is understandable that the behaviorist's main interest is the number of occurrences of a behavior, especially because events in the environment are the behaviorists' focus rather than events that take place inside the organism. From the behavioral perspective, studies of development look at the effect of particular happenings in the environment. This can be accomplished by distinguishing events in the environment that govern behavior and examining changes in behavior that may result from manipulation of the events (Salkind 1985).

Animal laboratory research supports behaviorist learning principles, showing that learning is best under specified conditions. Based on laboratory research, which is considered to have implications for human learning, behaviorists emphasize that a learning environment can lead students to certain responses. As mentioned earlier, the use of contracts, containing a structured set of course requirements and utilizing behavioral objectives to accommodate a student's learning of content, is one way that the environment can be helpful to learning (Fuhrmann and Grasha 1983). Mager (1984) speaks of behavioral objectives as statements that direct students' learning of content by informing them of the expected content learning and the manner in which the learning will take place. Observable behaviors are stressed. In alerting students to content objectives, the teacher's aim is to have clearly stated objectives for a particular course.

In addition to the already mentioned behavioristic principle that states the need for immediate feedback to the organism, another related behavioral perspective emphasizes the importance of students' mastery of information. To assist students in attaining this goal, teachers may allow students to retake an examination, give students comprehensible learning objectives, and offer course content separated into smaller components or modules. Modules allow students to learn at their own pace and advance in stages of difficulty. As discussed elsewhere, each module has its own learning objectives. A module can comprise a textbook, outside readings, or laboratory assignments. In using modules, teachers usually ask that a student be successful in finishing a minimum number of modules (Fuhrmann and Grasha 1983). Mastery of course content can then be measured by examinations.

Human Interaction Models

Interactive strategies are concerned with teaching approaches "that rely heavily on discussion and sharing among participants" (Seaman and Fellenz 1989, p. 119). In learning processes involving interaction, students are able to make their own thinking clearer and share their impressions with one another. Enhanced recall can result from students' ability to apply new problem-solving knowledge related to their interactions with peers, or from correlation of new knowledge with personal experiences (Seaman and Fellenz 1989). Furthermore, learning related to interactive strategies is advantageous to students in combining segments of information into a meaningful entity. With interactive approaches, teachers serve more in the capacity of a facilitator than a controller. Through their role as stimulator and resource, teachers help students to become self-directed in their learning (Crow 1980). Teaching techniques that use interactive methods include: "discussions and participation training, buzz groups, audience reaction and listening teams, brainstorming, colloquies, forums, critical incidents, problem-solving groups, committees and committee hearings, and learning teams" (Seaman and Fellenz 1989, p. 119).

The use of discussion as an interactive strategy has been well received in adult learning. For the most part, adults have daily experience participating in discussion on an informal basis. In a more formal learning situation in which discussion is used as a learning approach, the number of individuals in the group may be important, depending upon the purpose of the discussion. The ideal number of individuals in a group has been the topic of considerable research, and the number suggested varies from four to fifteen (Seaman and Fellenz 1989). Discussion groups of six or seven may be more practical (Crow 1980). However, the group should be composed of an adequate number of people to allow for different opinions (Seaman and Fellenz 1989). Discussions can be directed toward content learning under the direction of a strong leader; toward the sharing of discernments by the participants; or toward the solution of a problem or creation of a plan to carry out a charge. Participation training, that is, the fostering of communication and interaction in students, can be used to instruct them in the use of discussions to enhance learning effectiveness (Egan 1970).

Buzz groups comprise smaller learner units that focus briefly on a subject presented by a facilitator. This approach permits a number of students to probe ideas and correlate new concepts with previous experiences. Brainstorming is guided by a facilitator and is "an interaction strategy used to generate ideas or to help determine the exact nature of content to be discussed" (Seaman and Fellenz 1989, p. 134). Brainstorming is useful in cultivating different avenues of thinking and encouraging group members to be creative in enlarging upon their ideas.

Listening teams, comprised of four to seven individuals, can be utilized for the purpose of listening for specific information given during a presentation. Because the topic assignment is made previous to the presentation, listeners have the opportunity to plan the organization of the information presented. The audience reaction team involves an interaction strategy that can be used for difficult-to-follow material or when audience input is beneficial during the presentation. It differs from listening teams in that members can interrupt the speaker. The colloquy, another interactive strategy, can be employed as a format for members of a large audience to converse. It incorporates elements of the panel and forum. A forum allows participants to present their viewpoints as a reaction or in open discussion (Seaman and Fellenz 1989).

An educational strategy requiring acquisition of knowledge is seen in the committee, described as a "small group of people given an assigned task or responsibility by a larger group (parent organization) or person with authority" (Brilhart 1982, p. 3). Another means of extracting information is the committee hearing. Typically, the committee hearing is an interview that includes the dynamics of group interaction by permitting the group to question one or more individuals at a time or in a sequence (Seaman and Fellenz 1989).

Information-Processing Models

Effective learning, according to Eggen and Kauchak (1988), is the result of students' active engagement in organizing and detecting relationships in the information they receive. Teaching methods that view learners as active in examining their surroundings are based on an information-processing theory (Wingfield and Byrnes 1981).

As related earlier, information processing has as its basis the premise that behavior is decided by the internal flow of information within the organism. Because this flow cannot be seen directly, the procedures and methods used to deduce the features of this hypothesized information flow are complicated (Gazda and Corsini 1980). Information-processing models have been developed as a means of explaining this particular learning theory. Smith (1980) points out that individuals' education should include assistance in learning "how to diagnose their own situation, organize information, learn, and know what and how much they have learned" (p. 11) if information-processing skills are to be identified with them as educated persons.

Mastery Learning Models

Another teaching rationale, the mastery learning model, contends that practically all students are able to learn most of what is taught under appropriate instructional conditions (Block and Anderson 1975). The current scheme for mastery learning is a conventional model believed to be effective in helping students learn particular types of material. Feedback or evaluation is important in making the learner aware of components that have or have not been mastered. In this method, there should also be some means to determine the status of learning as well as criteria to define mastery of the specific learning elements. Differences in the rates at which individuals learn (Bloom 1971, 1974, 1976, 1981) and the fact that practically all individuals have the capacity to learn are fundamental assumptions identified with all mastery learning models.

Distinct instructional objectives are a necessary component of mastery learning programs. A course can be divided into small units with particular skills to be learned and the means for assessing them, on an individual basis. The already-mentioned Personalized System of Instruction (PSI), developed by Keller (1968), is an example of a mastery learning model; it allows students to progress through a set of learning sequences, mastering each step before moving to the next step. If the student has not mastered the sequence, he/she then restudies the material (Fincher 1985; Stipek 1988). A subject's mastery of a particular skill or competency is determined by the subject's performance (Fincher 1985). Educators such as Cox and Dunn (1979) contend that mastery of content in a specific course is not indicative of students' mastery of prior coursework. In addition, Cox and Dunn are concerned that retaking tests may result in students' memorizing instead of comprehending material.

With mastery learning, faster students are not impeded by slower students; they move at their own pace. In this instructional approach, errors are looked upon as normal steps of learning. Although it is important that teachers note students' errors, teachers do not stress that students avoid errors. It is felt that individuals who learn at a slower pace could have a negative reaction to errors (Stipek 1988). Despite the negative aspects of mastery learning, instructors should be aware that it does offer an alternative to the more conventional single examination approach (Fuhrmann and Grasha 1983).

SUMMARY AND CONCLUSION

Developmental factors, especially those in the psychosocial, perceptual, attitudinal, emotional, personality, and cognitive areas, when taken together, have a real effect on the learning of students in higher and continuing education. These and other factors underlying the learning process contribute to learning styles that educators need to understand and appreciate. In turn, instructors' working knowledge of teaching styles, including their own, and of teaching-learning models can result in better teaching.

REFERENCES

Anderson, J. R., and Bower, G. H. 1973. *Human Associative Memory.* Washington, DC: V. H. Winston.

Atkinson, J. 1964. *An Introduction to Motivation.* Princeton, NJ: Van Nostrand.

Axelrod, J. 1970. Teaching styles in the humanities. In *Effective College Teaching,* ed. W. H. Morris. Washington, DC: American Association for Higher Education.

Bernard, H. W. 1972. *Psychology of Learning and Teaching.* New York: McGraw Hill Book Company.

Block, J. H., and Anderson, L. W. 1975. *Mastery Learning in Classroom Instruction.* New York: Macmillan Publishing Company.

Bloom, B. 1971. Mastery learning and its implications for curriculum development. In *Confronting Curriculum Reform,* ed. E. W. Eisner. Boston: Little, Brown and Company.

Bloom, B. 1974. An introduction to mastery learning theory. In *Schools, Society, and Mastery Learning,* ed. J. H. Block. New York: Holt, Rinehart & Winston, Inc.

Bloom, B. 1976. *Human Characteristics and School Learning.* New York: McGraw Hill Book Company.

Bloom, B. 1981. *All Our Children Learning.* New York: McGraw Hill Book Company.

Botwinick, J. 1967. *Cognitive Processes in Maturity and Old Age.* New York: Springer.

Botwinick, J. 1973. *Aging and Behavior* (1st ed.). New York: Academic Press.

Botwinick, J. 1978. *Aging and Behavior* (2nd ed.). New York: Academic Press.

Bower, G. H. 1970. Analysis of a mnemonic device. *American Scientist* 58: 496–510.

Breslin, F. D. 1974. *The Adolescent and Learning* (2nd ed.). New York: Collegium Book Publishers, Inc.

Brilhart, J. K. 1982. *Effective Group Discussion* (4th ed.). Dubuque, IA: William C. Brown.

Campbell, R. L., and Bickhard, M. H. 1986. *Knowing Levels and Developmental Stages.* New York: Karger.

Catania, A. C. 1979. *Learning.* Englewood Cliffs, NJ: Prentice-Hall.

Chickering, A. W. 1969. *Education and Identity.* San Francisco: Jossey-Bass.

Claxton, C. S., and Ralston, Y. 1978. *Learning Styles: Their Impact on Teaching and Administration.* AAHE-ERIC/Higher Education Research Report No. 10. Washington, DC: Association for Higher Education.

Coles, R. 1970. Erik H. Erikson: *The Growth of His Work.* Boston: Little, Brown and Company.

Cooper, S. 1983. Independent and self-directed learning. In *The Practice of Continuing Education in Nursing,* ed. S. Cooper. Rockville, MD: Aspen Systems Corporation.

Cox, W. F., and Dunn, T. G. 1979. Mastery learning: A psychological trap? *Educational Psychologist* 14:24–29.

Craig, G. J. 1976. *Human Development.* Englewood Cliffs, NJ: Prentice-Hall.

Cronbach, L. J., and Snow, R. E. 1977. *Aptitudes and Instructional Methods: A Handbook for Research on Interactions.* New York: Irvington.

Cross, K. P. 1971. *Beyond the Open Door: New Students in Higher Education.* San Francisco: Jossey-Bass.

Cross, K. P. 1976. *Accent on Learning: Improving Instruction and Reshaping the Curriculum.* San Francisco: Jossey-Bass.

Crow, M. L. 1980. Teaching as an interactive process. In *New Directions for Teaching and Learning: Improving Teaching Styles* (no. 1), ed. K. E. Eble. San Francisco: Jossey-Bass.

Csikszentmihalyi, M. 1975. *Beyond Boredom and Anxiety.* San Francisco: Jossey-Bass.

Darkenwald, G. G., and Merriam, S. B. 1982. *Adult Education: Foundations of Practice.* New York: Harper & Row, Publishers.

Douglas, K. C., Hosokawa, M. C., and Lawler, F. H. 1988. *A Practical Guide to Clinical Teaching in Medicine.* New York: Springer Publishing Company.

Eble, K. E. 1980. Teaching styles and faculty behaviors. In *New Directions for Teaching and Learning: Improving Teaching Styles* (no. 1), ed. K. E. Eble. San Francisco: Jossey-Bass.

Egan, G. 1970. *Encounter: Group Processes for Interpersonal Growth.* Belmont, CA: Brooks/Cole Publishing.

Eggen, P. D., and Kauchak, D. P. 1988. *Strategies for Teachers. Teaching Content and Thinking Skills* (2nd ed.). Englewood Cliffs, NJ: Prentice-Hall.

Ellis, H. C. 1972. *Fundamentals of Human Learning and Cognition.* Dubuque, IA: William C. Brown Company.

Ericksen, S. C. 1984. *The Essence of Good Teaching.* San Francisco: Jossey-Bass.

Erikson, E. 1963. *Childhood and Society* (2nd ed. rev.). New York: W. W. Norton.

Erikson, E. 1968. *Identity. Youth and Crisis.* New York: W. W. Norton.

Erikson, E. 1982. *The Life Cycle Completed.* New York: W. W. Norton.

Feldman, K. A., and Newcomb, T. M. 1976. *The Impact of College on Students.* San Francisco: Jossey-Bass.

Fincher, C. 1985. Learning theory and research. In *Higher Education: Handbook of Theory and Research. Vol. I,* ed. J. C. Smart. New York: Anathon Press, Inc.

Foley, R. P. 1983. Instructional media and methods. In *Handbook of Health Professions Education,* eds. C. H. McGuire, R. P. Foley, A. Goor, R. W. Richards, and Associates. San Francisco: Jossey-Bass.

Fuhrmann, B. S., and Grasha, A. F. 1983. *A Practical Handbook for College Teachers.* Boston: Little, Brown and Company.

Fuhrmann, B. S., and Jacobs, R. 1980. *The Learning Interactions Inventory.* Richmond, VA: Ronne Jacobs Associates.

Gagne, R. M. 1974. *Essentials of Learning for Instruction.* Hinsdale, IL: The Dryden Press.

Garity, J. 1985. Learning styles: Basis for creative teaching and learning. *Nurse Educator* 10(2):12–16.

Gazda, G. M., and Corsini, R. J. 1980. *Theories of Learning. A Comparative Approach.* Itasca, IL: F. E. Peacock Publishers, Inc.

Gibson, E. J. 1969. *Principles of Perceptual Learning and Development.* New York: Appleton-Century-Crofts.

Grolnick, W., and Ryan, R. 1984. Self-regulation and motivation in children's learning: An experimental investigation. University of Rochester. Unpublished manuscript.

Hayslip, B., Jr., and Kennelly, K. J. 1985. Cognitive and noncognitive factors affecting learning among older adults. In *The Older Adult as Learner,* ed. D. B. Lumsden. New York: Hemisphere Publishing Corporation.

Heimstra, R. 1976. *Lifelong Learning.* Lincoln, NE: Professional Educators.

Hill, J. 1976. *The Educational Sciences.* Bloomfield Hills, MI: Oakland Community College Press.

Hill, J., and Nunney, D. N. 1972. Personalized educational programs. *Audio-Visual Instructor* 14:25–30.

Joyce, B. R., and Weil, M. 1980. *Models of Teaching* (2nd ed.). Englewood Cliffs, NJ: Prentice-Hall.

Katz, J., and Henry, M. 1988. *Turning Professors into Teachers. A New Approach to Faculty Development and Student Learning.* New York: American Council on Education & Macmillan Publishing Company.

Keller, F. S. 1968. Good-bye, teacher. . . . *Journal of Applied Behavior* 1:79–89.

Keller, J. M. 1983. Motivational design of instruction. In *Instructional-Design Theories and Models: An Overview of their Current Status,* ed. C. M. Reigeluth. Hillsdale, NJ: Lawrence Erlbaum Associates.

Kemp, J. E., and Smellie, D. C. 1989. *Planning, Producing, and Using Instructional Media* (6th ed.). Grand Rapids, MI: Harper & Row, Publishers.

Knowles, M. S. 1980. *The Modern Practice of Adult Education.* Chicago: Follett Publishing Co.

Kolb, D. A. 1976. *The Learning Style Inventory: Technical Manual and Self-Scoring Test and Interpretation Booklet.* Boston: McBer and Company.

Kuhlen, R. G. 1952. *The Psychology of Adolescent Development.* New York: Harper & Row, Publishers.

Lange, C. 1972. A study of the effects on learning of matching the cognitive styles of students and instructors in nursing education. Michigan State University. Unpublished doctoral study.

Lapp, D., Bender, H., Ellenwood, S., and John, M. 1975. *Teaching and Learning. Philosophical, Psychological, Curricular Applications.* New York: Macmillan Publishing Company.

Lorton, J. W., and Lorton, E. L. 1984. *Human Development through the Lifespan.* Monterey, CA: Brooks/Cole Publishing Company.

Mager, R. F. 1984. *Preparing Instructional Objectives* (rev. ed.). Belmont, CA: David S. Lake Publishers.

Mann, R. D., Arnold, J. L., Binder, J. L., Cytrynbaum, S., Newman, B. M., Ringwald, B. E., Ringwald, J. W., and Rosenwein, R. 1970. *The College Classroom: Conflict, Change, and Learning.* New York: John Wiley & Sons.

Maslow, A. 1954. *Motivation and Personality* (2nd ed.). New York: Harper & Row, Publishers.

Maslow, A. 1976. Education and peak experiences. In *The Person in Education: A Humanistic Approach,* ed. C. D. Schlosser. New York: Macmillan Publishing Company.

Mast, M. E., and Van Atta, M. J. 1986. Applying adult learning principles in instructional module design. *Nurse Educator* 11(1):35–39.

Mathis, B. C., and McGaghie, W. C. 1974. From theories for learning to theories for teaching. In *Theories for Teaching,* ed. L. J. Stiles. New York: Dodd, Mead & Co.

McKeachie, W. J. 1986. *Teaching Tips. A Guidebook for the Beginning College Teacher* (8th ed.). Lexington, MA: D. C. Heath & Co.

Melton, A. W. 1963. Implications of short-term memory for a general theory of memory. *Journal of Verbal Learning and Verbal Behavior* 2:1–21.

Mezoff, B. 1979. *Cognitive Style and Interpersonal Behavior: Implications for Human Relations Training Settings.* Amherst, MA: ODT Associates. (ERIC Document Reproduction Service No. ED 185 442.)

Myers, I. B., and Briggs, K. C. 1967. *The Myers-Briggs Type Indicator.* Princeton: Educational Testing Service.

Nicholls, J. 1979. Quality and equality in intellectual development. The role of motivation in education. *American Psychologist* 34:1071–1083.

Nicholls, J. 1983. Conceptions of ability and achievement motivation: A theory and its implications for education. In *Learning and Motivation in the Classroom,* eds. S. Paris, G. Olson, and H. Stevenson. Hillsdale, NJ: Lawrence Erlbaum Associates.

Norman, D. A. 1976. *Memory and Attention: An Introduction to Human Information Processing.* New York: John Wiley & Sons.

Perry, W. 1970. *Forms of Intellectual and Ethical Development in the College Years.* New York: Holt, Rinehart & Winston, Inc.

Pervin, L. A. 1984. *Current Controversies and Issues in Personality* (2nd ed.). New York: John Wiley & Sons.

Piaget, J. 1970. Piaget's theory. In *Carmichael's Manual of Child Psychology. Vol. I* (3rd ed.), ed. P. H. Mussen. New York: John Wiley & Sons.

Piaget, J. 1972. Intellectual evolution from adolescence to adulthood. *Human Development* 15(1):1–12.

Rezler, A., and French, R. 1975. Preferences of students in six allied health professions. *Journal of Allied Health* 4:20.

Rezler, A., and Rezmovic, V. 1981. The learning preference inventory. *Journal of Allied Health* 10(1):28–34.

Rich, J. M. 1988. *Innovations in Education* (5th ed.). Boston: Allyn & Bacon, Inc.

Riechmann, S., and Grasha, A. 1974. A rational approach to developing and assessing the construct validity of a student learning style scale instrument. *Journal of Psychology* 87:213–23.

Roberts, D. Y. 1977. Personalized learning processes. *Review Inter-Americana* 7: 139–43.

Rogers, C. 1969. *Freedom to Learn.* Columbus, OH: Merrill Publishing Company.

Rogers, C. R. 1983. *Freedom to Learn for the 80's.* Columbus, OH: Merrill Publishing Company.

Rogers, T. B., Rogers, P. J., and Kuiper, N. 1979. Evidence for the self as a cognitive prototype: "The false alarm effect." *Personality and Social Psychology Bulletin* 5:53–56.

Rotter, J. 1966. Generalized expectancies for internal versus external control of reinforcement. *Psychological Monographs* 1 (Whole no. 609).

Sahakian, W. S. 1976. *Learning: Systems, Models, and Theories* (2nd ed.). Chicago: Rand McNally College Publishing Company.

Salkind, N. J. 1985. *Theories of Human Development.* (2nd ed.). New York: John Wiley & Sons.

Sanders, D. P., and McCutcheon, G. 1986. The development of practical theories of teaching. *Journal of Curriculum and Supervision* 2(1):50–67.

Schmeck, R. R. 1988. Strategies and styles of learning. In *Learning Strategies and Learning Styles,* ed. R. R. Schmeck. New York: Plenum Press.

Schultz, D. (ed.). 1977. *Growth Psychology.* New York: Van Nostrand Reinhold.

Seaman, D. F. and Fellenz, R. A. 1989. *Effective Strategies for Teaching Adults.* Columbus, OH: Merrill Publishing Company.

Sheffield, E. 1974. *Teaching in the Universities: No One Way.* Montreal: McGill-Queens University Press.

Sims, D., and Ehrhardt, H. 1978. *Cognitive Style: Utilizing Cognitive Style Map-*

ping in Instruction. Manual used in workshop at Dallas County Community College District.

Skinner, B. F. 1968. *The Technology of Teaching*. New York: Appleton-Century-Crofts.

Skinner, B. F. 1971. *Beyond Freedom and Dignity*. New York: Alfred A. Knopf.

Smith, P. P. 1980. The new professional: Professor or facilitator? *Serving Lifelong Learners*, eds. B. Heerman, C. C. Enders, and E. Wine. San Francisco: Jossey-Bass.

Snow, R. E., and Peterson, P. L. 1980. Recognizing differences in student aptitudes. In *New Directions for Teaching and Learning: Learning, Cognition, and College Teaching* (no. 2), ed. W. J. McKeachie. San Francisco: Jossey-Bass.

Stipek, D. J. 1988. *Motivation to Learn. From Theory to Practice*. Englewood Cliffs, NJ: Prentice-Hall.

Tarpy, R. M. 1975. *Basic Principles of Learning*. Dallas: Scott, Foresman and Company.

Tennyson, R. D., Boutwell, R. C., and Frey, S. 1978. Student preferences for faculty teaching styles. *Improving College and University Teaching* 26(3):194–97.

Tobias, S. 1982. When do instructional methods make a difference? *Educational Researcher* 11(4):4–9.

Torrance, E. P. 1978. Healing qualities of creative behavior. *Creative Child and Adult Quarterly* 3:146.

Tough, A. 1978a. *The Adult Learner: Current Issues in Higher Education*. Washington, DC: American Association for Higher Education.

Tough, A. 1978b. Major learning efforts: Recent research and future directions. *Adult Education* 28(4):250–65.

Tyler, L. E. 1978. *Individuality: Human Possibilities and Personal Choice in the Psychological Development of Men and Women*. San Francisco: Jossey-Bass.

Wallhead, E. M. 1986. Developmental crises: Helping students grow. *Nurse Educator* 11(3):19–22.

Warren, J. R. 1974. Adapting instruction to styles of learning. *ETS Findings* 1:1–5.

Watson, J. B. 1924. *Behaviorism*. Chicago: University of Chicago.

Waugh, N. C., and Norman, D. A. 1965. Primary memory. *Psychological Review* 72:89–104.

Weiner, B. 1979. A theory of motivation for some classroom experiences. *Journal of Educational Psychology* 71:3–25.

Weiner, B. 1980. The role of affect in rational (attributional) approaches to human motivation. *Educational Researcher* 9(7):4–11.

Weiner, B. 1985. An attributional theory of achievement motivation and emotion. *Psychological Review* 92:548–73.

Weiner, B. 1986. *An Attributional Theory of Motivation and Emotion*. New York: Springer-Verlag.

Wilson, R. C., Gaff, J. G., Dienst, E. R., Wood, L., and Bavry, J. L. 1975. *College Professors and their Impact on Students*. New York: John Wiley & Sons.

Wingfield, A., and Byrnes, D. 1981. *The Psychology of Human Memory*. New York: Academic Press.

Witkin, H. A. 1976. Cognitive styles in academic performance and in teacher-student relations. In *Individuality in Learning*, eds. S. Messick and Associates. San Francisco: Jossey-Bass.

Witkin, H. A., et al. 1977. Field-dependent and field-independent cognitive styles and their educational implications. *Review of Educational Research* 47(1):7.

Witkin, H. A., Goodenough, D. R., and Oltman, P. K. 1977. Role of field-dependent and field-independent cognitive styles in academic evolution: A longitudinal study. *Journal of Educational Psychology* 69:197–211.

Yamamoto, K., and Dizney, H. F. 1966. Eight professors: A study on college student preferences among their teachers. *Journal of Educational Psychology* 57:146–50.

Chapter 3

Curriculum Development

Judith A. Rassi and Margaret D. McElroy

CURRICULUM IN COMMUNICATION SCIENCES AND DISORDERS

As a prelude to this chapter's theme on curriculum development, a discussion of curriculum in Communication Sciences and Disorders (CSD) is presented from several perspectives.

Historical Perspective

Distinctive chronological markers describe the evolution of higher education curriculum in CSD. Precursory references to continuing education curriculum also can be gleaned from an historical view.

Highland Park Conference. The first comprehensive examination of curriculum in speech pathology and audiology can be traced to the National Conference on Graduate Education in Speech Pathology and Audiology held in Highland Park, Illinois, in 1963. The need for such a conference grew out of a recognition that the profession had grown substantially and that the increasing number of university training programs demanded a thorough analysis of academic practices. In the previous year, 1962, the Professional Services Board of the American Speech and Hearing Association (ASHA) had begun its review of service facilities while, at the same time, the ASHA Education and Training Board was studying various aspects of training programs with an eye toward accreditation. In 1962, ASHA members had voted to require the master's degree as the minimal entry level for association membership. Curriculum matters, thus, were a key factor in the profession's evolving efforts in self-evaluation and self-regulation (ASHA 1963).

Of the five major issues considered at the Highland Park conference, one was devoted specifically to the development of graduate curricula in speech pathology and audiology. Questions related to this issue included: Should the curriculum have a common core for all students? What kinds of subject matter should provide the foundation for professional study, regardless of specialization area? What kinds of curricula are appropriate for certain areas of specialization? Should the curriculum be flexible so that students can have a diversified plan of study? Should the type and content of courses be designated? What kinds of external controls, e.g., certification and accreditation requirements, should influence the shaping of curricula? (ASHA 1963, p. 10.)

After deliberating the differing emphases and their corresponding labels, conference participants acknowledged that, although there are areas of common interest and study in the field, the specialization areas of speech pathology, audiology, and speech and hearing science should be recognized, and should be reflected in training programs (ASHA 1963, p. 44).

In another curriculum-related resolution, consensus was reached on the concept that there exists a common core of knowledge from which stem the diverse activities of teaching, research, and clinical work as well as areas of specialized content. Participants resolved that the fundamental core areas for students should include the biological, behavioral, physical, linguistic, and social foundations of communication (ASHA 1963, p. 46).

In addition, the group stated that there are three essential areas of study prior to specialization: (1) basic subject matter as a part of liberal education but having an emphasis in the sciences, e.g., physics, biological sciences, psychology, and mathematics; (2) information pertaining to normal speech and hearing processes, including anatomy, audition, developmental and experimental psychology, linguistics, measurement, physiology, voice and speech sciences, and the development of speech, language, and hearing functions; and (3) subject matter pertaining to disorders of speech and audition (ASHA 1963, p. 69).

Opinions varied greatly concerning the specific content and emphasis to be recommended for inclusion in these curriculum areas. It was decided that specific topic coverage should be stated in the form of guidelines rather than requirements and that course sequences should not be specified for training programs. It is noteworthy that some participants opposed any description of curriculum, stating that this matter should be left to the discretion of the respective graduate schools in which speech pathology and audiology training programs reside (ASHA 1963, pp. 47–48).

The majority of conference participants agreed that when students are in early stages of area specialization, they must acquire a comprehensive rather than a narrowly-focused knowledge of that particular area. Participants resolved that the so-called clinical laboratory experience should be an integral part of graduate professional training and should receive graduate credit. They acknowledged that this experience is necessary for the demonstration and teaching of certain principles just as is laboratory education in other fields (ASHA 1963, p. 48).

Conference participants were in general agreement that clinical and research objectives are appropriate at both the master's and doctoral levels. Then, as now, discussion and controversy surrounded the notion that there should be two kinds of degrees at the doctoral level, one a clinical degree and the other a research degree. The greatest number of participants finally endorsed the concept of the Ph.D. degree as being an academic scholarly degree that should not be changed to embrace a clinical emphasis. Fewer participants supported a resolution that the Ph.D. degree should be flexible enough to meet the training needs of both clinical and research objectives (ASHA 1963, p. 49).

A narrow majority of conference participants supported the idea that degrees should represent various levels of professional competence. However, there was a significant amount of disagreement with this proposition. Finally, it was decided simply to recommend to ASHA that steps be taken to study professional competence and its relation to graduate degrees (ASHA 1963, pp. 52–54). As evidenced in the first Requirements for the Certificate of Clinical Competence reported by the ASHA Committee on Clinical Standards (ASHA 1964b), professional competence later became linked with certification rather than with degrees. Meanwhile, authority to accredit master's degree programs in speech pathology and audiology at U.S. universities and colleges was being granted to ASHA by the National Commission on Accrediting (ASHA 1964a).

The resolutions of the Highland Park conference continued to have an impact for many years on the direction of training programs and, ultimately, on the profession (O'Neill 1987). Not until 1983 was there a second major conference dealing with education in the field. A search of the literature published during the two intervening decades reveals a modest number of articles on education but few of them relate directly to curriculum. A series of reports on undergraduate programs did include curriculum samples (Basinger 1968; Bloomer 1968; Norton 1968; Nuttall 1968; Powers 1968; Winitz 1968). And, in 1969, participants at the conference on Undergraduate Preparation for Professional Education in Speech Pathology and Audiology recommended that information on curriculum planning be made available to training programs (Villarreal and Lawrence 1970).

St. Paul Conference.   As indicated by its name, the 1983 National Conference on Undergraduate, Graduate, and Continuing Education, held in St. Paul, Minnesota, expanded on the mission of its 1963 predecessor, including undergraduate and continuing education as well as graduate education. Several phases of data collection preceded the conference. The first of these involved needs identification in which optimal clinical and educational service needs of communicatively handicapped persons were identified. Next, competencies required by speech-language pathologists and audiologists to provide appropriate services were defined in a series of regional study group meetings in the needs analysis phase. And, in the final phase, discrepancy identification, information about the competencies needed by speech-language pathologists and audiologists was collected from universities, service providers, and supervisors, and then analyzed (Rees and Snope 1983).

The conferees' deliberations culminated in 99 separate resolutions. Among those with curricular implications, one found unanimous endorsement for the need to strengthen undergraduate education in liberal arts and sciences. The group reaffirmed that the minimum entry level to the profession should be the master's degree or its equivalent. Not everyone agreed, although many did, that there should be some exposure to communicative disorders, including clinical observation and limited practicum, at the undergraduate level (Rees 1983).

For graduate education, there was general consensus on the need to strengthen the theoretical and scientific bases of education at that level. Strong support was received for the preparation of generalists rather than specialists in the two areas of clinical practice—speech-language pathology and audiology. Participants noted that there should be alternative models of clinical practicum and of the Clinical Fellowship Year. The professional doctorate still held interest for some participants, but the Ph.D. degree was affirmed as the appropriate doctoral degree for the discipline of human communication and its disorders (Rees 1983).

Conferees urged that there be a strengthening of interaction and interfacing with other disciplines in the areas of education, research, and service delivery. There was a recommendation that graduates be prepared to deliver services to persons with all types of disorders, regardless of work setting, and be equipped with a background of counseling and interviewing experience in each of these areas. Resolutions also reflected the importance of proficiency in oral and written language and the need to prepare students for delivery of services to different populations (Rees 1983).

The appropriate time for specialty training was considered by most conferees to be during the period following general professional education, that is, when continuing education becomes the primary learning vehicle. Continuing education and its role were strongly endorsed. The group urged that new "creative and innovative methods" for obtaining continuing education be pursued. They further recommended that the effectiveness of continuing education be studied. Voluntary continuing education was favored over mandatory continuing education (Rees 1983, p. 91).

The importance of research experience was underscored but more so for the Clinical Fellowship Year than for the period of study during master's education. There was strong support for increasing efforts in the areas of computers and advanced technology and for incorporating such information into both higher and continuing education (Rees 1983).

A multitude of association activities aimed at upgrading education at all levels have resulted from the deliberations of the St. Paul conference. In the form of committee, board, and task force efforts, curriculum matters have been addressed directly or indirectly by many individuals from a variety of perspectives. For example, a role delineation study and subsequent content validation study of the requirements for the certificates of clinical competence were conducted (Smith, Greenberg, and Lingwall 1986; Lingwall 1988; ASHA 1988e). The outcome of this evaluation, in turn, helped to shape revision of the national examinations in speech-language pathology and audiology and re-examination of other curriculum-related factors involving certification and accreditation (ASHA 1989d, 1990b). Conference resolutions also provided direction for the formation and/or deliberation of such groups as the Committee on Doctoral Education, the Ad Hoc

Committee on Undergraduate Education, the Continuing Education Board (ASHA 1989e); the Task Force on Audiology II (ASHA 1988d); and the Committee on Long Range Planning (ASHA 1988b, 1989e). Curriculum guidelines were presented in April 1989, at the Conference on Undergraduate Education: The Foundation of the Educational Continuum, held in conjunction with the annual meeting of the Council of Graduate Programs in Communication Sciences and Disorders (ASHA 1989a).

Throughout the years, periodic modifications of requirements (now standards) for certificates of clinical competence have influenced curriculum in speech-language pathology and audiology educational programs. Reflecting changes in the field over time, academic coursework and practicum requirements generally have become more stringent and, with some exceptions, more specific. (See Appendix A.) They, thus, have become more responsive to increasing demands for professional accountability and to changing and expanding scopes of practice (Ainsworth et al. 1972; ASHA 1972, 1981, 1983, 1984a, 1985b, 1986, 1988c, 1990b, 1991).

Curriculum requirements have also been addressed by the ASHA Education and Training Board, now the Educational Services Board (Matthews 1966; ASHA 1987d, 1989d, 1990a). (See Appendix B.) The change of name for this board in 1984 was significant, reflecting the views of the Council of Graduate Programs in Communication Sciences and Disorders and, ultimately, the views of the approving ASHA Legislative Council. In essence, these groups felt that the word "training" connotes preparation that is not of a scholarly nature and, further, that it applies more to technicians who carry out the orders of physicians or others (Cooper 1986; Aronson 1987).

The planned linking of certification with completion of graduate work carried out exclusively in ESB-accredited programs ensures total curricular influence by these regulatory mechanisms (ASHA 1990a). Nevertheless, it is important to note that stipulations have always been confined to areas of study rather than actual course content, thereby leaving the latter to the discretion of individual educational programs and their respective institutions (Ainsworth et al. 1972).

Historical evidence, thus, indicates that curriculum evolvement in speech-language pathology and audiology educational programs has been guided by actions of the ASHA through its governing bodies and its membership.

Professional and Philosophical Perspectives

Several issues related to curriculum are at the center of present-day discussions about the viability of the field. These include knowledge explosion, expanding scopes of practice, and changing health care delivery, as discussed below.

Knowledge Explosion. It is widely recognized that audiology and speech-language pathology practice requirements have changed dramatically in the past two decades (Aronson 1987; Schwartz 1987) and at an accelerated rate with each succeeding year. Attributed to unprecedented technological advances and ever-increasing knowledge bases, such changes demand continually updated and increasingly sophisticated curricula for both preprofessionals and practicing professionals. In the opinions of many individuals and groups in the profession, higher education is not keeping pace with the demand (Falck 1972; Minifie 1983; Feldman 1984; Brodnitz 1986; Aronson 1987; ASHA 1988c; Fowler and Wilson 1989; Goldstein 1989a, 1989b; AAA 1990; Goldstein et al. 1990).

This reported information gap leaves graduates responsible for acquiring current levels of expertise through on-the-job training, self-study, and other forms of continuing education. Even for those persons whose preprofessional preparation may be current and complete, the need for updating never ends. However, because continuing education is ordinarily voluntary and selective, it may be inferred that some graduates who are now practitioners or educators themselves, are not current in essential knowledge and/or skills. In other words, because there is no master curriculum plan required for continuing education, there can be no assurance that all who need information are obtaining it or that those who are getting it are getting all that they need. Nor is there any assurance that the students of continuing education are using what they are getting. Without such continuing education assurances, the major responsibility for depth, breadth, and currentness of appropriate curricula necessarily falls to educators in university programs.

Expanding Scopes of Practice. Parallel to, and partially as a consequence of, our broadening knowledge bases, the phenomenon of expanding scopes of practice has emerged (ASHA 1987a, 1989c; Cherow and Williams 1989, pp. 21–22). Again, curricular concerns become an issue as practitioners and educators alike seek to determine the boundaries of practice in audiology and speech-language pathology and the impact of these shifting lines on the shape and size of curriculum. Such deliberations have resulted in the publication of a number of area-specific guidelines and position statements (ASHA 1976; Muma, Webb, and Muma 1979; ASHA 1984b, 1984c; Raiford and Shadden 1985; ASHA 1985a, 1987b, 1987c, 1988a, 1989b, 1989c, 1989f). As the complexity of both audiology and speech-language pathology practices increases, boundary lines are not often clearcut because of marked philosophical differences among individuals. As a consequence, debates and controversy continue while related curricular content questions remain unanswered.

Changing Health Care Delivery. Inextricably interlinked to the factors of knowledge explosion and expanding scopes of practice is that of changing health care delivery. With the move of more practitioners into medical settings and private practices, many individuals feel that new and specific kinds of preprofessional preparation are needed. At issue, according to Spriesterbach (1989), is the question: "What kind of core curriculum is adequate for entry positions?" (p. 77). Indeed, it is this pivotal question that lies at the center of the professional doctorate controversy (Feldman 1984; Ringel 1984; Aronson 1987; AAA 1989; Goldstein 1989a, 1989b; Spriesterbach 1989).

Contextual Perspective

To gain insight into the curriculum issues of audiology and speech-language pathology, it is helpful to consider them from a contextual perspective, that is, from the vantage points of categorical or related domains.

Higher Education. A look at higher-education-curriculum history over time reveals gradual changes, change that is general and embraces all degree levels and change that is specific to various fields of study. Audiology and speech-language pathology educational programs can identify with several transformations that have taken place: the melding of graduate education and professional programs with the four-year undergraduate experience; the upgrading of professional curricula to the level of graduate study; and the professionalization of the Ph.D. degree (Menges and Mathis 1988).

Calls for change persist. Amidst the current reform movement in higher education, findings of national studies by such groups as the National Institute of Education (1984) and the Carnegie Foundation for the Advancement of Teaching (1986), for example, indicate an ongoing need to create change throughout curricula. Despite this recognized need, however, institutions, departments, and individual instructors reportedly have difficulty effecting change because they are uncertain about how to proceed and about the specific roles of administrators, curriculum committees, and faculty (Diamond 1989).

Health Professions Education. A review of certain trends in curriculum development and their impact on the health professions of medicine, nursing, pharmacy, and dentistry is instructive. During the 1950s, for example, nursing education began a changeover to collegiate programs; pharmacy education accelerated its move from four- to five-year programs; medical education began organizing subject matter by organ systems, a major departure from the traditional, discipline-based instruction in basic sciences during the preclinical years (Bussigel, Barzansky, and Grenholm 1988b); and dental education examined critically its educational objectives in light of changing professional practices, including the use of dental assistants and the advent of preventive dentistry (Rosinski 1983).

In the 1960s, curricula in existing medical schools underwent further change, while new medical schools developed curricula involving not only change in format but also in content and faculty organization. Although such changes were prevalent and often radical, little educational research was carried out at that time to evaluate their effectiveness. Furthermore, curriculum reform was often met with resistance by faculty who preferred more traditional approaches. In nursing education, where some of the changes paralleled those in medical education, there was similar resistance, especially to the new baccalaureate and associate degree programs. Nonetheless, this transition proceeded, curriculum was modified, and educational research, made possible because many nursing educators had advanced degrees in education, documented the details and effects of change. Curricular reforms in pharmacy and dental education during this period were less extensive and received little evaluative or research support (Rosinski 1983).

By the 1970s, curriculum reform in health professions education continued but at a slower pace. Scope-of-practice conflicts between clinical pharmacists and physicians, clinical pharmacists and clinical pharmacologists, physician assistants and nurse practitioners, physician assistants and physicians, and dental assistants and dentists, reduced the likelihood of substantial change. Among other influences on curriculum development during this time were the dwindling of available funds for institutional expansion; the decreasing number of patients seeking medical care at university centers; student and faculty demands for practice-relevant curricula including more elective courses to meet changing career goals; and scientific and technical advances. Consequent changes included the increasing use of off-site clinical facilities and teaching aids such as simulators, skills laboratories, and patient management problems. The most significant development in medical education, perhaps, was that of problem-based curriculum (Kaufman and Obenshain 1985). Competency-based curriculum in medical and nursing education also emerged. The problem-based approach has been subjected to extensive research, whereas evaluation of competency-based programs has been more limited (Rosinski 1983).

In a mode of reappraisal during this decade, most medical and dental programs in which three-year curricula had been instituted only several years earlier, decided to revert to four-year plans. In a number of studies (Greenberg 1976; Formicola 1978; Beran 1979; Kettel et al. 1979; Trzebiatowski and Peterson 1979), the reasons for failure of the shorter plan of study were documented, among them: time pressure and resultant stress on faculty and students alike; courses taught poorly in haste; lack of substance in programs where basic science material had been compressed; student deficiencies in problem-solving ability; limited contact between faculty and students; lack of flexibility in programs; and complaints by practitioners about the quality of graduates.

Present-day efforts to keep curriculum in the health professions current and responsive are continuing. As pointed out by Beaty (1989), practitioners of the next century, already in university classrooms, must be prepared now for the future. In order to meet the expected challenge of persistent economic pressures, continued advancements in knowledge and technology, and societal demands, medical faculties will need to draw on their creativity, even look toward the development of "a new paradigm for medical education" (p. 8).

Administrative Perspective

Administrators of educational programs in speech-language pathology and audiology are responsible ultimately for the delineation of curriculum structure and content. Operating in accordance with university policy and the aforementioned ASHA certification and accreditation requirements, administrators often appoint curriculum committees to assist in this effort. Faculty meetings provide a forum for reports and discussion of committee recommendations. Student as well as faculty contributions are important to thoughtful curriculum development and evaluation (Hardick and Oyer 1987).

CURRICULUM FOUNDATION

The soundness of an educational program's curriculum foundation can be identified by the integrity of its component parts. In their essay on the pursuit of excellence in an academic program, Adams et al. (1984) noted that:

> . . . a unit's program and curricula reflect excellence in several ways. For example, excellent programs and curricula clearly express the mission and philosophy of both the academic structures within which the unit is placed and the discipline that the unit represents. The programs and curricula should be comprised of an intellectually stimulating and de-

manding sequence of learning experiences (e.g., courses, field trips, experiments, lab assignments, practica, etc.) that follow some readily discernible, logical order. Thus, the student, moving from one experience to the next, should be able to see the unit's philosophy and mission unfolding. Excellence also finds expression in the well-rounded and meaningful character of each individual learning experience, as well as in the carefully developed interface between adjacent experiences in the sequence. Furthermore, the programs and curricula must be constructed with sufficient flexibility so that faculty and students share some latitude to exercise their curiosity, explore new ideas, and seek out different learning experiences. This flexibility is essential because it allows for qualitative growth and improvement in the learning experiences, and hence, in the programs and curricula. In turn, the programs and curricula then express the unit's mission and philosophy with greater depth and breadth and with greater wisdom and maturity (p. 27).

Theory

Underlying a well-planned curriculum are theoretical constructs that give it definition. It is an organizational rather than individual entity made up of various components that relate to one another in a pattern, e.g., goals, individual instructor roles, and institutional divisions. Each component has a definite, and often predetermined, function within the organizational structure (Bussigel, Barzansky, and Grenholm 1988b). Nevertheless, in comparative analyses among institutions of curricula in the same discipline, patterns and functions have been found to vary significantly. A case study of curriculum goals in four medical schools, for example, revealed differences in the substantive nature of goals, in the perceived importance of terminal and instrumental goals, and in the institutions' ability to focus goals on such themes as educational changes or innovations (Bussigel, Barzansky, and Grenholm 1988a, p. 121).

Politics

Because curriculum development involves individuals with different perspectives, competing interests sometimes affect final outcomes. To be supported, the conceptual framework underlying a curriculum plan needs to be accepted by its potential participants (Bellet 1981). Educational decision making can also be complicated by the hierarchical structure within an institution and the power, or lack of power, vested in the instructors who eventually carry out curriculum directives. Another determinant is the location of control for curriculum committee appointments and the approval of committee recommendations, that is to say, whether it lies in the hands of the department faculty, the general faculty, the department chair, or higher administrative officials.

Curriculum committee composition can also have a significant effect, as can a department's decision to seek the advice of an educator who specializes in curriculum development.

As alluded to earlier, an external factor, such as professional accreditation, wields considerable influence on curriculum development, perhaps too much so, according to some educators in the health professions. In nursing education, for example, it has been asserted that revisions in curriculum are often made in order to adhere to accreditation guidelines, thereby leading to curriculum patching (Quiring and Gray 1979). Moreover, the Carnegie Report on Governance of Higher Education (1982) states that specialized accreditation, when linked to state certification or licensure and to federal financial support, is tantamount to curriculum control.

Policies

Institutional curriculum policies can promote or hinder the efforts of departments seeking change, depending on the compatibility of policies with program goals. In addition, the actual absence of any formal policy for planning curriculum has its own adverse effect. This is illustrated in those instances where, in an attempt to fit increasing amounts of information into a fixed number of courses or program duration, educators sacrifice depth of learning for breadth of learning. Moreover, they may try to update program content by teaching only what they know or have recently learned or by constructing curricula on the basis of assumed certification-examination content. Such informality in the absence of specific curriculum policy often results in a directionless program and reduced teaching effectiveness (Drewry and Fiene 1985).

If institutional or departmental policies do not embrace teaching as a high priority among faculty activities, even the best of intentions in an otherwise sound curriculum plan may not be implemented satisfactorily (Bellet 1981). Policies concerning required and elective courses, course prerequisites, course distribution, residency requirements, theses and dissertations, and independent research studies have a further impact on curriculum planning. Finally, fiscal policy has a direct bearing on curriculum since the quality and quantity of course, laboratory, and practicum offerings are dependent, to a great extent, on supporting funds (Mennin and Martinez-Burrola 1985).

Resources

As reported earlier in this chapter, a recommendation for making educational information available to training programs was expressed as long ago as 1969 during an ASHA-sponsored conference on undergraduate preparation (Villarreal and Lawrence 1970). It is interesting that conferees then recognized the importance of obtaining such information from "experts in curriculum planning and teaching methods" (p. 70). They further advised that information be sought in disciplines or professions such as counseling, clinical psychology, social work, and medicine, where educational preparation involves "dealing with people, identifying and remedying disorders, and supervising clinical experience" (p. 70). Since that time, it would appear that speech-language pathology and audiology educators have not taken advantage of such resources to any great degree, at least not until more recent examinations of the professional doctorate and associated curricula in other fields began taking place. The extent to which curriculum consultants are used in CSD educational programs is not known.

A rich source of adaptable curriculum information is the educational literature in the fields noted above as well as in the nursing and health professions. Also, as might be expected, the field of education has extensive literature on every aspect of higher education curriculum. An excellent compendium of the latter may be found in the book, *Key Resources on Teaching, Learning, Curriculum and Faculty Development. A Guide to the Higher Education Literature*, by Menges and Mathis (1988). Other references listed herein will lead the reader to additional publication sources.

CURRICULUM CONSIDERATIONS

Curriculum developers must take into account a number of factors as they begin planning the stages of construction. The following discussion considers those that are most contributory.

Students' Learning Experience

What kinds of learning experiences have students had in the past and what kinds of learning experiences are desired in the educational program? The answers to these questions constitute an important source of data (Diamond 1989). As curricula are planned for students in speech-language pathology and audiology at the master's degree level, for example, the students' undergraduate academic coursework and clinical practicum experiences, or lack thereof, must be considered. Because some students, as undergraduates, major in speech and hearing sciences, while others do not, there is often a wide range of background experience in any group of individuals entering a master's program. Thus, even though a definite course of study, designed in conformance with ESB and CCC standards and institutional requirements, can be outlined readily for master's students, allowances for their individual differences may be problematic. For both academic coursework and clinical practicum assignments, proficiency examinations are helpful to individual instructional planning as well as to overall curriculum development.

Consideration of students' past and present learning experiences not only enters into curricular decision making but also into the admissions process itself. That is to say, criteria for admissions should relate to the kinds of achievements and characteristics that are deemed important for success in an educational program, whether undergraduate, master's, or doctoral, and for occupational success thereafter. In this regard, admissions and curriculum are interdependent educational components because admissions criteria seek to identify prospective students who can be expected to attain a program's curriculum goals.

Is this interrelationship acknowledged and practiced in CSD educational programs? Such data are not readily available although they may be embedded in ESB reports. A look at medical education, however, where admissions criteria have been questioned and studied, provides an enlightening parallel. As is typically the case in CSD programs, medical students traditionally have been selected on the basis of academic standing, that is, grade point averages and scores on the Medical College Admissions Test (MCAT). However, in a national survey of medical schools (American Association of Medical Colleges 1983), the following problems were uncovered: an overemphasis by admissions committees on scientific preparation, despite calls in the profession for more premedical emphasis on the social sciences and humanities; admissions criteria that did not address an acknowledged need for reading, writing, and communication skills; and overemphasis on the MCAT as an admissions criterion in the face of evidence that it evaluates test-taking ability rather than applicable knowledge and clinical performance potential. In short, admissions criteria were found to be incongruent with medical education (curriculum) goals.

In the views of a number of medical educators, among them, Martinez-Burrola, Klepper, and Kaufman (1985), admissions procedures should take into account a prospective student's problem-solving skills, interpersonal skills, self-motivation, and level of maturity, along with predicted achievement of the program's goals (p. 164). In fact, some medical schools have altered their admissions criteria and/or devised mechanisms for observing prospective students in situations that require demonstration of the desired qualities. Educational programs in audiology and speech-language pathology may want to consider their own alternative approaches to ensure that admissions criteria are consonant with curriculum and program goals.

Selection of Subject Matter

On the surface, selecting subject matter might appear to be a straightforward task, given that CSD is a professional discipline having accreditation and certification standards with already-established subject stipulations. However, due to several complicating factors, the task can be difficult and frustrating for educational planners. Part of the difficulty stems from the knowledge explosion, expanding scopes of practice, and changing health care delivery. Standards define only minimum requirements. Beyond this, a determination must be made as to the program's own maximum limits. How much and what kind of knowledge will make the educational program better than average or excellent? What material, what courses should be eliminated to make room for new information?

Educators must make choices filled with compromise. They are faced with the constraints imposed by time, number and expertise of available instructors, building space, laboratory and clinical equipment, size and diversity of clinical populations, program funding, and the hurdles of institutional bureaucracy. In addition, course and clinical instructors must be willing to update their own knowledge, change course content and clinical approaches accordingly, and take on new teaching assignments. Without such interest and cooperation, titles of courses and clinical practicum assignments may change, but actual course content and clinical approaches remain the same.

Breadth, Depth of Topic Coverage. The breadth and depth of course topics are linked to a philosophy of what constitutes sufficient preparation of students. If an educational program's philosophy is espoused by the curriculum planners and educators within, it is easier to determine the range of topics to be included in course offerings. If, however, individual philosophies differ, then, again, compromise becomes necessary. Even so, faculty and staff deliberations on such matters serve to broaden views and stimulate thinking, both necessary processes. Experimental curriculum, discussed later in this chapter, usually does not materialize in a climate of complacent satisfaction with the status quo or of unchallenging acceptance of any new topic.

Planners in universities, by reason of their proximity to research and clinical advances, have ready access to new areas of topic coverage. Nevertheless, input from non-university practitioners in the field and from students and former students also is valuable because these persons are in positions to see preservice educational needs from their respective vantage points. Keeping abreast of current developments in both the discipline and the profession is clearly essential for curriculum planners as they consider topic coverage.

Clinical and/or Research Emphasis. An important curriculum consideration for an audiology and speech-language pathology educational program, that of deciding whether to adopt a clinical and/or research emphasis, is directly related to the program's mission and goals. For what kinds of careers should the students be prepared? What kinds of skills and knowledge are required for these careers? What kinds of educational resources are available?

Related curricular decisions can be perplexing. In an ideal educational model, each topic and its correlates would be explored to the fullest so that clinical and research orientations would receive equal emphases within a curriculum and, insofar as possible, within individual courses. At least in part, this educational balance would contribute to the healing of the profession's long-standing and apparently widening schism between these two perspectives. However, in the present system where there is a vast amount of information to be taught in both a master's level clinical preparation program and a doctoral level research preparation program, a dichotomy along clinical and research lines often results. For many professionals, this clinic-research separation has seemed logical not only for the sake of preserving reasonable time lines for master's and doctoral degree programs, but also for preparing students with different preparation requirements for ostensibly different job markets.

The issue of emphasis for the clinical and research facets of education can be examined in other ways. Although it is generally assumed that clinical topics are less complex in nature than are research topics, as reflected in their respective ties to the master's and doctoral degrees, the levels of difficulty do not lend themselves necessarily to this type of differentiation. A simple analysis of certain clinical endeavors, for example, reveals some concepts that require higher levels of thinking, performance, or judgment than those required by certain research endeavors. Moreover, it is evident that a preponderance of research is embedded in underlying theory which is the prerequisite foundation for an individual's understanding of normal sensory processes, related disorders, and clinical remediation. Indeed, it is this order of curricular presentation that promotes clear conceptualization and conforms to accepted learning principles and orderly skill building.

Many research and clinical components of education are inseparable and, in some ways, even indistinguishable from one another. Because of this, curriculum planners must recognize that neither the "clinical" master's degree nor the "research" doctoral degree can or should be purely either. Career or job-market preparation then emerges as a major factor in the equation, and the question of emphasis dictated accordingly. Sources cited earlier suggest that not all persons responsible for curriculum planning in today's educational programs are paying enough attention to this external driving force.

Currentness of Information. As mentioned earlier in this chapter, information in our curricula is affected by the knowledge explosion, the changing system of health care delivery, and the expanding scopes of professional practice in audiology and speech-language pathology. Not only do courses need to be added to or deleted from a program for the purpose of keeping current, but the updating of existing courses may be indicated.

Requiring academic faculty and clinical supervisors to keep current through continuing education seems to be a reasonable expectation. However, when new or replacement topics are being considered for insertion into a program curriculum, it may be unrealistic to expect the typically small faculty groups found in CSD educational programs to have among them in-depth knowledge of all pertinent topics. Without the required expertise, hard decisions must often be made. If the subject matter in question is not required for program accreditation, certification preparation, or institutional requirement, then omitting it from the curriculum might be the resolution. Having decided this, curriculum planners may rationalize that there is too much information to teach in graduate school and that students can obtain the information after graduation through continuing education offerings. Critics contend that this attitude is irresponsible; defenders see it as being realistic.

Other remedies sometimes applied are the assignment of courses to faculty members with little or no knowledge of the topic area; or to clinical supervisors who have a working knowledge of clinical application, but may be lacking in theoretical knowledge in the topic area. With these kinds of compromises, curriculum planners reason that, even though the ideal has not been achieved, students nonetheless are receiving information in an area that otherwise would be uncovered. Even so, it is clear that students are being shortchanged by such arrangements.

Still other seemingly more appropriate solutions are possible but, depending on circumstances, may not be viable. Employing adjunct faculty who are experts in the topics to be covered, for example, can work well, but only if such individuals are available, accessible, and affordable. Bringing in guest lecturers from other geographical locations in a short-term arrangement sometimes succeeds in circumventing these problems. However, when such approaches are used, topics typically cannot be covered in depth, nor can students learn material on a gradual basis over an extended period. If local lecturers are available and willing to present information in otherwise uncovered topic areas, and without remuneration, an educational program clearly has the best chance of filling its curriculum gaps. As is understandable, however, such persons ordinarily are brought in only for a limited number of presentations. With any type of part-time instruction, whatever the arrangement, there is likely a lack of curriculum continuity, fewer opportunities for associated laboratory and/or clinical supplements, and limited instructor availability between classes.

Organization of Curricular Components

When curriculum planners consider their approach to organizing a program's various components, they must take into account curriculum balance, pace, sequence, and schedule. This is not an easy task, given the many limiting factors that are inherent in college and university systems are unique to a particular educational program, or are a consequence of professional accreditation and certification requirements.

Balance. There are a number of elements to balance within an overall curriculum, among them: required versus elective courses; departmental versus nondepartmental courses; professional-area versus related-area courses; and graduate-level versus undergraduate-level courses. Mixed into this array of offerings may be independent studies, seminars, research projects, and clinical practicum assignments.

What kinds of balance should planners strive to achieve? Depending on students' individual goals versus common or group goals, sample plans of study can be drafted to determine how they might fit into a projected curriculum framework. As this is done, and in light of such required curricular balances, planners should seek to balance: course demands on student time (for example, do some courses require a lengthy written paper and other ones not?); course difficulty; parallelism of course content; course instructors (do students take more than one course from the same instructor during a particular term?); and interface between clinical practicum and coursework and between research activity and coursework.

The objective of these and other kinds of curricular balancing is twofold: (1) to make course goals achievable for students within the allotted time and under a given set of circumstances; and (2) to maximize students' learning of the prescribed material in its entirety. Because of ongoing program changes, the balance in any curriculum should undergo periodic review. In order to be effective, both the planning and review phases demand cooperation and compromise from course instructors as well as curriculum planners.

Pace. Similar in purpose and effect to that described for balance, curriculum pacing has to do with the frequency and amount of information imparted to students. Here, too, curriculum planners need to look at individual courses, practica, and research projects within the larger context of a projected program curriculum. Do they meet criteria compatible with optimal learning? That is to say, are course, clinic, and research offerings presented at a pace that allows for understanding of all concepts and absorption of all material within the allotted time?

If it is determined that too much material (overwhelming for most students) or not enough material (lacking challenge for most students) is being offered, then adjustments need to be made. Experimentation, or the actual offering of certain curriculum-unit combinations, may be necessary initially to determine whether or not pacing changes are indicated.

Course difficulty levels figure prominently in pacing decisions. In general, the greater the difficulty, the slower the pace that is indicated. This can vary, however, depending on the stage within a curricular sequence. Pacing is also greatly affected by the duration of school terms, that is, whether they are based on a quarter, semester, or trimester system. In longer school terms, instructors can be more flexible in pacing the material within a given course, whereas shorter school terms allow for more pacing changes in course offerings from term to term.

Sequence. The sequencing of courses, practica, and research assignments is perhaps the most crucial of organizational maneuvers. And, frequently, it is the most difficult. The concept of sequencing is a simple one based on the learning principle that knowledge and skills should be acquired in a linear fashion from their bases to their manifestations, from theories to applications, from knowing to doing. But achieving this is quite another matter.

At the undergraduate level, the sequence of students' background and introduction courses for communication sciences and disorders may be rather straightforward in those cases where the major field of study is declared early. With a prescribed curriculum in place, students' schedules can be set accordingly. Although institutional distribution requirements sometimes interfere, they frequently and conveniently coincide with courses also required for professional certification.

For those students who have switched from another major area to CSD or for those who have entered the field late in the undergraduate program, however, the resultant curriculum patchwork may make appropriate sequencing difficult and, in some cases, impossible. Nevertheless, because the undergraduate level constitutes the earliest phase of the CSD sequence and, therefore, consists primarily of courses in the basic sciences, normal processes, and other fundamentals, progressive sequencing is not as important as foundation building. In other words, the groundwork pieces must be laid in place; this infrastructure, if solid, will provide firm support for a later course of study with more definite direction.

It is in the course of study for CSD students at the master's level that curriculum sequencing is needed the most and has the greatest impact. A graduate curriculum sequence, ordinarily based on the assumption that entering students will have completed basic coursework at the undergraduate level, should allow for a progression in the sequence of clinical practicum assignments as well as in the order of courses. An ideal knowledge- and skill-building sequence provides clinical work that parallels the coursework.

Faced with practical restrictions, curriculum planners find this ideal virtually impossible to achieve within the framework of a typical two-year (or shorter) master's degree program. University clinics, for example, cannot schedule clients with certain disorders only at those times dictated by students' learning needs. Nor can courses be scheduled in a completely linear pattern, given that several courses must be taken simultaneously. Even so, an approximation of the ideal sequence is achievable and worth striving for. To the extent that a curriculum design incorporates a carefully planned sequence, students' education will be more orderly and information more understandable.

For those students entering a master's program in CSD without undergraduate preparation in the field, individually designed courses of study must usually be undertaken. These students often do not fit into the graduate curriculum plan and must backtrack by taking courses their classmates have already completed. If the missing courses are taken along with other courses in the regular, planned sequence of graduate coursework and practicum, the frequent result is an orderless presentation of information that leads to confusion. An added stress may be that their lack of background in the field leaves these students less prepared for out-of-sequence learning. In most instances, such students are better served by being required to complete their foundation courses before enrolling in the regular CSD master's-level curriculum (Cunningham 1991), rather than trying to take the missed basic courses in the midst of this pre-programmed sequence.

At the doctoral level, general curriculum sequencing diminishes in importance because of the individualization of students' courses of study. However, the design of sample course sequences for different areas of emphasis can be very helpful to doctoral students and their academic advisors as, together, they chart a proposed plan. Within students' individual plans, sequencing can and should be considered both in coursework and in the orderly building of advanced research or clinical skills.

Schedule.   Invariably, scheduling considerations play a pivotal role in the implementation of any model curriculum plan. Scheduling conflicts can interfere with the best of balancing, pacing, and sequencing intentions. In programs with relatively small numbers of students, as is typical in audiology and speech-language pathology, there are correspondingly few instructors and few—often only one per academic year—offerings of a given course. When this limiting factor is coupled with the concurrent scheduling of clinical practicum assignments, which often are available only at the same times as certain classes, the task of curriculum scheduling becomes more complex. The scheduling of laboratory time for students working on research projects can be similarly complicated by multiple demands for the same piece of equipment or space at the same time.

How do curriculum planners circumvent these obstacles without compromising the quality of their educational program? There are several possible approaches, some more workable than others. Among the variations are the scheduling of classes during evening hours and clinical practica during regular daytime business hours, or setting aside certain days of the week for classes and the remaining days for clinical practica. These and other scheduling arrangements can create additional problems, some of them only an inconvenience, others more consequential. Often, experimentation with scheduling is necessary in order to arrive at workable compromises. Indeed, varying the schedule format from term to term in an academic year may even be incorporated into an overall master plan to allow maximum flexibility and minimum sacrifice for as many individuals as possible.

Meeting Special Requirements

Each program of study has its own set of special requirements that help to shape curriculum development. Those common to educational programs in CSD are reviewed in the following discussion.

Professional Certification. As already explained, because of their vital and integral roles in the educational preparation of audiologists and speech-language pathologists, practicum requirements have a great impact on balancing, pacing, and sequencing factors, and, ultimately, on the scheduling of courses. These requirements, along with coursework requirements, derive from the ASHA Standards for the Certificates of Clinical Competence (ASHA 1991), so they actually delineate the curriculum framework for master's degree programs. (See Appendix A.) Professional certification, thus, is the driving force behind curricular decision making at this level.

Although adherence to professional certification standards ensures that educational programs will meet minimal criteria in their coursework and practicum offerings, it can have a limiting effect as well. That is to say, curriculum planners may adhere only to the minimal criteria, putting forth little effort to develop activities that go beyond the minimum. When this kind of complacency coincides with a predetermined time frame for the master's degree program, creative curriculum planning may be curtailed further. Innovative curriculum is not likely to emerge in an atmosphere where new courses, new course content, or other revamped offerings are dismissed as being unachievable because of external factors. Curriculum planners, therefore, may need to find ways to overcome real or perceived barriers to imaginative curriculum (re)development.

Writing. Many educational programs in the field are housed in universities or departments having an undergraduate requirement for courses in writing or composition or for other courses involving the writing of a major paper. Some require that students pass a writing proficiency examination at the graduate level. In a number of fields, a writing course has become a certification requirement. That writing requirements are appropriate for students in audiology or speech-language pathology is beyond question. Nevertheless, because writing requirements are not universal and/or because students' skills may be lacking, curriculum planners must pay special attention to this area.

Should more courses be added to an existing curriculum? More papers required in existing courses? Should a certain level of writing proficiency be a prerequisite for clinical practicum assignments? For writing a dissertation proposal? Those in charge of individual programs must make individual determinations in this regard. But in all programs the pivotal role of writing needs to be recognized, particularly during curriculum planning.

Based on the premise that writing is a process through which information is shaped and understood, not just recorded, an innovative "writing to learn" paradigm was reported by nursing educators, Allen, Bowers, and Diekelmann (1989). The underlying assumption was that writing skills are thinking skills. Among the suggested activities were focused writing exercises wherein students are required to write, update, and critique "student journals"; write about their reactions to specific lecture material or clinical experiences; transfer information from one context to another; and abstract the contents from different sources into compact "microthemes."

Also proposed by Allen, Bowers, and Diekelmann (1989) were writing activities that would link courses across the curriculum: having students write a paper in a beginning course and, then, on the basis of added educational experiences (clinic, research, or courses), rewrite it in a subsequent course to reflect new knowledge, deeper understanding, and increased insight; having students keep a portfolio of their samples of sequential writing to give them evidence of how their writing and thinking skills have developed; and such student projects as writing instructions for patients or developing self-evaluation instruments through collaboration with classmates. Various other kinds of group writing projects were also suggested.

This group of educators further proposed short, in-class writing assignments: having students write short paragraphs on specific ideas, possibly to be used later in a longer paper; or having them write down a specified number of lecture points, then exchange papers with classmates to determine if the writing is understandable to others. Rosenthal and Sauer (1985) reported the many benefits to be derived from peer review by students.

It is clear from these examples that a unified approach to curriculum planning is necessary when special requirements can and should involve all components within a program. Not to view the curriculum as a whole in these matters usually results in oversight on the part of planners, hence the likelihood of curricular innovation is greatly reduced.

Thesis. Not a requirement of many programs in CSD, master's theses nonetheless are being completed by a number of students (Cooper, Helmick, and Ripich 1987). The thesis at this level is often an option; in some instances, students may take a comprehensive examination instead. Other programs require neither. Regardless of program policy differences, the completion of a thesis is acknowledged as an appropriate step for students interested in pursuing research interests. And, because its inclusion in curricula at the master's level is frequently a source of debate among educators—not only those in CSD but also educators in other health professions (May and Holzemer 1985)—the thesis demands special attention by program curriculum planners.

If it is included as an option, should the writing of a thesis be encouraged for all students, or only for those who appear to have the aptitude and interest? If the thesis is not required, should some other form of independent investigation or formal research project be required? These are the kinds of questions often asked by educational program administrators and faculty members as they contemplate whether or not competence in conducting research should be cultivated at the master's level.

The curriculum implications of the above questions give rise to another set of questions that must be considered in planning. Where will thesis preparation fit into a master's student's course of study? Will additional courses be required? Will the master's degree program for the thesis student need to be extended? If not, will coursework in other areas need to be sacrificed? For those students who desire clinical certification and the thesis option, can a reduction in the number of clinical practicum assignments be justified to allow more research time?

Curriculum balancing, as described in an earlier section, becomes essential here.

Comprehensive Examination. As indicated in the thesis discussion, master's students in some educational programs may take a comprehensive examination rather than write a thesis. Because some programs require neither, the challenge for curriculum planners is to decide whether or not to include a comprehensive examination requirement and, if they do, whether or not it will be an alternative to the thesis.

A comprehensive examination's purpose must be established before a decision can be reached about its appropriateness in a curriculum plan. There are some differences from program to program but, typically, the aim of the examination is to assess master's students' comprehensive knowledge of whatever was covered in their program of study. The examination, therefore, is administered usually near the end of a master's degree program. In some universities, the comprehensive examination is designed to help graduating students prepare themselves for the national examination in speech-language pathology or audiology. In other universities, there is an emphasis on students' abilities to integrate the knowledge and skill they have gained from their courses and their clinical practice. Practical and/or oral components are sometimes added to a written component, thereby providing a means to evaluate students' clinical abilities in specific areas (Rassi 1987). These components may be helpful for students who eventually take examinations for hearing aid dispenser licensure or certification.

Those who favor a comprehensive examination at the master's level believe it is advantageous for students to go through the integrative studying process required for examination preparation. Some educators believe that examination performance serves as a good indicator of a student's potential to pursue doctoral study. Another stated benefit is the feedback provided by students' group examination performance, signaling to a program faculty the strengths and weaknesses of academic and clinical offerings. According to some proponents, passing such an examination assures a minimum level of knowledge and skill if a practical component is administered. The latter can be an additional practical learning experience for students if administered interactively (Rassi 1987). In fact, medical educators recommend that "to optimize the value of evaluation to the student's future career, its methods should adequately assess those skills the student is expected to demonstrate in later practice" (West, Umland, and Lucero 1985, p. 144).

There may be as many reasons for not having, or for discontinuing, the comprehensive examination requirement as there are programs where this policy exists. Those educators in CSD programs who contend that the examination is unnecessary, argue that a truly comprehensive examination is not possible, that not all of the knowledge and skill gained in a master's degree program can be covered in a single test. If students have already demonstrated understanding of material at the conclusion of each course and if students have already performed satisfactorily in their clinical practicum assignments, then, the opponents say, a comprehensive examination is redundant.

The latter view supports *formative* evaluation, that which occurs throughout the students' program of knowledge and skill acquisition, in lieu of *summative* evaluation, that which occurs at the end of a program and looks at accumulated knowledge and skill. Proponents of the comprehensive examination, on the other hand, say that both formative and summative evaluations are important. Curriculum planners must decide which approach is more consonant with their program goals and proceed accordingly.

Qualifying Examination. The qualifying examination for admission to Ph.D. candidacy, taken at the end of a period of knowledge and skill acquisition, is summative. At this level, virtually all programs require a student to pass a qualifying examination before proceeding with the dissertation. Whether this practice will continue in the doctoral program variations being considered in the field of CSD remains to be seen.

Presently the primary task for curriculum planners is to decide, not if the examination should be administered, but how it will be administered. This entails such determinations as how and when the qualifying examination fits into a typical program of study for doctoral students; what the prerequisite requirements are; how the examination will be prepared; how content areas will be decided; and what the pass-fail criteria will be. To the extent that these determinations are decided in advance and presented to students at the beginning of their doctoral studies, the students will have the kind of information needed to make preparation plans.

Dissertation. A cornerstone of research-based Ph.D. study, the dissertation probably requires the least amount of advance curriculum planning. With consideration given to the desired time for completion, it simply needs to be included in the master curriculum plan. The method for selecting dissertation advisers and committees should also be determined and this information communicated to students. Most other rules and requirements concerning the dissertation are determined by the university graduate school, thereby leaving departmental curriculum planners with few decisions to make.

Special Students. Within the category of special students are those who may require a curriculum plan modified to meet their particular needs. These are the students who have little or no undergraduate background in CSD or other required coursework. Students changing their major area of study as they move from the undergraduate to the graduate level or from the master's to the doctoral level often fall in this category, as do many foreign students and nontraditional students (those who, at an age beyond that of most university students, begin or resume their educational preparation). Master's-level students, who want to pursue a nonclinical degree, may also need a special curriculum plan. Handicapped students may or may not need individualized curricula.

If, over time, a considerable number of special students are admitted to a particular program, curriculum planners will find it helpful to propose in advance some alternate plans of study for these people. Such planning allows more specific information to be sent to applicants and it lessens the burden for academic advisers when they try to design individual plans for students. The most important benefit to be derived from advanced alternate planning is the state of preparedness it affords the educational program before an impending difficulty arises: the availability of courses in other departments, the need to add courses, the resolution of class time conflicts, and the recalculation of program time frames.

In the case of special groups of students whom the educational program may wish to attract, curriculum planners may want to add *curriculum packages* to the regular design. Usually directed to already-employed nontraditional students who may only be able to attend the university during evening and weekend hours, classes can be scheduled expressly for the target group. They may be recast in the form of institutes, workshops, intensive courses, seminars, or summer courses. Offerings of this kind may or may not be part of a degree program. And, although the classes usually belong in the domain of continuing education, their inclusion in higher-education curricula frequently satisfies an unmet need and enhances the university's image in the professional community.

CURRICULUM APPROACHES AND PROGRAM TYPES

The literature on education in medical, nursing, and health professions, as well as that pertaining to higher education curriculum, contains numerous examples of curriculum approaches and program types. Some have features that are similar to others, but may have different applications or different names depending on the professional area of study they represent. Those considered to be applicable to education in CSD, either in whole or in part, are described in this section.

Competency-Based Curriculum

As the term suggests, competency-based curriculum stresses the attainment of competencies determined by educators in the field to be important for professional practice. In this context, competency encompasses the knowledge and skill required to accomplish a given task. The applicability of competency-based educational planning to speech-language pathology and audiology is apparent.

The identification of professional competencies to be targeted constitutes the first step in building a competency-based curriculum. Competencies can be delineated by compiling answers to basic questions such as "To become effective clinicians/researchers/teachers, what do our students need to know when they enter the profession following graduation?" and "To become effective clinicians/researchers/teachers, what do our students need to be able to do when they enter the profession following graduation?". Helpful in drafting competencies are the kinds of materials mentioned earlier in this chapter: area-specific guidelines, position statements, and other related materials such as the ASHA role delineation and content validation studies for the requirements for the certificates of clinical competence, and the new certification standards themselves.

Having determined the competencies to be learned, curriculum planners can then develop the courses, practica, and projects that will give students, in a logical sequence, the knowledge and skills required. In a curriculum that is entirely competency-based, written, oral and practical examinations are typically designed so that students' mastery of competencies can be evaluated on an ongoing basis. These checkpoints also provide curriculum planners with a built-in mechanism for periodically looking at the students' abilities to keep pace with the program. The critiques, in turn, allow regular curriculum adjustments to be made.

A competency-based curriculum is particularly well suited for preparation programs in the clinical health professions because it takes into account the competencies to be acquired in clinical practicum assignments along with those attained through coursework. A curriculum plan that considers these two primary components in one broad view is likely to be more cohesive and integrated. In other words, there ought to be fewer missing pieces of information between the classroom and the clinic. Ideally, a thorough and comprehensive competency-based plan would allow no holes in the curriculum.

Process- versus Product-Oriented Programs. Two different emphases characterize programs with a competency-based curriculum. The first is a process-oriented program in which the general processes of critical thinking, problem solving, and reasoning are stressed in the context of clinical decisions involving diagnosis, treatment, and management, or research decisions involving inquiry, hypothesis, and deduction. The second is a product-oriented program in which students' knowledge of facts and skills in performing tasks is stressed. The two types of programs are not mutually exclusive, of course, but the difference in emphasis can result in very different programs.

In a process-oriented program, for example, students might be involved in observing and analyzing behaviors in a disorder-based self-help group (Kreutz 1987). Or they might be learning to write scholarly discourse through a series of workshops and sequenced, course-related assignments emphasizing composition, concept analysis, locating resources, critiquing, editing, reviewing manuscripts, and publishing (Poteet, Edlund, and Hodges 1987).

In contrast, a product-oriented program might require students to conduct a literature search on an assigned or self-selected topic, then write a paper and make an oral presentation to classmates and teacher, with both products graded. Or there might be a skills-laboratory system consisting of audiovisual viewing rooms and practice rooms where, via simulated patient-care situations in equipped learning modules, students work with partners in developing and practicing clinical skills and are then tested on skill acquisition (Cook and Hill 1985). In another example, a clinical orientation module may require students to rotate through a specified number and type of clinical sites and to attend corresponding seminars, while their knowledge of pertinent facts is measured in pre- and post-module tests (Brown and Linzer 1988).

Experience-Based Curriculum

Another type of curriculum, referred to as experience-based, is also particularly suitable for the education and training of professionals in health and other professions. Incorporating the work-study concept, it stresses students' participation in real work environments, that is, field placements in whatever settings are appropriate to the professional preparation—hospitals, clinics, schools, industries, private practices, businesses. Interspersed among the work assignments are seminars specifically designed to parallel the students' experiences.

The difference between an experience-based curriculum and a more conventional curriculum with associated practicum requirements is the way in which the information is organized for teaching purposes.

Whereas the traditional approach divides material into traditional topic areas (for example, anatomy, psychoacoustics, and language) and offers classes in each area, the experience-based curriculum may include certain aspects of a variety of topic areas in a given seminar if they are considered relevant to the situations and experiences under discussion. Because this begins early in a preparation program, the student assimilates information that is both theoretical and applied, rather than learning the theory first, then integrating and applying it later.

Demonstration Programs. In a variation of the experience-based curriculum, demonstration programs stress the laboratory component of classes. In this arrangement, demonstrations of real and simulated clinical and research techniques become the focus of a particular course. Classroom lectures and discussions, secondary to the demonstrations, provide the forum for relating demonstration learning to corresponding concepts. Students as well as instructors participate in the demonstrations.

Module Approach. Already described as an example of a product-oriented program within a competency-based curriculum, the module approach can be either competency-based or experience-based. A unit of information, usually practical in nature—the unit in the above example was clinical orientation—becomes the focus of instruction and thus the basis for planning practicum or work assignments, classroom sessions, and pre- and post-testing. An entire curriculum can be constructed on the basis of these informational units or modules.

Exemplar Approach. Perhaps the most widely recognized application of the exemplar approach is seen in medical education where an attending physician, as educator, ministers to hospital inpatients at bedside, while simultaneously modeling for, and interacting with, the entourage of medical residents and students who accompany him/her on "rounds." The exemplar approach has a long history in medical education and has served as a model for clinical education in general.

It is likely that in the early days, the first clinician-teachers, then in speech therapy, patterned themselves after the medical exemplar model, blending their roles as clinicians, demonstrators, models, researchers, and teachers, as they engaged in "demonstration therapy." Today, this exemplar approach has diminished, even disappeared in some educational programs. With increasing specialization and the narrowing of professional roles, fewer educators regularly provide clinical service and teach classes, both in sufficient breadth and depth, to serve as exemplars in the traditional manner.

Although many individuals lament the passing of this know-all, be-all master, the sheer amount of knowledge and skill it now takes to be an expert has exceeded the capacity of most contemporaries. Nevertheless, a specialist can be an exemplar in his/her own particular area of interest, that is, if there is a commitment to total classroom-clinic-laboratory involvement. Indeed, it is evident that more of these kinds of persons are needed in university educational programs. The generalist as exemplar, on the other hand, is no longer a viable role for educators in audiology or speech-language pathology. And, finally, the clinical supervisor, although a frequent demonstrator of clinical techniques, is often not in a position to bridge classroom, clinic, and laboratory teaching.

Learner-Controlled Programs

Although there are, at all educational levels, examples of programs that are learner-controlled to varying degrees, their use in graduate education is the focus of this discussion.

   Innovative, Individualized Education Plans. As suggested earlier, individualized education plans are often indicated for master's and doctoral level students with special curriculum needs. It should be noted further, however, that virtually all doctoral students—whether or not they qualify as special students with special needs—are candidates for individualized education plans. Indeed, a core curriculum usually does not exist at this level, particularly if clinical certification is not being sought. By the very nature of its purpose, a doctoral student's plan of study is one that affords him/her new opportunities to explore topic areas within or outside the discipline in pursuit of specific expertise and research goals. A customized plan is, therefore, in order.

   A faculty member familiar with university, graduate school, and departmental requirements usually serves as an academic adviser to assist the doctoral student in developing a suitable individual plan and in modifying it when necessary. The role of curriculum planners here is to design an overall plan that will accommodate students' individual plans. Are the needed and desired courses available in the CSD department and in other departments of the university? Are there scheduling conflicts that need to be resolved? Can some required courses be changed to elective status? Which courses can be audited? Are there prerequisite requirements for certain courses in other departments? These and other questions can be addressed by curriculum planners through consultation with university officials and with students as well as advisers.

   Notwithstanding university-imposed constraints, an individualized education plan can be as innovative as the thinking of its planners, that is, the student and adviser. Flexibility is the key to designing a plan that will uniquely meet a student's needs and, at the same time, ensure quality preparation of sufficient scope.

Independent Study.   Also intended to meet a student's individual interests and/or needs, and therefore a kind of learner-controlled component, the independent study is available on both the master's and doctoral levels. This format pairs a student with a faculty member for the purpose of facilitating the study of a specific topic under individual tutelage and guidance. In many cases, the student writes a paper based on a literature search of the chosen topic or conducts a research project and then writes a corresponding paper.

Because it can be used for the study of any topic, the independent study format becomes the mechanism frequently employed to implement individual education plans and to provide the necessary flexibility in a program curriculum. Students who have missed opportunities to take certain required courses can substitute independent studies in the area of need. For those students interested in areas not covered by available courses, if there is an interested and qualified instructor, independent study can also be used. Because master's students usually follow the pattern of a core curriculum and doctoral students have more room in their plans of study for choices, the independent study is likely to be used more often by doctoral students.

Curriculum planners need only make independent study registrations available in a program curriculum; academic advisers and students are responsible for choosing this teaching-learning format wisely and appropriately.

Discovery- and Inquiry-Based Programs

Perhaps the most widely used and best known of the discovery- and inquiry-based programs in allied disciplines is the innovative problem-based curriculum found in medical education. In a problem-based curriculum, designed to prepare students to become problem-solvers and self-directed lifelong learners, the traditional lecture-format class and the rote memory of facts are discarded in favor of small tutorial groups where students, in search of answers to real patient problems, study, read, and otherwise acquire information with the help of an instructor who serves as a facilitator. Lecturing is supplemental and secondary.

Using real patient problems as the curriculum core, say the proponents, gives the medical student a natural learning stimulus. The subject matter is relevant. The learning pace, to a certain extent, is controlled by the student. (Thus, problem-based curriculum may also be viewed as a learner-controlled program as discussed above.) Moreover, the student's reasoning ability is developed at the same time that new factual knowledge is acquired (Barrows 1975; Kaufman 1985).

Problem-based curricula have been incorporated successfully into the educational planning of other health professions as well. For example, in studying the link between content mastery and problem solving in a curricular framework for a physical therapy educational program, Arand and Harding (1987) found that students' critical thinking skills significantly increased as a result of taking a problem-solving course. Similarly, in nursing education, management and ethical case studies were used to improve decision-making skills in students (Huston and Marquis 1987). Although case studies and problem solving are part of many speech-language pathology and audiology courses, it appears that traditional lecturing continues to be the primary method of classroom teaching in this field (Rassi and McElroy 1988) and thus remains the basis for curriculum development.

Interdisciplinary Programs

With ever-broadening knowledge bases and consequential overlapping of disciplines, the need for interdisciplinary study becomes increasingly important. Although enrollment in courses from other disciplines was mentioned previously in conjunction with individualized education plans for doctoral students, there also exist entire interdisciplinary programs, planned on a larger scale and targeted to groups of students. In order to advance research in heretofore undeveloped subspecialty areas, university departments combine their resources in these cooperative, collaborative intra- or inter-institutional endeavors. From such joint ventures, new hybrid disciplines are often born, a phenomenon not unlike that which engendered audiology and speech-language pathology.

By design, an interdisciplinary curriculum plan encompasses the systematic study of one discipline along with one or more others. Many courses within an interdisciplinary curriculum are themselves interdisciplinary. Even so, an established core curriculum is not uncommon. Furthermore, in many cases, a student may obtain a degree in the new discipline, granted by the host department.

This kind of advanced study seems most appropriate for students at doctoral or postdoctoral levels who are seeking research specialization in a developing area such as neuroscience (Land 1989). Efforts are also being made to institute clinically oriented interdisciplinary studies in areas such as geriatric specialization (Shepard, Yeo, and McGann 1985), or the training of "multicompetent" allied health professionals (Roush et al. 1986). Moreover, the need for greater involvement of audiology and speech-language pathology students in clinical interdisciplinary study is another reason, say some individuals, that a professional doctorate or clinical Ph.D. degree in this field is warranted.

Diversified Curriculum.   A diversified curriculum effects new growth within a particular program. That is to say, when curriculum planners identify a need for new direction or infusion, they may interject fresh topics, primarily or secondarily derived from other disciplines. By planning a course or courses to be taught to program students by resident faculty who may have previously untapped expertise and/or by faculty from other university departments or neighboring universities, they may be able to achieve the desired diversification. Examples of diversification can be found in education in the health professions (Laatsch, Milson, and Zimmer 1986) and in audiology and speech-language pathology where courses in such new areas as business management, clinic administration, and private practice have been added to the program curriculum. Obtaining the funding required to support a diversified curriculum may be a problem for some CSD educational programs, thus necessitating the exploration of other planning options.

Integrated Curriculum

When program administrators, faculty, clinical supervisors, researchers, and any others who participate in curriculum planning, development, or implementation succeed in putting together all of the components to form an intact and meaningful whole, then, and only then, is the curriculum truly integrated. (The clear intent here is to minimize the fragmentation of education, a circumstance that Kent [1989–1990] has analyzed and related to the fragmentation of clinical service and clinical science in communicative disorders.) The curriculum plan must be coherent and the end product must have internal consistency: content without gaps or redundancy; bridging activities that tie together theory and application in the classroom, clinic, and laboratory; a logical sequence of learning units; parallelism and balance in the learning strands within as well as throughout courses; and cooperative team and co-teaching efforts by staff and faculty. Curriculum integration is the ultimate goal in planning and development because it represents the achievement of a program's educational goals. Unified planning efforts are essential to its success.

The incorporation of specific goals, objectives, or competencies into curriculum planning provides the means for achieving integration. Thus, a detailed accounting of the knowledge and skills to be gained by students rather than a general consideration of topic areas to be covered facilitates integrative planning. It also provides a revealing glimpse into program operations, which otherwise might not be open to scrutiny, and thus serves as a valuable program evaluation tool.

CURRICULUM OBJECTIVES

As suggested earlier, a systematic approach to curriculum planning is necessary. An essential step in the planning process is the statement of objectives (Barrows 1985), not only those that are stated in the form of competencies, but others as well. The two categories of curriculum objectives used in the planning process and described in this section formalize many of the ideas discussed previously in this chapter and introduce a few new ones.

Design Objectives

Members of the curriculum planning and design team must be carefully selected and the procedures to be followed must be established (Diamond 1989). A statement of design objectives facilitates this initial part of the planning process. These might be formulated as follows:

Select team members who can provide the most meaningful input and who can be expected to participate actively. This may include an instructional developer, whose role is that of a process person; an evaluation specialist, at the appropriate time; faculty members, one of whom will serve as the key content expert and coordinator; and key administrators. Graduate students also might be invited to contribute ideas, but not to participate in team deliberations. (Diamond 1989)

Conduct a needs assessment on the institutional level and the disciplinary or departmental level. This involves a review of the general philosophic and specific professional bases (critical concepts) on which the educational plan is to be based.

Formulate program goals that define the overall purpose of the educational experience and instructional goals that represent the competencies students are expected to achieve at the end of a unit of study. (Knopke 1981)

Review goals and scope of curriculum project, anticipated time lines, and team members' responsibilities. (Diamond 1989)

Educational Objectives

After the preliminary design objectives have been accomplished, the delineation and actual achievement of educational objectives can be addressed next. These can be categorized and described in the following manner:

Delineate specific learning objectives that identify what students are expected to know and to do at the end of a unit of study. These should be separated into minimal competence objectives (specific knowledge, skill, ability, or attitude that all students are expected to develop) and developmental competence objectives (complex behaviors that may be developed by students to differing degrees). (Knopke 1981, pp. 41, 47–48)

Organize the teaching-learning process by determining which activities, experiences, resources, and materials are necessary and appropriate for students to achieve the learning objectives. (Knopke 1981, p. 41)

Determine the roles played by clinical and laboratory experiences in accomplishing educational objectives and include these as integral, rather than separate, parts of the teaching-learning process.

CURRICULUM DESIGN, IMPLEMENTATION, AND EVALUATION

Curriculum Design

After curriculum considerations and approaches have been reviewed and the organization of components and formulation of objectives completed, curriculum design begins to take shape. Because the collection of these data takes place over a period of time, so, too, does the process of designing the curriculum. It is likely that, as the pieces are put into place gradually, a change will occur in the desired sequence or content, or in fiscal and staff constraints, thereby changing the original "ideal" concept into what is eventually offered (Diamond 1989). Thus, planners must move from the ideal to the actual operational design (Diamond 1989).

Curriculum Implementation

After the operational design has been completed and necessary approval given, implementation can begin. New curriculum components, including new courses, should be put into operation on a trial basis and monitored to determine if adjustments need to be made. Each new component must be given time to succeed, however, before a thorough evaluation is undertaken.

Curriculum Evaluation

Continuing the trial phase for new components and then adding the systematic monitoring of all remaining curriculum components are actions that signal the beginning of the curriculum evaluation phase. As most individuals involved in the process know, this phase is somewhat circular in that curriculum review and change, although frequently conducted in steps, are ongoing. If the educational program is to be responsive to new students every year, to new faculty, changing content, and the availability of new educational methods, constant evaluation is to be expected (Diamond 1989).

Needs Assessment Studies. Cited in earlier discussions as resources for selecting subject matter or building a competency-based curriculum, area-specific guidelines, position statements (summarized annually in *Asha*; and now available in *Asha* supplements), results of the validation study, and other similar materials can also be used by educational program planners to determine which areas in their curriculum need to be bolstered or revised. Textbooks, journal articles, and convention and workshop presentations, along with input from resident faculty members who have expertise in specific content areas, are obvious sources. Especially useful are surveys of practitioners and of educational programs, such as those by Martin and Sides (1985), and Martin et al. (1987); and reports of unmet critical needs, for example, McCarthy, Culpepper, and Lucks (1986); Lenich, Bernstein, and Nevitt (1987); Oyler and Matkin (1987); Woodford (1987); Lass et al. (1989); Stone and Olswang (1989); and Luterman (1990). One such report in the latter category, concerning the need for multicultural professional education in CSD programs, actually provides detailed blueprints for four different curriculum approaches—the Pyramid Approach, the Unit Approach, the Infusion Approach, and the Course Approach (ASHA 1987c).

All such providers of content information—if it is current, reliable, and representative—serve collectively as indicators of curriculum content needs. Furthermore, educational programs can, and do, conduct their own surveys of other selected educational programs (for example, Crais and Leonard 1990) or of colleagues in common specialty areas with or without educational affiliations (for example, Jacobson, Kileny, and Ruth 1988). Comparable inquiries of graduates and practitioners have been conducted for the same purpose in discipline areas such as medical education (Mangione 1986; Garrett 1987). Thus, needs assessment material, related to process as well as content, is abundant.

Curriculum Evaluation Design. The heart of curriculum evaluation lies in the collection of data to determine whether or not the appropriate objectives are being met: educational—instructional, learning, or competency-based; organizational—institutional, departmental, or programmatic; and by discipline—accreditation or certification. In other words, the entire curriculum body, either as a whole or in units, is assessed operationally. On the basis of this information, revisions are made, then re-application occurs, and re-assessment follows. According to Diamond, before a program is functioning completely satisfactorily, several design/field-test/revision sequences can be expected (1989, p. 169).

Curriculum evaluation can be accomplished in different ways. Pretests and post-tests, for example, can be administered to students, and the results then analyzed. The university's instructional center may assist in interpreting results and making recommendations. Faculty members can be invited to attend others' classes periodically to collect specific information. Involved faculty can be interviewed as can students. Questionnaires, surveys, and other types of written evaluations can be designed for all participants and observers. Data can be collected at predetermined intervals and/or at midterm and end-of-term junctures. Throughout the program evaluation process, it is helpful and prudent to keep students informed of outcomes and remedial actions (Diamond 1989).

Although curriculum and course evaluation designs should correspond to individual programs, there is a core of questions common to most instructional units. Such a list, compiled on the basis of work done at several universities by Sudweeks and Diamond (1989, pp. 247–253), is shown in Appendix D. It should be noted that these are categories and questions considered during evaluation planning, but that actual question selection and adaptation, evaluation design, and evaluation methodology must be decided by individual program evaluators.

Curriculum Validation.   The validation of curriculum, that is, establishing whether or not it has accomplished what planners had intended, is tantamount to program evaluation, and thus an actual extension of that discussed above. Nevertheless, validation depends, for the most part, on more formal tools to be more objective, more quantitative, and more precise. It, therefore, can be used to compare students' performance in different curricular tracks, in different educational programs, or in the same educational program at different levels, pre- or postgraduation.

Experimental Curriculum.   One of the most efficient and effective ways to explore new educational methods or content areas is to incorporate them into existing curricula on an experimental basis. Experimentation necessarily includes ongoing monitoring and evaluation. Moreover, experimentation implies a temporary test so that skeptical faculty and staff might be more willing to attempt something new. It has a definite beginning and end. In addition, individual concerns, such as those frequently expressed regarding the added amount of time, effort, and expertise a new project might require, may be allayed in an experimental venture where the participants' responses on these and other related matters are being sought.

It should also be noted here that experimental curriculum is not the same as the trial phase of curriculum development discussed earlier. Experimental curriculum, like any other planned experiment, has predetermined methods of inquiry, data collection, analysis, and interpretation. Participants who themselves are part of the investigative team have a stake in the outcome of an experiment and are likely to be more cooperative and enthusiastic than are individuals who have a curriculum imposed on them.

Because experimental curriculum may be more acceptable to faculty, staff, and administrators, there is a greater probability that it will be innovative. Those involved in experimental curriculum design have greater latitude for trying ideas that depart substantially from standard formats when they know that there will be more cooperation than resistance.

CONCLUSION

Curriculum development, a complex, demanding process that requires careful planning and a great deal of expertise, is central to the preparation of audiologists and speech-language pathologists, and to the future of the field. Given the many available approaches to the task along with external indicators for curriculum change, CSD higher education programs have both reasons and opportunities to move forward with curriculum innovation.

REFERENCES

Adams, M. R., Aker, J., Bruce, M., Dowling, S., Falck, F., Fox, D., and Waryas, P. 1984. What constitutes excellence in an academic unit? *Asha* 26(5):27–28.

Ainsworth, S. H., Diedrich, W. M., Graham, J. K., Herer, G. R., Sutton, E. L., and Hardy, J. C. 1972. Principles underlying the requirements for the certificate of clinical competence adopted. *Asha* 14:139–41.

Allen, D. G., Bowers, B., and Diekelmann, N. 1989. Writing to learn: A reconceptualization of thinking and writing in nursing curriculum. *Journal of Nursing Education* 28(1):6–11.

American Academy of Audiology. 1989. The professional doctorate? *Audiology Today* 3.

American Academy of Audiology. 1990. Special issue: Graduate education in audiology. *Audiology Today* 2(5).

American Association of Medical Colleges. 1983. *Emerging Perspectives on the General Professional Education of the Physician.* Washington, DC: Author.

American Speech and Hearing Association. 1963. *Graduate Education in Speech Pathology and Audiology.* Washington, DC: Author.

American Speech and Hearing Association. 1964a. ASHA receives accrediting privilege. *Asha* 6:166–68.

American Speech and Hearing Association. 1964b. Committee on Clinical

Standards. Requirements for the certificate of clinical competence. *Asha* 6: 162–64.

American Speech and Hearing Association. 1972. Proposed revision to the requirements for the certificate of clinical competence. *Asha* 14:141–46

American Speech-Language-Hearing Association. 1976. Task Force on Learning Disabilities. Position statement of the American Speech and Hearing Association on learning disabilities. *Asha* 18:282–90.

American Speech-Language-Hearing Association. 1981. Requirements for the certificate of clinical competence. *Asha* 23:287–91.

American Speech-Language-Hearing Association. 1983. Proposed changes in the requirements for the certificate of clinical competence. *Asha* 25:65.

American Speech-Language-Hearing Association. 1984a. Changes in the requirements for the certificates of clinical competence. *Asha* 26(3):41.

American Speech-Language-Hearing Association. 1984b. Definition of and competencies for aural rehabilitation. Position statement. *Asha* 26(5):37–41.

American Speech-Language-Hearing Association. 1984c. Guidelines for graduate training in amplification. *Asha* 26(5):43.

American Speech-Language-Hearing Association. 1985a. Learning disabilities: Issues in the preparation of professional personnel. A position paper of the National Joint Committee on Learning Disabilities. *Asha* 27(9):49–51.

American Speech-Language-Hearing Association. 1985b. Proposed requirements for the certificates of clinical competence. *Asha* 27(7):57–61.

American Speech-Language-Hearing Association. 1986. Proposed requirements for the certificates of clinical competence. *Asha* 28(7):53–57.

American Speech-Language-Hearing Association. 1987a. Committee on Interperprofessional Relationships. Scope of practice. A position statement. (Draft). *Asha* 29(6):43.

American Speech-Language-Hearing Association. 1987b. Committee on Language, Subcommittee on Cognition and Language. The role of speech-language pathologists in the habilitation and rehabilitation of cognitively impaired individuals. A position statement. (Draft). *Asha* 29(6):43.

American Speech-Language-Hearing Association. 1987c. Committee on the Status of Racial Minorities. Curriculum approaches to multicultural professional education in communicative disorders. (Draft). *Asha* 29(6):49–52.

American Speech-Language-Hearing Association. 1987d. *ESB Educational Standards Board 1987 Accreditation Manual.* Rockville, MD: Author.

American Speech-Language-Hearing Association. 1988a. Committee on Augmentative Communication. Competencies for speech-language pathologists providing services in augmentative communication. (Draft). *Asha* 30(1):55–58.

American Speech-Language-Hearing Association. 1988b. Committee on Long Range Planning. Long range plan: 1988–1989–1990. *Asha* 30(3):52–54.

American Speech-Language-Hearing Association. 1988c. Council on Professional Standards. Certificates of clinical competence: Standards Council requests member comment. *Asha* 30(6/7):71–78.

American Speech-Language-Hearing Association. 1988d. Report of the Task Force on Audiology II. *Asha* 30(11):41–45.

American Speech-Language-Hearing Association. 1988e. *Supplementary Report. Professional Domains, Tasks, Knowledges and Skills in the Practice of Speech-Language Pathology and Audiology.* Rockville, MD: Author.

American Speech-Language-Hearing Association 1989a. Ad Hoc Committee on Undergraduate Education. Advisements for undergraduate/preprofessional education. Rockville, MD: Author.

American Speech-Language-Hearing Association. 1989b. Committee on Audiologic Evaluation, Working group on auditory evoked potential measurements. Competencies in auditory evoked potential measurement and clinical applications. (Draft for peer review). *Asha* 31(5):39–41.

American Speech-Language-Hearing Association. 1989c. Committee on Infant Hearing. Guidelines for audiologic screening of newborn infants who are at risk for hearing impairment. *Asha* 31(3):89–92.

American Speech-Language-Hearing Association. 1989d. Council on Professional Standards. Accreditation of educational programs. *Asha* 31(6/7):41–46.

American Speech-Language-Hearing Association. 1989e. Executive Board report. Annual reports of vice presidents. *Asha* 31(3):39–52.

American Speech-Language-Hearing Association. 1989f. Task Force on Dysphagia. Knowledge and skills needed by speech-language pathologists providing services to dysphagic patients/clients. (Draft for peer review). *Asha* 31(5):35–38.

American Speech-Language-Hearing Association. 1990a. Standards for accreditation of educational programs. *Asha* 32(6/7):93–94, 100.

American Speech-Language-Hearing Association. 1990b. Standards for the certificates of clinical competence. *Asha* 32(3):111–12.

American Speech-Language-Hearing Association. 1991. Standards for the certificates of clinical competence. *Asha* 33(3):121–22.

Arand, J. U., and Harding, C. G. 1987. An investigation into problem solving in education: A problem-solving curricular framework. *Journal of Allied Health* 16(1):7–17.

Aronson, A. E. 1987. The clinical Ph.D: Implications for the survival and liberation of communicative disorders as a health care profession. *Asha* 29(11):35–39.

Basinger, W. 1968. Preprofessional education in speech pathology and audiology, III. The University of Puget Sound. *Asha* 10:375.

Barrows, H. S. 1985. *How to Design a Problem-Based Curriculum for the Preclinical Years.* New York: Springer Publishing Company.

Beaty, H. N. 1989. Educating the physician of the 21st century. *Building Together* 2(2):8.

Bellet, P. S. 1981. Primary medical care education as an institutional endeavor. In *Approaches to Teaching Primary Health Care,* eds. H. J. Knopke and N. L. Diekelmann. St. Louis: C. V. Mosby Company.

Beran, R. L. 1979. The rise and fall of three-year medical school programs. *Journal of Medical Education* 54(3):248–49.

Bloomer, H. H. 1968. Preprofessional education in speech pathlogy and audiology, I. The University of Michigan. *Asha* 10:255–56.

Brodnitz, F. S. 1986. Academe and the clinic. *Asha* 28(12):25–26.

Brown, J. T., and Linzer, M. 1988. Description and preliminary evaluation of an orientation module to teach general internal medicine. *Journal of Medical Education* 63(8):645–47.

Bussigel, M. N., Barzansky, B. M., and Grenholm, G. G. 1988a. *Innovation Processes in Medical Education.* (Comparative analysis of the innovation processes). New York: Praeger Publishers.

Bussigel, M. N., Barzansky, B. M., and Grenholm, G. G. 1988b. *Innovation Processes in Medical Education.* (Introduction). New York: Praeger Publishers.

Carnegie Foundation for the Advancement of Teaching. 1982. *The Control of the Campus.* Lawrenceville, NJ: Princeton University Press.

Carnegie Foundation for the Advancement of Teaching. 1986. *College: The Undergraduate Experience in America.* New York: Author.

Cherow, E., and Williams, J. (eds.) 1989. *Audiology Update* 9(1).

Cook, J. W., and Hill, P. M. 1985. The impact of successful laboratory system on the teaching of nursing skills. *Journal of Nursing Education* 24(8):344–46.

Cooper, E. B. 1986. Preprofessional and continuing education. In *Speech-Language Pathology and Audiology: Issues and Management*, ed. R. M. McLauchlin. Orlando, FL: Grune & Stratton, Inc.

Cooper, E. B., Helmick, J. W., and Ripich, D. N. 1987, October. Council of Graduate Programs in Communication Sciences and Disorders: 1986–87 National Survey. Council of Graduate Programs in Communication Sciences and Disorders.

Crais, E. R., and Leonard, C. R. 1990. PL 99-457: Are speech-language pathologists prepared for the challenge? *Asha* 32(4):57–61.

Cunningham, D. R. 1991. Observations on preprofessional education: Is there a "major" difference? *Asha* 33(1):39–41, 53.

Diamond, R. M. 1989. *Designing and Improving Courses and Curricula in Higher Education. A Systematic Approach.* San Francisco: Jossey-Bass.

Drewry, S., and Fiene, M. A. 1985. Cost-effective curriculum planning in health education. *Journal of Allied Health* 14(1):109–117.

Falck, V. T. 1972. The role and function of university training programs. *Asha* 14:307–310.

Feldman, A. S. 1984. In support of the professional doctorate. *Asha* 26(11):24, 26, 28, 30, 32.

Formicola, A. J. 1978. Reflections on the three-year program. *Journal of Dental Education* 42(10):572–75.

Fowler, C. G., and Wilson, R. H. 1989. More degrees, but no more degrees. *Audiology Today* (special issue) 3:22–23.

Garrett, C. R. 1987. Ratings by practicing internists and faculty members of the importance and use of selected procedural skills. *Journal of Medical Education* 62(5):433–35.

Goldstein, D. P. 1989a. Au.D. degree. The doctoring degree in audiology. *Asha* 31(4):33–35.

Goldstein, D. P. 1989b. Au.D. degree: The doctoring degree in audiology. Purdue University, 90–91. Unpublished article.

Goldstein, D. P., Anderson, C. V., Binnie, C. A., Kricos, P.B., Lesner, S. A., Oyer, H. J., Roser, R. J., and Spriestersbach, D. C. 1990, November. The Au.D. degree: University perspective. Miniseminar presented at the annual convention of the American Speech-Language-Hearing Association, Seattle.

Greenberg, R. M. 1976. It takes four years. *Journal of the American Medical Association* 235(16):1689.

Hardick, E. J., and Oyer, J. J. 1987. Administration of speech-language-hearing programs within the university setting. In *Administration of Programs in Speech-Language Pathology and Audiology*, ed. H. J. Oyer. Englewood Cliffs, NJ: Prentice-Hall.

Huston, C., and Marquis, B. 1987. Use of management and ethical case studies to improve decision-making skills in senior nursing students. *Journal of Nursing Education* 26(5):210–12.

Jacobson, J. T., Kileny, P. R., and Ruth, R. A. 1988. Auditory evoked potentials: A survey of educational and practice patterns. *Asha* 30(4):49–52.

Kaufman, A. (ed.). 1985. *Implementing Problem-Based Medical Education. Lessons from Succcessful Innovations.* New York: Springer Publishing Company.

Kaufman, A., and Obenshain, S. S. 1985. Origins. In *Implementing Problem-Based Medical Education. Lessons from Successful Innovations*, ed. A. Kaufman. New York: Springer Publishing Company.

Kent, R. D. 1989–1990. The fragmentation of clinical service and clinical sciences in communicative disorders. *National Student Speech-Language-Hearing Association Journal* 17:4–16.

Kettel, L. J., et al. 1979. Arizona's three-year medical curriculum: A postmortem. *Journal of Medical Education* 54(3):210–16.

Knopke, H. J. 1981. A framework for systematic educational planning. In *Approaches to Teaching Primary Health Care,* eds. H. J. Knopke and N. L. Diekelmann. St. Louis: C. V. Mosby Company.

Kreutz, R. 1987. Self-help groups as a teaching strategy. *Nurse Educator* 12(1):6.

Laatsch, L. J., Milson, L. M., and Zimmer, S. E. 1986. Use of interdisciplinary education to foster familiarization among health professionals. *Journal of Allied Health* 15(1):33–42.

Land, D. J. 1989. Neuroscience institute established. *Northwestern Observer* 4(10):1, 8.

Lass, N. J., Woodford, C. M., Pannbacker, M. D., Carlin, M. F., Saniga, R. D., Schmitt, J. F., and Everly-Myers, D. S. 1989. Speech-language pathologists' knowledge of, exposure to, and attitudes toward hearing aids and hearing aid wearers. *Language, Speech, and Hearing Services in Schools* 20(2):115–32.

Lenich, J. K., Bernstein, M. E., and Nevitt, A. 1987. Educational audiology: A proposal for training and accreditation. *Language, Speech, and Hearing Services in Schools* 18(4):344–56.

Lingwall, J. B. 1988. Evaluation of the requirements for the certificates of clinical competence in speech-language pathology and audiology. *Asha* 30(9):75–78.

Luterman, D. M. 1990. Audiological counseling and the diagnostic process. *Asha* 32(4):35–37.

Mangione, C. M. 1986. How medical school did and did not prepare me for graduate education. *Journal of Medical Education* 61(9):3–10.

Martin, F. N., and Sides, D. G. 1985. Survey of current audiometric practices. *Asha* 27(2):29–36.

Martin, F. N., George, K. A., O'Neal, J., and Daly, J. A. 1987. Audiologists' and parents' attitudes regarding counseling of families of hearing-impaired children. *Asha* 29(2):27–33.

Martinez-Burrola, N., Klepper, D. J., and Kaufman, A. 1985. Admissions into a problem-based curriculum. In *Implementing Problem-Based Medical Education. Lessons from Successful Innovations,* ed. A. Kaufman. New York: Springer Publishing Company.

Matthews, J. 1966. Essentials of an acceptable program of training for speech pathologists and audiologists. *Asha* 8:231–36.

May, K. M., and Holzemer, W. L. 1985. Master's thesis policies in nursing education. *Journal of Nursing Education* 24(1):10–15.

McCarthy, P., Culpepper, N. B., and Lucks, L. 1986. Variability in counseling experiences and training among ESB-accredited programs. *Asha* 28(9):49–52.

Menges, R. J., and Mathis, B. C. 1988. *Key Resources on Teaching, Learning, Curriculum, and Faculty Development. A Guide to the Higher Education Literature.* San Francisco: Jossey-Bass.

Mennin, S. P., and Martinez-Burrola, N. 1985. Cost of problem-based learning. In *Implementing Problem-Based Medical Education. Lessons from Successful Innovations,* ed. A. Kaufman. New York: Springer Publishing Company.

Minifie, F. D. 1983. Knowledge and service: Does the foundation of the profession need shoring up? *Asha* 25:29–32.

Muma, J. R., Webb, P. H., and Muma, D. B. 1979. Language training in speech-language pathology and audiology: A survey. *Asha* 21:467–73.

National Institute of Education. 1984. *Involvement in Learning: Realizing the Potential of American Higher Education.*

Norton, M. C. 1968. Preprofessional education in speech pathology and audiology, V. Stanislaus State College. *Asha* 10:473–74.

Nuttall, E. C. 1968. Preprofessional education in speech and hearing, IV. University of Oklahoma. *Asha* 10:442–44.

O'Neill, J. J. 1987. The development of speech-language pathology and audiology in the United States. In *Administration of Programs in Speech-Language Pathology and Audiology,* ed. H. J. Oyer. Englewood Cliffs, NJ: Prentice-Hall.

Oyler, R. F., and Matkin, N. D. 1987. National survey of educational preparation in pediatric audiology. *Asha* 29(1):27–33.

Poteet, G. W., Edlund, B. J., and Hodges, L. C. 1987. Promoting scholarly work among graduate students. *Nurse Educator* 12(1):6, 18.

Powers, G. R. 1968. Preprofessional education in speech pathology and audiology, VI. The University of Connecticut. *Asha* 10:507.

Quiring, J., and Gray, G. 1979. Is baccalaureate education based on a patchwork curriculum? *Nursing Outlook* 27(11):708–713.

Raiford, C. A., and Shadden, B. B. 1985. Graduate education in gerontology. *Asha* 27(9):37–43.

Rassi, J. A. 1987. Comprehensive examination of audiology graduate students: A competency-based practical component. In *Clinical Supervision: A Coming of Age,* ed. S. S. Farmer. Proceedings of a conference held at Jekyll Island, GA. Las Cruces, NM: New Mexico State University.

Rassi, J. A., and McElroy, M. D. 1988. Classroom teaching in ESB-accredited programs: A survey of instructors. Paper presented at the annual convention of the American Speech-Language-Hearing Association, Boston.

Rees, N. S. 1983. Summary and implications. In *Proceedings of the 1983 National Conference on Undergraduate, Graduate, and Continuing Education* (Report No. 13), eds. N. S. Rees and T. L. Snope. Rockville, MD: American Speech-Language-Hearing Association.

Rees, N. S., and Snope, T. L. (eds.). 1983. *Proceedings of the 1983 National Conference on Undergraduate, Graduate, and Continuing Education* (Report No. 13). Rockville, MD: American Speech-Language-Hearing Association.

Ringel, R. L. 1984. In support of the practitioner-scholar. *Asha* 26(11):25, 27, 29, 31–32.

Rosenthal, T. T., and Sauer, R. 1985. Helping students write. *Journal of Nursing Education* 24(9):384–85.

Rosinski, E. F. 1983. Curricular trends. Critical review and analysis. In *Handbook of Health Professions Education,* eds. C. H. McGuire, R. P. Foley, A. Gorr, R. W. Richards, and Associates. San Francisco: Jossey-Bass.

Roush, R. E., Fasser, C. E., DeBell, R. H., Jr., and Nathanson, J. M. 1986. The training of multicompetent allied health professionals using a combined-fields method. *Journal of Allied Health* 15(1):23–31.

Schwartz, D. M. 1987. Philosophical controversies in audiology: An allegory. *Ear and Hearing* 8(Suppl 4):55S–57S.

Shepard, K., Yeo, G., and McGann, L. 1985. Successful components of interdisciplinary education. *Journal of Allied Health* 14(3):297–303.

Smith, I. L., Greenberg, S., and Lingwall, J. B. 1986, November. Content validation of the requirements for the certificate of clinical competence. Paper presented at the annual convention of the American Speech-Language-Hearing Association, Detroit.

Spriesterbach, D. C. 1989. Professional education and communication disorders. *Asha* 31(6/7):77–78.

Stone, J. R., and Olswang, L. B. 1989. The hidden challenge in counseling. *Asha* 31(6/7):27–31.

Trzebiatowski, G. L., and Peterson, S. 1979. A study of faculty attitudes toward Ohio State's three-year medical program. *Journal of Medical Education* 54(3): 205–209.

Villarreal, J. J., and Lawrence, C. F. 1970. Undergraduate preparation for professional education in speech pathology and audiology. A summary report of a conference. *Asha* 12:67–70.

West, D. A., Umland, B. E., and Lucero, S. M. 1985. Evaluating student performance. In *Implementing Problem-Based Medical Education. Lessons from Successful Innovations,* ed. A. Kaufman. New York: Springer Publishing Company.

Winitz, H. 1968. Preprofessional education in speech pathology and audiology, II. University of Missouri. *Asha* 10:294–95.

Woodford, C. M. 1987. Speech-language pathologists' knowledge and skills regarding hearing aids. *Language, Speech, and Hearing in Schools* 18(4):312–22.

SECTION II
Educational Environment

Chapter 4

Higher Education

John E. Bernthal and Nicholas W. Bankson

HISTORICAL BACKGROUND

Academic programs in Communication Sciences and Disorders (CSD) have come into existence relatively recently when compared to many other areas of college/university study. In the United States, academic programs related to the study of speech disorders can be traced to the late teens and early 1920s. At this time two events occurred that were critical to the development of academic programs in CSD: (1) the initiation and publication of data-based studies in the area of speech disorders; and (2) the establishment of coursework at colleges and universities dealing with the nature and treatment of speech disorders.

The first presence of "speech correction" on college and university campuses was often the development of a "speech clinic," designed to serve college students with speech disorders. The first such clinic was developed at the University of Wisconsin in 1914, with the first Ph.D. degree in the field being granted at the same institution in 1921 (Paden 1970). By 1923, courses concerned with speech disorders were also being offered at the University of Iowa and the University of Illinois. From this time on, there was a steady increase in the number of programs. The most significant increase occurred during the 1960s due to federal financial support for program development and student aid. Since 1970, relatively few new educational programs in CSD have come into existence.

Audiology, as an area of professional practice, came into being during the 1940s as a result of World War II hearing rehabilitation efforts. The development of "hearing centers" during this period served to spawn audiology (hearing testing and aural rehabilitation) as an area of professional practice related to the practice of "speech correction." In 1947, the American Speech Correction Association changed its name to the American Speech and Hearing Association, reflecting the fact that "hearing" was recognized as related to but separate from speech correction as a professional practice. Similarly, speech clinics began to be called speech and hearing clinics as their scope of practice included audiological services.

By the late 1980s, there were approximately 235 programs in the United States offering the master's degree in speech-language pathology and/or audiology, and about 60 offering the doctoral degree. Approximately 40 other colleges/universities offered undergraduate degrees only.

It is appropriate that a few comments be made relative to the development of academic programs in speech and hearing in Canada. Just as in the United States, speech and hearing programs in Canada were developed on college campuses and in schools and clinics before professionals organized themselves and developed certification standards

(Doehring and Coderre 1989). In 1964, the Canadian Association of Speech-Language Pathologists and Audiologists was established.

The first academic program in speech and hearing was developed at the University of Montreal in 1956, 30–35 years after the first such program in the United States. By 1991, seven master's level academic programs in speech-language pathology and/or audiology were offered at Canadian colleges and universities; but because of the earlier introduction of educational programs in the United States, plus their more extensive proliferation, a significant percentage of speech-language pathologists and audiologists in Canada have been and continue to be educated in the United States. Educational programs and professional certification in Canada are similar to that in the United States, undoubtedly a reflection of common roots and background.

Programs in speech and hearing typically emerged from and became a part of the arts and sciences faculties of colleges and universities. This occurrence was probably a reflection of the speech and drama background of many of the early academicians who were instrumental in the development of programs in speech and hearing disorders on their campuses. These early founders often established CSD as sections or program areas of the speech departments in the colleges of arts and sciences. To this day, approximately half of the programs in the field are housed in colleges of arts and sciences (liberal arts).

The second largest location of programs in CSD is colleges of education. The next most common location for programs is colleges of health and/or medicine. Decisions about where to house programs are often based on the organizational structure of an institution, history and tradition of an institution, faculty interests, needs of the department, finances, and politics. While advantages and disadvantages for each administrative location can be identified, much depends on the characteristics of the faculty and the institution. What seems most important is that the program be located in an environment where it will receive adequate support to achieve its goals and purposes. In spite of differences in administrative location, it is probably safe to say that CSD programs have many similarities from campus to campus in terms of curriculum and faculty.

ACCREDITATION OF EDUCATIONAL PROGRAMS

As is typical with the development of many professional organizations in the early years, what is now the American Speech-Language-Hearing Association (ASHA) was organized and influenced primarily by academicians. The membership, likewise, reflected a high percentage of individuals with college or university appointments. As the years passed, the percentage of membership from the academic ranks diminished, and practitioners' memberships increased. The demographic profile of the ASHA members at the beginning of the 1990s showed that only about 7.5% of the members listed college or university as their primary employer (Shewan 1989). This profile of ASHA membership is important when considering the development of accreditation standards for academic programs.

Accreditation of postsecondary educational institutions and programs is a topic of concern to college and university administrators and faculty. In spite of its importance and the interest it generates, accreditation is not fully understood by many faculty members, administrators, boards of trustees, and even less well by the general public (Selden 1960). Some administrators question the value of the accreditation process. The recommendations that come from accreditation boards are sometimes viewed as attempts by outsiders, lacking an appreciation for the constraints of the institution, to dictate educational policies. Defenders of accreditation point out that, if done properly, accreditation should serve the interests of the general public, including students, by assuring a certain level of educational quality and commitment. A basic premise underlying accreditation is that it improves educational quality.

Postsecondary accreditation is a process whereby groups of educational institutions, professional practitioners, and/or educators, form voluntary, nongovernmental associations to (1) develop standards reflective of quality educational programs, (2) encourage and assist institutions or programs in the evaluation and improvement of their educational endeavors, and (3) identify publicly those institutions or specialized units that meet or exceed the accepted standards of the accreditation organization.

Types of Accreditation

There are two types of accreditation: (1) institutional accreditation and (2) specialized accreditation. Institutional accreditation is a status accorded an institution of postsecondary education to verify that the institution meets the standards set by an accrediting body. The Council on Postsecondary Accreditation (COPA), a private, nongovernmental organization comprised of representatives of regional and specialized accreditation agencies and the public, currently recognizes six regional institutional accrediting bodies (Middle States, New England, North Central, Northwest, Southern, and Western). Specialized accreditation is a status accorded a specialized unit (college, school, division, department, program, or curriculum) within an institution. Specialized accreditation bodies (such as the Educational Standards Board of ASHA) review the relationship of the program to the institution and its mission, review the organization of the program and the resources available for development and maintenance, and seek evidence that the program is meeting its objectives. Specialized accrediting bodies are frequently concerned with details of program organization, management, resources, and curriculum. They usually require that programs be a part of institutions that have been accredited by the appropriate regional accrediting body.

The need for specialized accreditation of educational programs in speech-language pathology and audiology was recognized in 1963 when the National Commission on Accrediting (forerunner of the COPA) designated the American Speech and Hearing Association as the appropriate agency to develop and administer the accreditation of programs in speech-language pathology and audiology. Curtis (1984) has pointed to this recognition as a significant event in the history of the profession. Such recognition demonstrated that speech- language pathology and audiology had reached a level of maturity that justified the accreditation of its educational programs, and further that ASHA was the organization that should be entrusted with this responsibility. The ASHA requested and received recognition for the accreditation of master's degree programs only, and the focus of ASHA's accreditation program has been and continues to be on the master's degree. It follows, then, that undergraduate and doctoral degree programs are excluded from ASHA accreditation. The rationale for seeking recognition for accreditation of master's degree programs only was that the master's degree is the entry level degree for professional practice in the field.

ASHA Accreditation Program

The ASHA has designated a semi-autonomous body called the Council on Professional Standards in Speech-Language Pathology and Audiology (Standards Council) to establish and monitor standards for the profession. This council is composed of members of the profession but also includes a representative of the public. There are three sets of standards that concern this body: (1) accreditation standards for college and university programs administered by the Educational Services Board (ASHA 1990), (2) accreditation standards for agencies that provide speech, language, and hearing services administered by the Professional Services Board (1989), and (3) standards for the certification of members in the profession administered by the Clinical Certification Board (ASHA 1991). It should be noted that the standards set by the Council on Professional Standards are not subject to approval by either the Legislative Council or the Executive Board of ASHA. The Educational Standards Board (ESB) interprets the standards for educational programs in CSD set by the Council on Professional Standards and administers the accreditation program. This board reviews the applications or reapplications for programs seeking accreditation, assigns site visitors to verify that the program is, or is not, doing what it purports to be doing, reviews the report of the site visitors, and makes decisions regarding accreditation.

Beginning January 1, 1993, in order for individuals to be eligible for the Certificate of Clinical Competence (CCC), they must be graduated from an ESB-accredited program in CSD. (See Appendix A.) In the past, graduates of master's programs could obtain ASHA certification without graduating from an accredited program if they met the academic and practicum requirements for the CCC. This new policy makes program accreditation essential.

NCATE Accreditation

A second accrediting body is the National Council for Accreditation of Teacher Education (NCATE). The NCATE has been recognized by COPA as the agency to evaluate and accredit units that prepare professional personnel for employment in schools. The NCATE established a Specialty Areas Studies Board that charged the Council for Exceptional Children (CEC) to develop standards and review procedures for curriculum folios in special education, including speech-language pathology and audiology. Programs with ESB accreditation need only submit a copy of their ESB accreditation letter of approval in lieu of curriculum folios. For master's degree programs without ESB accreditation, CEC will review curriculum folios using the same standards set by the ASHA Standards Council. Undergraduate-only programs, with no master's degree and seeking NCATE approval, must submit curriculum folios for review by CEC (ASHA 1989).

UNDERGRADUATE EDUCATION

It is usually difficult to separate undergraduate education in CSD from graduate education at the master's degree level because of the continuum of knowledge and skill development that occurs across the two degree programs. Undergraduate education is treated as a separate topic in this chapter primarily for organizational purposes. In reality, undergraduate education in CSD is best viewed as the entry point for an educational continuum, leading to a master's degree, possibly a doctoral degree, and follow-up continuing education.

The Role of Liberal Arts

Historically, undergraduate education in CSD has been rooted in a strong liberal arts and sciences tradition. This position was reaffirmed at the 1963 ASHA Highland Park Conference on Graduate Education; the 1969 ASHA New Orleans Conference on Undergraduate Education; the 1983 ASHA St. Paul Conference on Undergraduate, Graduate, and Continuing Education; the 1984 St. Louis Annual Conference of the Council of Graduate Programs in Communication Sciences and Disorders; and the 1989 ASHA Tampa Conference on Undergraduate Education. Whereas no specific arts and sciences curriculum has been recommended in the reports from these conferences, discussions during the 1980s at the Council of Graduate Programs in Communication Sciences and Disorders' annual conferences have strongly urged that undergraduate students majoring in CSD emphasize courses in the sciences and mathematics. The requirements for the Certificates of Clinical Competence call for a broad general education background and mandate 27 hours of coursework in basic sciences. (See Appendix A.) Often the arts and sciences background that students in CSD receive is part of the institutional general education requirements. Many programs recommend arts and sciences courses that not only meet general education requirements at their institution but also have particular relevance to students in CSD.

Professional Education in the Preprofessional Undergraduate Program

The preprofessional curriculum, currently advocated at the undergraduate level, has a liberal arts orientation (Naas and Flahive 1991). This liberal arts component includes 27 semester hours designed to meet ASHA certification standards in the "basic sciences." These basic sciences credits required for the ASHA Certificate of Clinical Competence are further subdivided into the following areas: (1) six semester credit hours (s.c.h.) in biological/physical sciences and mathematics; (2) six s.c.h. in behavioral and/or social sciences; and (3) 15 s.c.h. in basic human communication processes to include the anatomic and physiologic bases, the physical and psychophysical bases, and the linguistic and psycholinguistic aspects. In addition to the basic science coursework, most undergraduate programs offer 21–30 semester credits of professionally oriented courses, including 25 clock hours of clinical observation, and in some programs, an initial practicum experience.

The position espoused by ASHA, and reaffirmed at several conferences over the past three decades, is that undergraduate education is to be preprofessional and thus does not prepare students to enter professional practice at the baccalaureate level. While this position is widely accepted and advocated by academicians and professionals in the field, the reality is that in some states individuals may be employed to work in schools with only a bachelor's degree. This situation has led some educational programs to provide sufficient coursework and practicum opportunities at the undergraduate level to prepare individuals with a baccalaureate degree for employment in school settings. In these undergraduate programs, some of the professional coursework typically included at the graduate level is offered at the undergraduate level, with the result that the liberal arts education of such students is diminished. Bachelor's degree preparation programs typically do not include the breadth and depth of coursework and practicum opportunities found at the graduate level. This leads to concern for the clients, particularly those with more complex problems, who are served by bachelor's degree level practitioners.

Council of Graduate Programs'
Position Regarding Undergraduate Education

In 1989, a task force, appointed by the Council of Graduate Programs in Communication Sciences and Disorders (Wiley et al. 1989), endorsed the concept that undergraduate preparation should be broad rather than narrow, and should include coursework in the following areas: English and communications, physical sciences, biological sciences, social sciences, philosophy, and communication sciences and disorders. They further recommended that undergraduate education should provide:

1. Effective preparation for graduate education in the field;
2. Adequate preparation to follow other educational or career paths (i.e., the undergraduate experience should have a general educational relevance for all students including those who do not pursue graduate work in the field); and
3. Promotion of the profession through course offerings of interest (e.g., an introductory course on human communication) to students in related specialties and perhaps even to the student population at large.

It should be pointed out that these guidelines are only recommendations of the Council of Graduate Programs in Communication Sciences and Disorders (Wiley et al. 1989).

ASHA Position Regarding Undergraduate Education

A set of advisements relative to undergraduate education in CSD was adopted by ASHA. These advisements indicate that undergraduate education should be consistent with the philosophy of a liberal education and that students studying speech-language pathology and/or audiology should demonstrate:

1. Introductory knowledge of human anatomy and physiology, specifically those systems involved in communicative function.
2. Introductory knowledge of articulatory and acoustic phonetics, including transcription skills and appropriate experience in auditory discrimination.
3. Introductory knowledge of the physics of sound and the use of instrumentation essential to the measurement of sound.
4. Introductory knowledge of the normal development of speech and language.
5. Introductory knowledge of the diversity of normal communication behaviors and developmental patterns found in a multicultural society.
6. Introductory knowledge of the nature and prevention of language delays/disorders.
7. Introductory knowledge of the nature and prevention of hearing loss.
8. Introductory knowledge of the measurement of auditory sensitivity and acuity.
9. Introductory knowledge of those principles commonly used by professionals for the re/habilitation of persons with hearing impairments.
10. Introductory knowledge of the nature and prevention of speech delays/disorders.
11. Awareness of those principles commonly used by professionals in the assessment of communication differences, delays, or disorders.
12. Awareness of those principles commonly employed by professionals working with persons demonstrating differences, delays, or disorders of communication.

When a practicum is a part of the undergraduate curriculum, the following are recommended:

13. Twenty-five (25) hours of supervised observation of assessment and intervention with a variety of cases selected from more than one clinical setting must be provided prior to a student's first clinical practicum experience.

14. In addition, all practicum experiences must be in compliance with ASHA accreditation standards for supervision and practicum. (ASHA 1989)

MASTER'S DEGREE EDUCATION

Ever since the ASHA Highland Park Conference in 1963 (ASHA 1963), the master's degree has been the offically recognized degree for entry into the profession. Thus, the master's degree has become the degree of focus for students interested in professional practice in speech-language pathology or audiology.

In order to meet the requirements for the ASHA Certificate of Clinical Competence (and licensure in most states) in Speech-Language Pathology or Audiology, students are required to have coursework at both the undergraduate and graduate levels. Thus, the undergraduate coursework for most students is inextricably bound to the master's degree curriculum. For those students who begin study of the field at the master's degree level, it is common for undergraduate prerequisite coursework to be required.

Curriculum

The ASHA certification requirements at the master's degree level have remained much the same since the master's degree or its equivalent was adopted in 1965 as the level of academic preparation required to enter the professions of speech-language pathology and audiology. As a result, curricula at the master's degree level have remained fairly stable for three decades. Implicit in this statement is the recognition that certification standards tend to drive some of the undergraduate and much of the master's degree coursework in the field.

In the section above describing undergraduate education, the coursework required for certification usually taken at the undergraduate level was delineated. As stated, 27 s.c.h. of basic science coursework, including 15 s.c.h. in basic communication processes and six s.c.h. of disorders-related coursework are typically taken at the undergraduate level. Thirty (30) s.c.h. of professional coursework (speech-language pathology or audiology) are required at the graduate level. Within these 30 hours are some specific categories of required coursework. Three hundred fifty (350) clock hours of practicum are also required, 250 of which must be accrued at the graduate level. Of these hours, there are specific requirements as to type of service performed (evaluation/treatment), age of clients (children/adults), and the number of practicum settings (three) (ASHA 1991). (See Appendix A.)

Professional coursework at the master's degree level for those majoring in speech-language pathology includes the traditional areas of voice, fluency, phonology, language (child and adult), audiology, and aural rehabilitation. Courses in hearing evaluation of children and adults, amplification and assistive devices, and treatment of hearing disorders are typically included in audiology curricula. Master's degree programs in both areas often include speech science/hearing science as well as statistics and/or research methods as a part of their degree requirements. In addition, curricula in speech-language pathology typically include disorders courses, such as augmentative communication, supplemental to the traditional areas.

Of particular interest to a discussion of curriculum is the changing demographics of the United States. In almost all areas of the country, it is increasingly common for many individuals to be from a culture other than the traditional white middle-class population. These individuals bring with them perspectives, values, and speech and language patterns that must be accepted, appreciated, and accommodated in the larger culture. Speech-language pathologists and audiologists must learn to be sensitive to and competent in dealing with this cultural diversity. Preparing students for this sensitivity and competence represents a major challenge to most academic programs. Many institutions are seeking to address deficiencies in this area through curriculum modification and practicum experiences.

The scope of professional practice has expanded over the last two decades, and this development has had an impact on the courses offered in graduate programs. For example, courses in augmentative communication, dysphagia, closed-head injury, and literacy were developed in the 1980s, largely in response to an expanded scope of practice in the field. A dilemma for college and university educational programs is how to incorporate such topics into an already burgeoning curriculum. Many master's degree programs require two years of full-time graduate study, and adding more course requirements is difficult. One possible solution is to defer certain content areas to the post-graduate level. It may also be that program faculty will need to combine traditional course topics into a single course. Each educational program must determine what is to be included in its core degree program, what courses are to be elective, and what is to be relegated to post-master's education. Several programs have initiated a system of different tracks or branches so that students, while meeting certification requirements, can have some specialization through elective courses to prepare themselves for specific employment settings, specific populations, or particular disorders.

ASHA Standards Validation Study

In 1988, the ASHA reported the results of a study (Lingwall 1988) to determine (validate) the professional domains, tasks, knowledges, and skills in the practice of speech-language pathology and audiology. Of most relevance to master's degree programs were the knowledge and skills needed for professional practice, since many of these are acquired during the master's degree program. Once an extensive list of such knowledge and skills had been identified, professionals were asked to rate the point of acquisition for each.

Audiologists and speech-language pathologists who participated in the study reported spending about 20% of their time on administration. Respondents recommended that practicum clock hour requirements in speech-language pathology and audiology should be increased to insure that graduates have a variety of experiences with individuals with various disorders and of differing levels of severity and age. Another recommendation was that most skills and knowledge needed for professional practice should be acquired by the time the student has completed academic and practicum requirements for the Certificate of Clinical Competence.

Matriculation of Part-Time Students

A final topic that merits some discussion relative to master's degree programs is the issue of part-time degree students. Historically, it was common for developing programs not only to allow for, but to encourage, part-time students. As programs expanded with a large pool of students, emphasis was placed on full-time programs. The advent of federal funding for full-time students during the 1960s enhanced the trend toward full-time study. In addition, in states where the master's degree became the minimum entry level for practice, programs were more likely to have full-time students because graduates with only a bachelor's degree had few employment opportunities in the field. The fact that for over a decade the ASHA accreditation self-study guidelines specifically asked whether or not the program could be completed on a part-time basis was interpreted by some faculty as indicating that full-time study was preferable to part-time.

As we move toward the twenty-first century, demographics suggest that part-time programs should receive more attention. As the number of high school graduates declines, programs may not easily fill their student quotas with full-time students. A possible source to fill this void may be individuals who are seeking a career change, former professionals who wish to update their skills, or students who do not have the financial resources for full-time study. Another factor that may encourage programs to develop ways for students to obtain master's degrees on a part-time basis is the qualified provider clause in PL 99-457. The passage of PL 99-457 Part H in 1986 required state education agencies to establish and maintain personnel standards that are based on the highest personnel requirements in the state. This means that for states requiring a master's degree for licensure, a lower standard for practitioners in schools would not be in compliance with the "qualified provider" aspect of this legislation. This statute, therefore, may require people in certain states who work in school settings to obtain additional education leading to a master's degree. Creative efforts to develop quality programs for part-time students have the potential not only to help academic programs survive but to provide a much needed pool of talent for the profession.

DOCTORAL DEGREE EDUCATION

The Ph.D. Degree

Doctoral degree programs in CSD were developed in the tradition of the Doctor of Philosophy degree. The traditional thrust of the Ph.D. degree has been to prepare individuals to conduct research in a given area. The Ph.D. degree is viewed as a robust or open research degree, appropriate for all fields of learning, and including both basic and applied research training.

A review of Ph.D. degree requirements in CSD at various institutions reveals that most students and their planning committees have considerable flexibility in developing a course of study. Logemann (1987) stated that the Ph.D. "is as flexible as we choose to make it" (p. 61) and can be used to prepare the academic teacher/investigator, the clinical teacher/investigator, and the hospital clinician/investigator as well as the basic scientist.

Individuals with a variety of interests and professional goals, including research, teaching, administration, and clinical practice or a combination of these, have sought the Ph.D. degree in CSD. One reason for the diversity of these goals is that the Ph.D. degree has traditionally been the only degree available to individuals who wished to pursue a doctoral degree. Moll (1983) reflected this practice when he stated that "doctoral education in our field cannot be a singly focused entity but must vary to accommodate diverse student objectives in regard to both career goals and disciplinary specialization" (p. 33).

Components of the Research Doctoral Degree

Most research-oriented Ph.D. degree programs include at least four components: (1) theory mastery and knowledge of the field; (2) knowledge and skills to conduct research; (3) a written and/or oral comprehensive examination; and (4) a major original research project (dissertation) sometimes described as a "culminating research experience." In addition, a residency of one or two years is required by most universities. While the specifics of these requirements have evolved and changed over time and vary from one program to another, these components have traditionally been the core of most doctoral programs.

Doctoral coursework in CSD has changed to reflect the greater depth of knowledge in the field and to allow for greater specialization. In addition, doctoral students have increasingly taken work in areas related to CSD, for example, psychology, linguistics, neurosciences, and engineering. There is also more emphasis on conducting research projects at earlier stages of the doctoral program, usually with the student serving as a co-investigator with a faculty member. This procedure is followed to help students develop research skills leading to the dissertation. The goal of such programming is that by the time the student has completed the Ph.D. degree, he or she will have presented and published research findings, and, it is hoped, will have begun to establish a line of research inquiry.

During the decade of the 1970s, the Ph.D. degree research tool requirements changed as institutions allowed programs to determine appropriate tool requirements for their disciplines. Prior to this, most institutions required some level of competence in the translation of foreign languages, plus some background in statistics. With the flexibility to modify tool requirements, most doctoral programs in CSD elected to require a sequence of courses in statistics and/or research methods to meet all or part of the tool requirements for the degree.

The dissertation typically consumes a relatively large portion of the time devoted to the doctoral degree—usually one to three years—but there have been suggestions and alternative proposals to the traditional dissertation. One suggested alternative is a series of research investigations that would begin even before the comprehensive examination. Such a series of successive projects is proposed in part because: (1) the experience is assumed to be similar to research in the work environment; and (2) the student has the opportunity to develop a line of inquiry.

For individuals who wish to pursue a research-oriented career, post-doctoral study prior to accepting a research/academic appointment is increasingly prevalent. Demand for scholarly productivity, including external funding, at research-oriented institutions seems to indicate that post-doctoral research training is highly desirable.

Alternative Degree Tags

While most doctoral degrees granted in CSD are Ph.D.s, there are other doctoral degrees available in the field. The two most common are the Doctor of Education (Ed.D.) and the Doctor of Science (Sc.D.). Although these degrees are available at some institutions, they continue to be the exception rather than the rule. When one looks carefully at specific components of these degrees and compares them with those found in Ph.D. degree programs, one is struck by the great similarity in requirements. The philosophy behind the degrees is similar, and frequently the name of the degree is the result of affiliation of the department in the university rather than the content of the degree program. For example, the Ed.D. degree, both at the University of Georgia and at Columbia University, reflects the fact that CSD departments at these institutions were located in the school or college of education. Likewise, the Sc.D. degree is issued by Boston University because the program is housed administratively in the college of allied health where departments are authorized to grant a Sc.D. degree but are not authorized to grant the Ph.D. degree. A current concern is whether the Ph.D. degree is appropriate for those who wish to pursue a career in clinical service or administration as opposed to a research and/or academic career.

Professional Doctorate

The traditional Ph.D. degree has been oriented toward preparing students for academic careers. Individuals who earn the Ph.D. degree are educated as scholars with the expectation that they will disseminate knowledge and add to the knowledge base of the field. For close to three decades, discussions have occurred within our field regarding the need for a second type of doctorate designed specifically for those individuals who wish to pursue, at the post-master's level, a career of treating patients and/or administering clinical programs. This type of degree has been identified as a professional or clinical doctorate and modeled after professional degrees in medicine, dentistry, optometry, and clinical psychology.

Two basic arguments support the idea of a professional doctorate in speech-language pathology and audiology: (1) proliferation of knowledge, advances in technology, and an expansion of the scope of practice, including professional interactions, make it difficult to prepare independent practitioners at the master's degree level; and (2) professional image, recognition, and acceptance, particularly in medical settings, would be significantly enhanced if practitioners had a clinical doctoral degree.

The concept of a clinical doctorate has had both strong proponents

(Feldman 1981; Loavenbruck 1983, 1990; Goldstein 1989, 1990) and detractors (Koenigsknecht 1983; Ringel 1982, 1990). As discussed above, there are those who indicate that present Ph.D. degrees are robust and flexible enough to allow for doctoral study that emphasizes professional practice (Ringel 1990). Others argue that the Ph.D. degree is a scholarly degree with clinical practice assuming a position of secondary importance to research. For example, Saxman (1991) concluded in an historical review of doctoral education, "I am not convinced that the traditional Ph.D. model is appropriate for the education of top-flight clinicians" (p. 36). By separating advanced clinical knowledge from research preparation and experience, it has been suggested, both research and professional types of doctoral education can be strengthened.

The recommended length of time required to earn a professional doctoral degree has been discussed. Goldstein (1989) has proposed a degree based on six years beyond high school. Others, such as Feldman (1984), have suggested two to three years beyond the master's degree or three to four years beyond the bachelor's degree. Hood (1989) pointed out that foundation courses, specialized courses, and time needed for maturation of students into professionals are factors that should be considered in determining the length of time for the degree.

For the most part, academics have not supported the need for a professional doctorate while those in professional practice have been more enthusiastic. At conferences focusing on graduate education, the notion of a professional doctorate has been discussed but not approved (ASHA 1963; Rees and Snope 1983). A clinical doctorate proposal that has received considerable attention is the Au.D. (Audiology Doctorate) degree proposed by David Goldstein (1989). This proposal not only identifies a specific degree, but outlines a matriculation sequence and curriculum that varies considerably from existing Ph.D. degree programs.

A few academic programs have begun to offer professional doctorates or a clinical doctoral track to complement a research track. Professional organizations such as the ASHA have task forces studying the topic. The Academy of Dispensing Audiologists has even endorsed a specific proposal. Issues yet to be resolved are whether or not the doctoral degree should be the entry requirement for certain types of clinical practice, whether variations related to the professional doctorate should exist between speech-language pathology or audiology, and how division of labor might be organized among individuals prepared at the master's degree, the doctoral degree, and other levels of preparation. The American Academy of Audiology supports the principle that a doctoral degree should be the appropriate minimal entry level degree for the practice of audiology and that "the Au.D. is an appropriate designator for the professional doctorate in audiology" (AAA 1990, p. 10).

The hope of those individuals who embrace advanced clinical education at the doctoral level is that the professional practice of speech-language pathology and audiology will achieve a level of effectiveness and recognition that has heretofore not been achieved in most centers. It is assumed that the preparation of doctoral-level practitioners will translate into better assistance for the communicatively handicapped and more rewarding careers for those who serve this population.

Further Issues Related to Doctoral Education

Quality of Research Training. As mentioned above, the quality of research training in current Ph.D. degree programs has been called into question. One factor leading to this concern has been the paucity of grant applications from speech-language pathologists and audiologists to the National Institute of Neurological and Communication Disorders and Stroke (NINCDS), when compared to other disciplines. Ludlow (1987) pointed out that the numbers of grant applications in the neurosciences have increased more rapidly during the last decade than have those in hearing, speech, and language. She also reported that, in a study of NINCDS principal investigators, formal post-doctoral study was much more common among graduates in the neurosciences than those in speech and hearing. Much of the research in CSD is conducted by individuals in disciplines other than CSD. Comments such as these lead to questions about the quality of research preparation of doctoral students in CSD.

As stated above, individuals with the Ph.D. degree who assume academic/research positions in universities can expect to find increasing expectations for scholarly publication and external funds to support their research. It may be postulated that some graduates from Ph.D. degree programs are not on a par with graduates from other disciplines because of (1) less-than-adequate research preparation in their graduate education, (2) an overabundance of professional coursework in their doctoral program, and (3) lack of post-doctoral research experience.

Faculty Shortage. There are a number of studies predicting a shortage of qualified faculty members during the 1990s and into the twenty-first century. These projections anticipate that the rate of faculty retirement during this period, together with a slight growth in the number of professorial positions, will create a shortage of university professors. The reason for the large number of anticipated retirements is that an exceptionally large number of professors were hired in the 1960s and will be retiring in the 1990s. Already there are scattered reports of shortages of doctoral level individuals in certain areas. While these projections are based on the demographics of the entire professorial population, one might expect that this phenomenon will apply to CSD. However, it appears that the field of CSD will not experience the large number of retirements projected for education, humanities, and agriculture in the 1990s. In a study reported by Cooper, Bernthal, and Creaghead (1989), it was found that only 18% of the faculty in CSD are age 56 or older while 64% are between 36 and 55.

FURTHER COMMENTS AND CONCERNS
REGARDING GRADUATE EDUCATION IN CSD

A major concern of program administrators and faculty in CSD relates to whether or not academic units have sufficient resources, ongoing support, and talented faculty and students to maintain a quality education program, including the advancement of scholarly knowledge. It should be recognized that education of students in CSD is expensive relative to that in most other disciplines. Programs in CSD require one-to-one teaching/supervision in addition to specialized space and equipment demands. Historically, the largest and most prestigious programs (based on faculty size, student numbers, laboratory facilities, and scholarly output) have been in public institutions. One reason that programs have tended to flourish in public institutions is that state legislatures and university administrations have supported programs to meet statewide manpower needs for speech-language pathologists and audiologists. Financial support through the states has assisted and sustained most of the programs in our field.

One factor that enhances a program's viability is to be perceived favorably on campus. While there are many variables that influence such perceptions, student quality, external support, scholarly productivity, teaching excellence, and faculty contributions to the campus and external community are important. Quality programs are those that contribute significantly to the education of students and to the mission of the institution. The stronger the links between CSD and other productive units on campus, the more indigenous our specialty becomes to the institution. Factors such as these add to the viability and effectiveness of the program.

Of concern in college and university programs is the recruitment and retention of quality students. Typically, CSD has drawn students with strong academic ability, good interpersonal skills, and a desire to serve humanity. In the 1990s, certain factors regarding student enrollments in the field merit attention. The first is the decline in the number of males entering the field. In 1990–1991, almost 94% of undergraduate students in the field were female (Creaghead, Bernthal, and Gilbert 1991). Although the specific impact of this trend may be uncertain, most would agree that fields are enhanced with a more balanced gender work force. The second concern relates to the small number of minority students in CSD educational programs. For example, in 1990–1991, only 8.7% of the undergraduate students in CSD, 7.8% at the master's level, and 10.9% at the doctoral level were minority students. Likewise, it was reported in the same survey that percentages of minority faculty members were under-represented in CSD academic programs; only 5.2% of the full-time and 3.5% of the part-time faculty were from minority groups. Given the projected future demographics in the United States, much greater emphasis needs to be given to minority and multi-cultural issues.

Another area of concern is the status of the Graduate Record Exam scores for master's degree applicants. Recent comparison indices suggest that our students have scores below those of students in many disciplines. Some have postulated that the salaries in the field and the women's movement have contributed to the pursuit of other disciplines. Regardless of the reason, both academic programs and the profession at large must mobilize their energies to recruit capable students. Quality of clinical services provided and the caliber of the research base underlying practice will be jeopardized if the profession/ discipline lacks bright and talented practitioners.

Job opportunities for graduates are many. The field of speech-language pathology and audiology offers numerous options for employment of individuals at the master's degree or doctoral degree levels. Clinical positions are available in hospitals, schools, clinics, and private practices, and include direct intervention, consultation, and supervision. At the doctoral degree level, some positions combine teaching and/or research at universities, medical settings, and government agencies. The employment picture for the 1990s shows plentiful jobs and increasing diversity of roles and specialization among professionals in the field.

REFERENCES

American Academy of Audiology. 1990. American Academy of Audiology: Graduate education. *Audiology Today* 2(5):10.

American Speech and Hearing Association. 1963. *Graduate Education in Speech Pathology and Audiology.* Washington, DC: Author.

American Speech-Language-Hearing Association. 1989. Ad Hoc Committee on Undergraduate Education. Advisements for undergraduate/preprofessional education. Rockville, MD: Author.

American Speech-Language-Hearing Association. 1990. Standards for accreditation of educational programs. *Asha* 32(6/7):93–94, 100.

American Speech-Language-Hearing Association. 1991. Standards for the certificates of clinical competence. *Asha* 33(3):121–22.

Creaghead, N., Bernthal, J., and Gilbert, H. 1991. *The Council of Graduate Pro-*

grams in Communication Sciences and Disorders 1990–91 National Survey. Minneapolis, MN: Council of Graduate Programs in Communication Sciences and Disorders.

Curtis, J. F. 1984. An emeritus looks at graduate education. In *Proceedings of the Fifth Annual Conference on Graduate Education, St. Louis,* ed. J. E. Bernthal. Council of Graduate Programs in Communication Sciences and Disorders.

Doehring, D., and Coderre, L. 1989. The development of Canadian university programs in communication disorders. *Journal of Speech Language Pathology and Audiology* 13(4).

Feldman, A. S. 1981. The challenge of autonomy. 1981 presidential address. *Asha* 23:941–45.

Feldman, A. S. 1984. In support of the professional doctorate. *Asha* 26(11):24–32.

Goldstein, D. P. 1989. Au.D. degree: The doctoring degree in audiology. *Asha* 31(4):33–35.

Goldstein, D. P. 1990. Au.D. degree in doctoral level audiology: Demographic and statistical considerations. *Audiology Today* 2(5):14–16.

Hood, L. J. 1989. A professional doctorate in audiology—some issues to consider. *Audiology Today* 3:10–12.

Koenigsknecht, R. 1983. Issue III: What is the need for a professional doctorate in communication disorders? In *Proceedings of the 1983 National Conference on Undergraduate, Graduate, and Continuing Education* (Report No. 13), eds. N. S. Rees and T. L. Snope. Rockville, MD: American Speech-Language-Hearing Association.

Lingwall, J. B. 1988. Evaluation of the requirements for the certificates of clinical competence in speech-language pathology and audiology. *Asha* 30(9):75–78.

Loavenbruck, A. 1983. Issue V: How may we better prepare clinicians for the realities of providing services to the communicatively disordered in a variety of settings? In *Proceedings of the 1983 National Conference on Undergraduate, Graduate, and Continuing Education* (Report No. 13), eds. N. S. Rees and T. L. Snope. Rockville, MD: American Speech-Language-Hearing Association.

Loavenbruck, A. 1990. Standards of clinical competency: M.A. to Au.D. degree. *Audiology Today* 2(5):20–21.

Logemann, J. A. 1987. Future directions in graduate education: Quo Vadis? The doctoral program. In *Proceedings of the Eighth Annual Conference on Graduate Education,* eds. S. Steiner, R. L. Erickson, and J. Montague. Council of Graduate Programs in Communication Sciences and Disorders.

Ludlow, C. 1987. The need for integrating the communication sciences and disorders with the neurosciences in training and research. In *Proceedings of the Eighth Annual Conference on Graduate Education,* eds. S. Steiner, R. L. Erickson, and J. Montague. Council of Graduate Programs in Communication Sciences and Disorders.

Moll, K. 1983. Issue II: What should be the content and objectives of graduate education in communication disorders? In *Proceedings of the 1983 National Conference on Undergraduate, Graduate, and Continuing Education* (Report No. 13), eds. N. S. Rees and T. L. Snope. Rockville, MD: American Speech-Language-Hearing Association.

Naas, J. F., and Flahive, M. J. 1991. Preprofessional-only programs: A fruitful endeavor. *Asha* 33(1):39–41, 53.

Paden, E. 1970. *A History of the American Speech and Hearing Association 1925–1958.* Washington, DC: American Speech and Hearing Association.

Professional Services Board. 1989. American Speech-Language-Hearing Association. *1989 ASHA PSB Accreditation Manual.* Rockville, MD: Author.

Rees, N. S., and Snope, T. L. (eds.). 1983. *Proceedings of the 1983 National Confer-*

ence on Undergraduate, Graduate, and Continuing Education (Report No. 13). Rockville, MD: American Speech-Language-Hearing Association.

Ringel, R. L. 1982. Some issues facing graduate education. *Asha* 24:339–403.

Ringel, R. L. 1990. Doctoral education in speech-language pathology and audiology. *Audiology Today* 2(6):12–16.

Saxman, J. H. 1991. Doctor or doctor? A choice of guilds. *Asha* 33(1):34–36.

Selden, W. 1960. *Accreditation: A Struggle over Standards in Higher Education.* New York: Harper.

Shewan, C. M. 1989. Omnibus survey—quality is not a four letter word. *Asha* 31(8):51–55.

Wiley, T. L., Andrews, J. R., Kent, R. D., and Lieberman, R. J. 1989. Report of the task force on undergraduate education, Council of Graduate Programs in Communication Sciences and Disorders. In *Proceedings of the Tenth Annual Confernce on Graduate Education,* ed. J. M. Pettit. Tampa, FL: Council of Graduate Programs in Communication Sciences and Disorders.

Chapter 5

Education in the Classroom

Margaret D. McElroy and Judith A. Rassi

THE CLASSROOM AS A LEARNING ENVIRONMENT

As a learning environment, the classroom incorporates both physical and psychological components. Communication can be fostered or inhibited by the interplay of these factors.

Classroom Physical Environment

Physical environment can facilitate communication in a classroom (Fuhrmann and Grasha 1983). A teacher's understanding of the arrangement of people and objects in relation to communication, referred to by Steele (1973) as environmental competence, can lead to improved interactions between teachers and students.

Seating Arrangements. A classroom seating arrangement can encourage or discourage social contact by creating for students a feeling of being pushed apart or together. Sommer (1969) found, for example, that the placement of chairs across the corner of a table fosters conversations between two seated individuals. An effective alternative for small group discussions is a circle in which opposite chairs are placed five to seven feet apart. Both of these arrangements allow visual contact, thereby enabling participants to be responsive to each other. Fuhrmann and Grasha (1983) have found the circle arrangement to be optimal for classroom interpersonal communication either in a grouping of chairs placed at a round table or in a circle without a table.

Front-to-back rows with people seated side by side, although popular, often is the poorest arrangement because it encourages one-way communication between the teacher, located in the front of the classroom, and the students seated near the front of the room. In another common arrangement, where people are seated at each end and along the sides of a rectangular table in a seminar room, conversations tend to flow toward the leader at one end of the table and between persons sitting opposite each other. Moreover, people seated next to each other may communicate less (Fuhrmann and Grasha 1983).

Class Size. Audiology and speech-language pathology instructors who teach communication disorders students at the graduate level usually find themselves teaching small classes in which enrollment does not exceed 20 or 25; in fact, classes with ten or fewer students are not uncommon. Classes that include nonmajors and/or undergraduates, on the other hand, may be substantially larger.

Differences in class size have certain educational implications. Over the years, the findings of many studies (Cheydleur 1945; Macomber and Siegel 1957, 1960; Siegel, Adams, and Macomber 1960) have consistently supported smaller classes over larger classes in a variety of comparisons. In the light of these and other comparative data, large class enrollments should be resisted.

Classroom Psychological Environment

The impact of a classroom's psychological environment on learning is as great as that of the physical environment or class size.

Psychological Well-Being. A socially and emotionally healthy classroom is one that promotes ingenuity and creativity, embraces nonconformity, imagination, humor, light-heartedness, acceptance, and sensitivity (Torrance 1962; Taylor 1964; Cropley 1967). Conversely, in classrooms where there is an emphasis on grading and group conformity along with teacher-centered authority and discouragement of student questions, the psychological atmosphere mitigates against creativity and independent thinking (Read and Greene 1980). An atmosphere that allows student freedom and creativity helps to lessen student apprehension concerning oral class participation and to establish high, yet realistic, expectations for learning. An increase in student productivity and trust is the usual outcome.

The psychological well-being of individual students within a classroom naturally extends to the class as a whole, thereby contributing to and influencing class morale. The morale of the group, in turn, is affected by other factors as well. It can fluctuate, for example, before and after exams and at high and low points in the school term. The interaction of students and instructor further influences class morale (Lowman 1984). Instructors need to be aware of prevailing group attitudes and their reasons for being. With this awareness, the need for modification of the psychological learning environment is more likely to be recognized (Gordon 1974).

Psychological Size. Psychological size, a concept discussed by Richard Wallen in workshops on interpersonal interactions, refers to the effect one person has on another, whether it be negative or positive (Fuhrmann and Grasha 1983). In a communication system where a difference in psychological size between individuals is perceived, the potential exists for manipulation by the person(s) perceived to be psychologically bigger and, if realized, open communication may be suppressed (Fuhrmann and Grasha 1983).

Boyer and Bolton (1971) point out that this frequently happens in the classroom where, because of their status difference, teachers are typically considered to have a greater psychological size than their students. As a consequence, the teacher is often assumed to be the problem solver, the caretaker, and the person who tells students what to do. This kind of dependence in a classroom can lead to indifference and lack of initiative on the part of students (Fuhrmann and Grasha 1983).

A teacher's greater psychological size, according to Fuhrmann and Grasha (1983), is reinforced by such teacher actions as:

- Use of high status and titles
- Inappropriate use of criticism, sarcasm, ridicule, and humor
- Use of terminal statements permitting no disagreement
- Use of very formal manner
- Use of punishing remarks
- Display of a great amount of detailed knowledge
- Use of language that is too complicated for the listener
- Failure to use the name of a student
- Overemphasis on grades and grading (pp. 144–45)

Self-assessment of the teacher's psychological size relative to that of the students in a particular classroom situation constitutes the first step toward open communication. If a difference in size is reflected by the presence of any of the above factors, the teacher should seek to eliminate them. Next, the teacher can take steps to expand the students' psychological size by showing regard for their views and giving them more responsibility for what happens in the classroom through such activities as selecting topics for class discussion or serving as small-group discussion leaders. Not only does this kind of active participation by students serve to reduce the difference in psychological size between them and their teacher, but the teacher can benefit from gaining added insight into issues or situations from the contributions of students (Fuhrmann and Grasha 1983).

Classroom Communication

Research by Leavitt (1951) has shown that the instructor controls the communication climate in a class, thereby affecting the extent of student involvement. Messages in the classroom can be sent and received in different ways, depending on the communication circumstances within a particular classroom environment. The manner in which people interact and the kind of information they bring to a task can be related to the communication form established.

Communication Direction. Leavitt (1951) found that with movement of communication from an open, free exchange to more restrictive one-way patterns, mistakes increase and people are less satisfied with their contributions. A major advantage of one-way communication is that it permits the teacher to manage the amount, rate, and course of the information. The major disadvantage of one-way communication is that it provides students with little opportunity for prompt and direct response to the teacher's comments, thus discouraging student questions and discussion (Fuhrmann and Grasha 1983).

Two-way communication allows a flow of communication among and between people, especially in discussions. It provides immediate feedback and, therefore, allows for less dependence on the instructor, resulting in more accountability and greater initiative on the part of students. Participating students appear to be more involved and interested. Conversely, the time required for transmission of messages and the lack of control on the teacher's part are viewed by some educators as disadvantages. The value of two-way communication is reinforced by Anderson (1979) on the basis of his observations of students. He believes that students can become depersonalized because of noncommunication in the classroom which occurs, for example, when they have no say in decisions affecting the class or when they are given no means for discussion of lectures or evaluation of tests. A more caring and reciprocal approach, he asserts, is one that allows a positive exchange of information and feelings from both the students and the teacher, thus promoting two-way patterns of communication. A focus on relationships between people helps to clarify the meaning of words in student-teacher classroom communication.

A classroom instructor can tell the direction in which communication is flowing by tape recording a class session, then determining the amount of student- and teacher-talk (Greive 1984). Comparisons can also be made between those who initiate talk and those who speak only in response to another person. Following this kind of analysis, the instructor can seek to shift the balance of participation according to individual and class needs.

Communication Messages. Although intended primarily for elementary and secondary school teachers, Gordon's teacher effectiveness training suggestions (1974) concerning communication are applicable at higher-education levels as well. Especially noteworthy is his delineation of teachers' statements that convey messages open to misinterpretation or negative reception by students. To minimize such risks either inside or outside the classroom, instructors are advised to avoid, temper, or practice judiciously the following:

- Ordering, commanding, directing
- Warning, threatening
- Moralizing, preaching, giving "shoulds and oughts"
- Advising, offering solutions or suggestions (without student input)
- Teaching, lecturing, giving logical arguments (without student participation)
- Judging, disagreeing, blaming
- Praising, agreeing, giving positive evaluations (if incongruous with student self-esteem; if stated insincerely; if expressed in vague terms)
- Name-calling, stereotyping, ridiculing
- Interpreting, analyzing, diagnosing (i.e., a student's problems)
- Reassuring, sympathizing, consoling, supporting (if done without a clear understanding of a student's problems)
- Questioning, probing, interrogating, cross-examining
- Withdrawing, distracting, being sarcastic, humoring, diverting (pp. 80–86)

Nonverbal Communication. Always evident in the classroom, nonverbal communication, through its many expressions, shapes messages and influences their interpretation. An instructor's use of body language such as gesturing or walking back and forth in front of the class can enhance instruction or be a source of distraction. Facial expression, frequently indicative of an instructor's approval or disapproval (Greive 1984), can reflect thoughtful consideration and acceptance if carefully self-monitored.

Classroom Instruction

Presentation Organization. Organization facilitates learning: it distinguishes between major and minor points and helps to convey ideas. Most classroom instructors recognize the importance of organizing material for teaching purposes. They know that it is beneficial not only to student understanding but also to their own preparation for teaching. Instructors can determine their success in making their lectures into logical, well-organized presentations by comparing their lecture notes to class notes taken by students. This kind of comparison will reveal whether or not more attention should be given to the students' understanding of the specific intent of the oral presentation (Weimer 1988c).

According to Weimer (1988b), several factors contribute to the significant differences that are often evident between organization on paper and organization as it is transmitted orally. Written language is characterized by discrete signals. Although spoken language also contains directional cues, most are nonverbal rather than verbal, hence more variable. A new, spoken paragraph, for example, is not signaled by a gesture. Even if there were a paragraph indicator, this in itself might be confusing because not all paragraphs are intended to convey a change of thought. There simply are no rules of syntax to designate nonverbal directional cues.

Verbal cues, on the other hand, can be used to relate explicit messages as, for example, "This is an important point; be sure to remember it."

Most teachers do not compensate for the transitory nature of oral communication. Writing notes and listening to the instructor at the same time is difficult for many students. Or a student may become distracted during a class lecture with resultant note-taking gaps. In either case, the original material cannot be retrieved unless it has been tape-recorded. Choosing to use another student's notes may or may not be helpful. Finally, the disparity between teacher and student familiarity with the format, as well as the content, of lecture material may not be taken into account. As a consequence, the presentation of information is not modified appropriately, and causes confusion and frustration among those students who need the full benefit of complete lecture notes (Weimer 1988b).

Recognition, on the teacher's part, of these kinds of distinctions between spoken and written language is very important. The delivery of the lecture must be considered as carefully as the preparation of the lecture. In the periodical publication, *Teaching Professor* (Weimer 1988c), can be found methods for communicating structure. These suggestions include:

A listing on the board, prior to beginning the class, of the three main points to be covered in the class for that specific day with a check-off of each point following its discussion; or use of an abbreviated outline shown on an overhead projector. The list or outline can be utilized for review or summary of the presentation

Intermittent use of lecture checkpoints to highlight important points made during a lecture. With this method, the class can be asked to repeat the important points. Routine use of this technique is not advised, however, because some students may not take notes until the important points are reviewed

Conscious use of effective nonverbal cues to present points from a specific location and to provide directional cues and thought structures

The building of relationships between ideas, lectures, and content segments, and encouragment of students to make similar kinds of associations

Allowance of timeouts periodically to permit students to catch up with note-taking, request clarification, or ask for repetition of a previous point. At these times the teacher stops talking and listens. Such a technique encourages students and teachers to contemplate content

Structural Clarity. The importance of structural clarity is emphasized by Pagliocca (1988). Learning is facilitated when students are aware of the structure of the instructor's presentation.

In the literature on effective teaching methods, the organization and structuring of lessons is constantly stressed. Brophy and Good (1986) assert that "achievement is maximized when teachers not only actively present material, but structure it by: beginning with overviews, advance organizers, or review of objectives; outlining the content and signaling transitions between lesson parts; calling attention to main ideas; summarizing subparts of the lesson as it proceeds; and reviewing main ideas at the end" (p. 362).

Objectives and overviews highlight pertinent points for students, whereas structuring and lesson planning provide a sense of direction for the student as well as the teacher. Such approaches enable the teacher to remain on track. Outlines are a form of organization that can be learned and retained by students. They include, in visual format, the primary points to be covered by the teacher and offer an understanding of relationships among and between ideas (Pagliocca 1988).

The review of a lesson includes two fundamental phases: "recapitulation . . . and extension of learning to related areas" (Pagliocca p. 188). Lesson review, therefore, is useful in summarizing a topic and in encouraging more in-depth understanding of a topic. It can also be employed between presentations of different topics as a means of organizing recently learned information and speculating upon the next area of presentation or study.

STUDENT INVOLVEMENT IN THE CLASSROOM

Constructive teacher-student relationships are indispensable to effective classroom teaching. In his model designed to assist elementary and secondary teachers in working with problems related to classroom behavior, Gordon (1974) stresses the importance of "openness, caring, interdependence, separateness, and mutual needs meeting" (p. 24). These same factors also serve the teaching-learning process in higher education. Because of their inherent humaneness, they invite student involvement and participation in classroom learning. An open, stimulating classroom climate can imbue in both the instructor and students a sense of commitment and responsiblity that reaps untold educational benefits.

In order to cultivate in students the kinds of attitudes and behaviors that invite and welcome learning, a classroom instructor needs to model at least two roles, one as exemplary learner, the other as exemplary teacher. Superimposed on this expression of self, moreover, there must be an understanding of, and accommodation for, a number of interdependent student and classroom influences.

Student Characteristics

Any group of students, although clearly heterogeneous, displays identifiable characteristics having educational implications.

Personality. In a study conducted by Flocken (1980), Cattell, Eber, and Tatsuoks' *Sixteen Personality Factor Questionnaire* (1970) was administered to graduate students in a communication disorders program. Scores on all sixteen factors were neither extremely high nor extremely low, indicating that these students in communication disorders courses had personality factors not much different from those in the general population. Even so, these students "tended to be reserved, bright, mature, assertive, enthusiastic, uninhibited, sensitive, imaginative, unpretentious, self-assured, and experimenting" (p. 13), findings that were similar to those for elementary school teachers and nurses. Educators working with students in communication disorders programs may want to look at nursing and teacher education for parallel teaching strategies.

Age. Burrill and Ryan (1983) describe students in higher education as being self-directed, demanding as consumers, exposed to life experiences, desirous of being treated as adults, demanding of relevant and prompt application of information, and eager to participate in the development of their learning activities. Some of these traits are more evident in the older than the younger higher-education student. One might speculate, therefore, that CSD graduate students, whose age range often falls between those of the typical older and younger higher-education study groups, are represented in some but not all facets of this profile.

Findings by Steitz (1985) indicate that older, nontraditional students may respond differently in the classroom, thereby necessitating changes in the instructional approach. This is another factor, then, for the instructor in CSD education to consider—for older students at the graduate level and for all students at the continuing education level. Andragogy applies to them, not pedagogy.

Learning. The proficient teacher is aware of the differences among learners, discerning in students their rates of learning, ways of learning, and responses to learning (Coolican 1988).

Confluent Education

The interdependence of student and environmental variables is directly addressed in the teaching method known as confluent education, which has been defined by Brown (1971) as "the integration of cognitive learning with affective learning" (p. 4). The confluent approach is flexible enough to be adapted to classroom teaching in virtually all fields including health education and CSD education.

Confluence in the educational domain embraces the view that learning is best achieved by integrating the intellectual environment (facts) with feelings (values, decision making) (Read and Greene 1980). By its very nature, then, confluent methodology individualizes learning for classroom students which, as previously mentioned, is an important step.

Affective Component. The affective emphasis calls for sensitivity training in which learners identify their feelings and discover how to deal with them. Opportunities are presented for learners to examine values and attitudes while, at the same time, learners' concerns are given the same respect as are teachers'. The process of coping with these feelings, values, attitudes and concerns is then stressed. Self-actualization, that is, the attainment of "full humanness" is the final goal (Read and Greene 1980, p. 122).

Followers of humanistic education—another term for the affective component in confluent education—create environments that allow questions, answers to questions, openness, and creativity. Integration of intellect and feelings in any classroom is possible, they contend. Acceptance of students as "real, feeling, worthy, responsible, and valuable human beings" (Read and Greene 1980, p. 123) is the foundation of humanistic education.

Application of a humanistic educational approach to professional preparation in any field, including that of health and communication disorders, involves acceptance of students as they are rather than as their instructors might like them to be. By assisting students in defining their strengths, teachers can help them develop stronger self-concepts. Humanistic education further stresses withholding judgment while encouraging individual differences; permitting various life styles and values by encouraging openness in the classroom; and permitting various work styles by promoting creativity and individuality. The humanistic teacher is open to fresh and creative answers to questions and cultivates trust in the classroom by encouraging individuals to trust themselves, as well as each other. The teacher also participates by trusting others and accepting others' trust (Read and Greene 1980).

Cognitive Component. In 1948, the American Psychological Association presented the view that a classification of educational objectives could be beneficial and applicable to education across a wide spectrum. The classification includes three broad categories, or domains, and encompasses a number of objectives. In the cognitive domain, attainment of an objective is accomplished through successive levels that involve such activities as remembering, reasoning, problem solving, concept formation, and creative thinking (Read and Greene 1980). Objectives in this domain pertain to the resolution of an intellectual task in which the basic problem must be determined. The learner must then rearrange or synthesize given material with previously learned concepts or procedures. Cognitive objectives vary from simple recollection to extremely unique and productive ways of blending concepts and materials (Read and Greene 1980).

The Combination. The affective domain, an active expansion of the several subcategories of the cognitive domain, is associated with "values, attitude, feeling, and appreciation objectives" (Read and Greene 1980, p. 51). Because the observable behaviors for this domain are given wide interpretations, the teacher may need to infer whether or not learning has occurred (Eiss and Harbeck 1969).

A student's learning cannot be calculated simply by determining how information is interpreted and utilized; indeed, some behavior cannot be observed and some cannot be explained until the student functions in circumstances outside the college environment. A student can have exposure, however, "to a body of information (cognitive), realize and place its implication within his individual character (affective), and also show that the values inherent in the information can be expressed in actual behavior (action)" (Read and Greene 1980, p. 53).

Steitz (1985) points out that cognitive ability is not a factor of age. In other words, cognitive ability does not decrease with age. However, adults do need reassurance, more time in evaluating circumstances, and increased opportunities to witness the practical applicability of theoretical information. As alluded to earlier, the classroom instructor should be aware of the variations among older students in processing and learning information (Greive 1984); in experience and psychological set; in their ability to recall stored information; and in degree of motivation.

Positive self-image or esteem, a psychological need that is important to the learning process, can be addressed through teaching strategies. Indeed, it is the claim of some learning theorists that motivation (affective) and learning (cognition) result from success itself, thus increasing the learner's esteem and self-image. Greive (1984) offers some suggestions for classroom teachers in helping students experience success and thus build status or esteem: make students aware of expectations by providing them with written course objectives; inform students of what is expected of them in terms of work and time; provide students, whenever possible, with non-verbal encouragement through eye contact and gestures; give students, whenever possible, reinforcement through written comments and notes; create a comfortable but structured situation while inviting student participation; and encourage discussion of outside exeriences and resources. Enabling students to grow or to increase their self-concept or self-image, says Greive (1984), can be achieved by creating a classroom environment that is challenging, especially through problem solving. This can be enhanced by making time available for individual student-instructor conferences and providing opportunities for students to know one another and the teacher; by being cautious not to stereotype students; by recognizing students' wishes to be treated as adults; by considering, when appropriate, students' personal problems and using flexibility in addressing issues; and by giving opportunities for flexibility in the classroom (Greive 1984). These guidelines for building success and the self-concepts of students can be rewarding and exciting for both the teacher and the students.

Socioemotional Factors in the Classroom

That there are a number of socioemotional factors with an impact on classroom teaching and learning is recognized by almost everyone who has experienced the educational process. Several of these factors are examined in this section.

Attitudes.   Students demonstrate variability in their approaches to assignments and the degree of effort they put forth. This variability is often attitude-dependent. As noted by Lowman (1984), some students are dutiful, while others are suspicious and belligerent. Their attitudes vary as much as their approaches.

It is fortunate that, in most situations, students anticipate that teachers will be warm and outgoing, and teachers expect the same of students. The attitudes one advocates are often reciprocal in others (Jones et al. 1972; Altman and Taylor 1973). Classroom instructors need to recognize not only the differences in intellect and motivation among students but also the kinds of emotional interactions in the classroom that heighten motivation and learning.

Psychological research on college-level students indicates that they derive some degree of pleasure from satisfying their intellectual inquisitiveness and from learning. At the same time, they can master challenges, whether in the academic or nonacademic realm, even in the presence of competition. Nonetheless, students need affection and acceptance as learners and as persons, particularly from individuals in authority. They also demonstrate a need for peer acceptance and approval (Lowman 1984).

Not unlike their teachers, students display dissatisfaction with their academic lives. Frustrations arise for different reasons. Students may wish, for example, to establish a personal relationship with their teachers but factors, such as class size and the teacher's inability to call the student by name, are obstacles. Or, if a teacher's organizational skills are so poor that objectives for the course are not stated and students are not informed when assignments are due, student frustration is a frequent result (Lowman 1984).

Another attitude shaper is criticism. For the most part, students can accept criticism when it is given tactfully. Even so, it is more acceptable when specific than general. Good interpersonal rapport between teacher and student increases the chances for criticism to have a constructive rather than destructive consequence (Lowman 1984).

Students' behaviors communicate to the teacher their feelings and expectations as well as attitudes. The implications of students' intentions and feelings are demonstrated through their questions, classroom demeanor, and responses to the teacher. The adept teacher is skilled in interpreting and handling student communication subtleties both inside and outside the classroom.

Classroom Climate. The socioemotional climate in a classroom may not always be what it appears to be. College classes usually begin with anticipation characterized by optimistic and positive attitudes. Even so, underlying fears may be present. Students may be fearful of an authoritarian instructor and of failure to perform well on tests. At the same time, instructors are aware they must meet the needs of yet another new group of students. But, overall, the initial feeling usually is positive on the part of both teacher and students (Lowman 1984).

Developing events can quickly decrease satisfaction and develop anxiety. An examination, for instance, may accelerate student dissatisfaction because the teacher's evaluative role comes into play. This sudden drop in morale may be followed by a more natural period of satisfaction, according to Lowman (1984), in which participation in class discussion and independent thinking become evident.

The conclusion of a course can be emotional for the teacher and students. Students may become more uneasy about exams, grades, and the fact that the course is ending. Teachers may be dissatisfied, too, that they were unable to present the amount of material they had planned and that they did not provide enough assistance for the students to learn the material better. At the same time, concern that the personal relationship between teacher and student, whatever its level, is ending may be a concern. During this period, the teacher and students may need to express the way they feel about each other (Lowman 1984).

Lowman (1984) believes that the emotional needs of the last class meeting should take precedence over presenting a final topic or scheduling an exam. This time should be reserved for the students' emotional and intellectual reflection concerning the end of the semester. It is also an appropriate time to administer course evaluations.

Conflicts are a part of human relationships, and there is no exception in the relationship between teacher and student. Both parties have some degree of responsibility in conflicts; both own the problem, according to Gordon (1974). In his book on teacher effectiveness training, he suggests a problem-solving technique for resolving conflict. The method, a step-by-step procedure based on the problem-solving process advocated by John Dewey, addresses conflicts between individuals or groups. The six separate steps are: (1) defining the problem; (2) generating possible solutions; (3) evaluating the solutions; (4) deciding which solution is best; (5) determining how to implement the decision; and (6) assessing afterwards how well the solution solved the problem (Gordon 1974, p. 228). Joint student-teacher participation in these problem-solving steps expedites conflict resolution.

Classroom Competition

Competition is frequently associated with classroom settings. Usually, competition is related to grades and honors. It can be healthy if moderate, unhealthy if excessive.

Classroom Motivation. Renowned for his extensive research and publications on teaching, Eble (1988) indicates that a primary concern is that of motivating students in the learning process. Eble recommends that the teacher provide an environment in which intrinsic motivation becomes more important than extrinsic motivation. "Among education's highest aspirations is the development of the self-motivating and continuing learner" (Eble 1988, pp. 185–186).

An intrinsic source of motivation is simply performing a task well. Although a student may obtain a high mark on a paper, he/she is motivated even more when given the additional reward of a complimentary (re)mark other than just the letter grade. Such an indication confirms the student's own feeling about the accomplishment and serves as an impetus for repeat performance.

Motivation increases for the student if the teacher is able to gain and hold the student's attention. And motivation rises when students are respected by teachers. Such acts as the teacher's being on time for class and appointments demonstrates respect for students.

Having clear and appealing goals and objectives is another way of promoting motivation, as when an instructor sets achievable goals at specific stages of the semester. For students who experience difficulty in reaching goals, the teacher can offer assistance as students encounter problems. Mutual reinforcement and motivation among students can be promoted through increasing opportunities for cooperation among students.

People can motivate people. One can be inspired to do well simply on the basis of having witnessed someone else perform the same activity well. In a similar way, the teacher can be a source of motivation just by the example he/she sets for students.

Reinforcement in the Classroom. Behavioral techniques can be useful to teachers. Instructors should be aware of the effects of behaviors as reinforcers. Essentially, a reinforcer is "any stimulus or event that follows a response and increases the occurrence of that response in the future" (Cohen and Hearn 1988, p. 45). The most relevant kind of reinforcer for the classroom is positive reinforcement. For example, as indicated in the discussion of motivation, if a teacher writes complimentary comments on a student's paper, the student is likely to try repeating the same performance.

Instructor Expectations

Studying the effects of interpersonal expectation has been a main interest in human communication research. Studies on perception indicate that we frequently attend to and see that which we expect. In Rosenthal's research (1973) on the positive and negative effects of expectation, students whose teachers expected them to do well did well, and students not expected to do well, did not do well. The success of the high-expectation students was related to four teacher provisions: a climate characterized by supportive and emotional warmth; explicit and active feedback; more effort; and more encouragement of student responsiveness.

Expectations can have a significant effect on student-teacher interactions. Teachers need to encourage interactions among students as well as between students and teachers. Student participation on university or college committees and inclusion in deliberations with teachers and administrators are important steps in furthering interpersonal communication. The higher the positive expectations are for a given student, the more likely he/she will be to interact with peers and teachers.

Student Rights

Although students' rights were bigger issues in the 1970s, they still have relevance today. Teachers and administrators should not lose sight of the fact that students do have rights as learners. This is especially important because students must depend on specific faculty members to uphold these rights in the classroom. In his discussion regarding the rights of students in college classrooms, Strickland (1975) offers the following list:

- The student has the right to be recognized as an individual
- The student is entitled to a faculty member interested in teaching
- The student is entitled to instruction based on adequate preparation
- Students have a right to express opinions and to challenge those of the instructor
- Instruction should be individualized
- The student is entitled access to the teacher at hours other than class time
- The student is entitled to know the system by which he is to be graded
- The student has the right to attend or not to attend class
- Students have the right to evaluate their courses and teacher (pp. 81–85)

Strickland (1975) explains that students are at a disadvantage in teacher-student relationships because power is not equitable for the two groups. Thus, it may be helpful to call teachers' attention to a list of rights such as this for use in their classroom teaching.

THE ROLES OF THE INSTRUCTOR IN CLASSROOM TEACHING

Whether teaching at the level of elementary, secondary, postsecondary, or adult education, an instructor has more than one role to assume in carrying out classroom instruction. Several roles considered to be especially important for instructors in higher and continuing education are presented here.

The Expert Role

The most outstanding teachers are regarded as experts. The expert role is perhaps more easily attained than retained. In audiology and speech-language pathology a lag in skill can emerge when an instructor is no longer actively involved with clinical work or research.

There are many other possible ways in which classroom instructors risk losing expertise through interruption or termination of skill application and/or knowledge acquisition. There is the person, for example, who might continue to be active as a clinician or researcher but does not participate in continuing education of any type. Another may participate in clinical education yet fail to apply it. Still others may find that, regardless of their attempts to keep current, through clinical, research, or continuing education, they are no longer specialists. In these times of exponentially increasing skill and knowledge, specialties have become generic, and subspecialties have become specialties. Conversely, an educator who has continued to specialize may no longer be in touch with the broad scope of course content for which he/she is responsible. As these examples illustrate, it is not difficult for the educator's role as expert to come into question.

A conscientious teacher recognizes that material must be presented in a clear and convincing manner and that the teacher must, therefore, be well informed in his/her own area. Class preparation, just to be adequate, requires constant study and continual updating of information. An added bonus for the classroom instructor is that "teachers teach and learn simultaneously—to teach is to learn twice. Teachers' understanding of the information or skill to be taught is increased substantially by having to organize, plan, and present it to someone else" (Douglas, Hosokawa, and Lawler 1988, p. 39).

The Master Clinician/Master Researcher Role

Even though the importance of clinical and research experience was discussed as part of the instructor's expert role, the instructor as master clinician and/or master researcher constitutes a separate and distinct role.

The classroom instructor who is also a master clinician and/or master researcher can model through demonstration in the clinic and laboratory settings, respectively, and in class laboratory sections involving projects associated with these roles. By demonstrating, the instructor provides a bridge between classroom and clinic or laboratory teaching. Such proficiency, modeled and discussed in a teaching-learning context, lends credibility to the instructor's words and evokes respect from students. Moreover, in seeing the instructor as a doer, students may be motivated to emulate this person as a professional. Indeed, the master clinician/master researcher role is not uncommon for those instructors who are also mentors, to be discussed in a later section.

The Facilitator Role

The teacher's role as a learning facilitator is preferred by humanistic theorists over the role of expert (Fuhrmann and Grasha 1983). Indeed, when practiced on a full-time basis, this role is transformed into an entire approach to classroom teaching. As a facilitator, the teacher is both a stimulus and a resource for student-learning. Mann et al. (1970) describe this role as one in which the teacher fosters growth and creativity in the student. Responsiveness to student needs is encouraged as a means of advancing students' self-discovery. Although there may be differences between students' goals and those of the teacher, the primary responsibility of a facilitator is to assist students in recognizing these differences and in developing strategies to achieve their goals (Douglas, Hosokawa, and Lawler 1988).

When a teacher is functioning as a facilitator, interactions in the teacher-student relationship depend upon the teacher's support for the students' learning (Rogers 1983). Students may have choices in class projects and other aspects of the course. The teacher encourages students to make choices, and, at the same time, makes students aware that they are responsible for specific choices. Rogers contends that procedures identified with the facilitator role are effectual in a classroom atmosphere where students feel confident in making choices related to their learning.

Active student involvement in learning is necessary to the success of facilitated learning. Inclusion of discussion groups or journals in this kind of teaching forum also contribute to its effectiveness. Helping people to inquire is a primary responsibility of the teacher-facilitator (DeLay 1971). The teacher provides opportunities for students to use resources, to seek information for themselves, and to form their own ideas concerning content. Demonstrations, research assignments, position papers, and discussion groups led by students are some of the classroom activities recommended. Others include student-teacher contracts and mechanisms for peer teaching, role playing, and student feedback (Fuhrmann and Grasha 1983). Teachers who plan to serve in a facilitator role are advised to spend as little time as possible lecturing so that these other student-involved activities might be pursued.

The (Career) Counselor Role

Classroom instructors in higher education are frequently assigned an advisory role or are sought out by students to serve in this capacity. This is appropriate because such faculty members can provide guidance to students in the planning and implementation of a specific course of study (Ericksen 1984). As both professionals and educators, faculty also have knowledge of specific academic and professional regulations and the manner in which these regulations affect the students' educational progam. According to Judge (1981), an adviser can help students contemplate their reasons for being in school, which is not an inconsequential issue for many preprofessionals. In addition, through individual conferences with students, the adviser can directly dispense honest information and give students the individual interest and attention they may need while attending a large, and often impersonal, institution.

More information on counseling and advising may be found in Chapter 14. It has been mentioned here because of its prominent role in the work of a classroom instructor.

The Mentor Role

In response to students' needs for individual instruction, using mentors became especially popular in the late 1960s and 1970s (Bradley 1981). As conceived then, instructional mentors hardly exist today, but many kinds of significant mentoring relationships do exist. A blending of tutor, exemplar, and counselor, mentor relationships have particular value for both the mentor and the student. Doctoral students, whose educational programs are individualized and whose goals include the completion of a research-based dissertation, are but one example of students who stand to benefit from such a relationship.

Daloz (1986) describes a mentor's function as that of providing support, challenge, and vision (p. 212). Eble (1988) elaborates on Daloz' concept by stating that the mentor must be caring, that he/she must be concerned about the student's achievements and, at the same time, have the desire to be successful in bringing out the best in the student.

In a mentor relationship, the mentor's availability is a necessity.

Listening is important. Support of a student's efforts and interests outside a given course is required. Daloz asserts that, in teacher-student relationships, teaching and learning take place outside the classroom. According to him, students learn as much from the way in which teachers relate to them as they do from what teachers tell them. Mentors also are needed, he relates, as part of continuing adult education, even in such situations as interactive teaching.

Because of teacher diversity, Eble (1988) believes it is difficult for any teacher not to be regarded as a mentor by some students. In seminars and small group discussions as well as tutoring and advising sessions, teachers and students find themselves in situations that nourish mentor relationships. A number of the traits associated with mentors are also identified with effective teachers.

Another use of mentors is associated with relationships between senior and junior faculty. Each can benefit from the other, thus improving their classroom teaching (Weimer 1988a). The more experienced teacher may gain new information and knowledge from a junior colleague, and infuse courses with new ideas. In a similar way, the junior associate can benefit from the teaching expertise of an older colleague.

THE CLASSROOM INSTRUCTOR AS A PERSON

To be a positive force in the classroom and assist students in learning more about themselves, a teacher should make a practice of learning students' names, being courteous to students, being available to students, giving individual attention to students, and noticing matters that are personally important to students. Although these actions clearly deal with students on a personal level, they do affect the students' environment and, therefore, become important in a classroom learning situation (Purkey 1970).

Carl Rogers (1969) maintains that these teacher qualities faciliate the learning process: genuineness; awareness of one's own feelings; avoidance of role playing; awareness of the expectations a teacher has for him/herself and others have for him/her; valuing the learner and his/her feelings; having concern for the learner; trusting the person; having empathy; and having the capability of placing one's self in the learner's situation. Acceptance of certain feelings in one's self is necessary if one is to be responsive to students' feelings (Read and Greene 1980). Also important is the students' recognition of the value of relieving tension through sharing concerns with the teacher. It is a mutual building of trust on the part of both individuals.

Students' awareness of a teacher's knowledge about a particular subject is a source of gratification to many teachers. Being in charge of the classroom is pleasurable to other teachers, while some enjoy serving in the capacity of recruiter and guide to students who are interested in entering a teacher's specific field. Formation of personal relationships with students as a group gives satisfaction to other teachers (Lowman 1984). Teachers may elect to share information regarding their careers or interests. Such disclosures may make teachers more human in the eyes of students. In other situations, teachers may encourage supportive relationships, some of which may endure, with individual students.

Students appear to remember teachers who have had genuine respect for them in their learning. The building of positive self-images in students is facilitated by teachers who listen to students and encourage them to express their feelings. This building process is helpful also to the students' development of decision-making. The teacher uses humanness in the classroom to assist students in evolving their value systems of self and environment.

The Effect of Personal Values on Classroom Teaching

Rollins (1988) points out that teaching has been devalued by teachers themselves. According to him, teachers have discouraged evaluations of themselves and have not sought the helpfulness of colleagues and peers. More emphasis has been given to publications than to teaching, and teachers' approaches to teaching have been complicated by personal and private motives. Rollins maintains that teachers put too much responsibility on learners to learn and have no regard for the manner in which material is presented. Moreover, he says, teachers do have a responsibility for students' learning, and their teaching is pointless if learning does not take place (pp. 12–14). In essence, Rollins is questioning the priority of teachers' personal values in their work.

Some teachers feel that their only obligation is to teach their specific classes and not become involved with their students' value systems (Gordon 1974). However, some conflicts over values cannot be ignored and, indeed, must be addressed. Of the various approaches available to resolve conflicts between teachers and students, many incorporate teacher modeling as the key element. In order to use this method, it is necessary for the teacher to maintain a good relationship with the student. Davis (1978) maintains that teachers devote little time to assessing values that are important to the teacher-student relationship. The teacher can look at his/her own value system, recalling values adopted from others, and, at the same time, be cognizant of whether anyone may have modeled the teacher by adopting these same values. Such an approach requires flexibility on the teacher's part because of the possible need to change some behaviors that are more acceptable as models for students (Gordon 1974).

Another effect of personal values on college teaching can be seen in the teacher's commitment to the classroom versus commitments to other areas, such as conducting research, serving on committees, publishing papers and books, and keeping abreast of the field (Kozma, Belle, and Williams 1978). Although a teacher may be able to manage the time element of these commitments relatively well, there is always a time during which teaching must become the primary focus. On a personal level, the teacher wants to be recognized by students and associates as an outstanding teacher. Whether one is teaching for the first time or renewing enthusiasm for teaching, questions must be confronted daily regarding personal feelings about one's teaching approach, the ability of students to learn from this teaching, and problems related to individual students in the learning process.

Motivation is of primary importance in the teacher's personal value system. The teacher must be motivated to believe in him/herself and in what he/she is doing (Eble 1988). The love of teaching itself can be a motivation derived from the students, from commitment to a specific area of interest, and from identification with an institution.

The Effect of Personal Characteristics on Classroom Teaching

Like values, an instructor's individuality influences what happens in the classroom. Such factors as personality, gender, and social background help to shape personal values and thereby affect classroom teaching. Several others are discussed briefly below.

Instructor Expectations. Teachers' expectations range from having little confidence in students' intellectual ability and commitment to being overzealous in the belief that the students possess capability, motivation, and enthusiasm for the teacher's particular course (Lowman 1984). As suggested before, teachers' expectations of students are often fulfilled, that is, low expectations are met by low student performance and high expectations by high student performance. Inasmuch as expectations are not a direct cause of outcomes, the link appears to be the teacher who teaches according to his/her expectations. And students then respond to the teaching.

Instructors' Teaching/Clinical/Research Experience. An instructor's clinical and research experience, when related to course content, is very important to effective teaching. So, too, is teaching experience, although there is no hard evidence to support the notion that experienced teachers are better than inexperienced ones, or vice-versa.

Personal Constraints Within the Classroom Instructor. Resistance to change in teaching methods is common to all teachers. Personal opinions and behaviors can constrain a teacher's ability and interest in investigating new possibilities. It is not unusual for individuals to blame external entities for their own problems (Kelley 1971; Nisbett and Valins 1971; Jones 1976). A teacher may attribute lack of student involvement to the students, the classroom logistics, the time the class is scheduled, and other such factors rather than look at his/her own personal responsibility in the matter. Personal factors and the situation itself may be the source of the problem. Ellis (1973a, 1973b) contends that people's actions can be affected strongly by what they say to themselves. Their skill in adapting or not adapting to situations can be influenced by their self-concepts. In addition, one can have irrational beliefs that control behavior. Such thoughts or beliefs are represented by illogical or expanded thoughts which then are reflected in words like "all, every, always, awful, terrible, horrible, totally, and essential" (Fuhrmann and Grasha 1983, p. 138). In Ellis' system, there are words that are indicative of no alternatives (e.g., "must, should, have to, need and ought" (Fuhrmann and Grasha 1983, p. 138). Such words can direct actions and keep people from seeing choices in a situation.

Irrational beliefs of this nature can prevent teachers' investigation of new ideas for teaching and, in turn, affect student involvement. These beliefs influence the ability to change behaviors. It is easier to continue with old behaviors. Students and colleagues may be affected, and, in particular, students may become passive. In order to surmount irrational beliefs, especially the opinion that nothing can be done to improve teaching, an instructor must first recognize and then seek ways to overcome them, possibly with the help of a colleague or instructional consultant.

Another approach to breaking personal constraints and improving teaching methods is to heed feedback from students and associates. However, one must be open and exercise a willingness to explore its application to classroom problems (Argyris 1976).

SUMMARY

The dynamics of classroom teaching, which are varied and complex, reflect the physical and psychological environment. The type and direction of communication between an instructor and students and among the students is a contributing factor, as is the clarity of instruction itself. A classroom instructor should create a climate that is conducive to students' involvement in their own learning. Competition and motivation influence attitudes and expectations, all of which are important in the classroom teaching-learning process. The roles and personal values of an instructor also influence classroom events.

REFERENCES

Altman, I., and Taylor, D. A. 1973. *Social Penetration: The Development of Interpersonal Relationships*. New York: Holt, Rinehart & Winston.

Anderson, R. 1979. *Students as Real People*. Rochelle Park, NY: Hayden Book Company, Inc.

Argyris, C. 1976. Theories of action that inhibit individual learning. *American Psychologist* 31:636–54.

Boyer, R. K., and Bolton, C. 1971. One and two way communication in the classroom. *Faculty Resource Center Monograph Series*. Cincinnati: University of Cincinnati.

Bradley, A. P., Jr. 1981. Mentors in individual education. *Improving College and University Teaching* 29(3):136–40.

Brophy, J., and Good, T. L. 1986. Teacher behavior and student achievement. In *Handbook of Research on Teaching* (3rd ed.), ed. M. C. Wittrock. New York: Macmillan Publishing Company.

Brown, G. I. 1971. *Human Teaching for Human Learning: An Introduction to Confluent Education*. New York: Viking Press.

Burrill, D., and Ryan, J. 1983. Student motivation. In *Teaching in College: A Resource for Adjunct and Part-Time Faculty*, ed. D. Greive. Cleveland: Info-Tec, Inc.

Cattell, R. B., Eber, H. W., and Tatsuoks, M. M. 1970. *Handbook for the Sixteen Personality Factor Questionnaire*. Champaign, IL: Institute for Personality and Ability Testing.

Cheydleur, F. D. 1945. Criteria of effective teaching in basic French courses. *Bulletin of the University of Wisconsin* August.

Cohen, S. B., and Hearn, D. 1988. Reinforcement. In *Guide to Classroom Teaching*, ed. R. McNergney. Boston: Allyn & Bacon, Inc.

Coolican, J. 1988. Individual differences. In *Guide to Classroom Teaching*, ed. R. McNergney. Boston: Allyn & Bacon, Inc.

Cropley, A. 1967. *Creativity*. London: Longmans, Green.

Daloz, L. A. 1986. *Effective Teaching and Mentoring*. San Francisco: Jossey-Bass.

Davis, J. W. 1978. Must teachers love their students? The value structure of the teacher-student relationship. *Teaching-Learning Issues* 36:1–16.

DeLay, D. 1971. Preliminaries of a learning theory. In *Tough and Tender Learning*, ed. D. Nyberg. Palo Alto, CA: National Press Books.

Douglas, K. C., Hosokawa, M. C., and Lawler, F. H. 1988. *A Practical Guide to Clinical Teaching in Medicine*. New York: Springer Publishing Company.

Eble, K. E. 1988. *The Craft of Teaching* (2nd ed). San Francisco: Jossey-Bass.

Eiss, A. F., and Harbeck, M. 1969. *Behavioral Objectives in the Affective Domain*. Washington, DC: National Science Teachers Association.

Ellis, A. 1973a. *Humanistic Psychotherapy: The Rational-Emotive Approach*. New York: Julian Press.

Ellis, A. 1973b. Rational-emotive therapy. In *Current Psychotherapies*, ed. R. Corsini. Itasca, IL: Peacock.

Ericksen, S. C. (1984). *The Essence of Good Teaching*. San Francisco: Jossey-Bass.

Flocken, J. M. 1980. Personality characteristics of communicative disorders graduate students. *Asha* 22:7–16.

Fuhrmann, B. S., and Grasha, A. F. 1983. *A Practical Handbook for College Teachers*. Boston: Little, Brown and Company.

Gordon, T. 1974. *T. E. T.: Teacher Effectiveness Training*. New York: Peter H. Wyden, Publisher.

Greive, D. 1984. *A Handbook for Adjunct and Part-Time Faculty*. Cleveland: Info-Tec, Inc.

Jones, E. E. 1976. How do people perceive the causes of behavior? *American Scientist* 64:300–305.

Jones, E. E., Kanouse, D. E., Kelley, H. H., Nesbitt, R. E., Valins, S., and Weiner, B. 1972. *Attribution: Perceiving the Causes of Behavior*. Morristown, NJ: General Learning Press.

Judge, C. A. 1981. The academic counseling office of the college of literature, science, and the arts. *Memo to the Faculty*, No. 69. Ann Arbor, MI: Center for Research on Learning and Teaching, University of Michigan.

Kelley, H. H. 1971. *Attribution in Social Interaction*. Morristown, NJ: General Learning Press.

Kozma, R. B., Belle, L. W., and Williams, G. W. 1978. *Instructional Techniques in Higher Education*. Englewood Cliffs, NJ: Educational Technology Publications, Inc.

Leavitt, H. J. 1951. Some effects of certain communication patterns on group performance. *Journal of Abnormal and Social Psychology* 46:38–50.

Lowman, J. 1984. *Mastering the Techniques of Teaching*. San Francisco: Jossey-Bass.

Macomber, F. G., and Siegel, L. 1957. A study of large-group teaching procedures. *Educational Research* 38:220–29.

Macomber, F. G., and Siegel, L. 1960. Experimental study in instructional procedures. *Final Report*. Oxford, OH: Miami University.

Mann, R. D., Arnold, S. M., Binder, J. L., Cytrynbaum, S., Newman, B. M., Ringwald, B. E., Ringwald, J. W., and Rosenwein, R. 1970. *The College Classroom: Conflict, Change, and Learning*. New York: John Wiley & Sons.

Nisbett, R. E., and Valins. S. 1971. *Perceiving the Causes of One's Own Behavior*. Morristown, NJ: General Learning Press.

Pagliocca, P. 1988. Clarity of structure. In *Guide to Classroom Teaching*, ed. R. McNergney. Boston: Allyn & Bacon, Inc.

Purkey, W. W. 1970. *Self Concept and School Achievement*. Englewood Cliffs, NJ: Prentice-Hall.

Read, D. A., and Greene, W. H. 1980. *Creative Teaching in Health*. (3rd ed.). New York: Macmillan Publishing Company.

Rogers, C. R. 1969. *Freedom to Learn*. Columbus, OH: Merrill Publishing Company.

Rogers, C. R. 1983. *Freedom to Learn for the 80s*. Columbus, OH: Merrill Publishing Company.

Rollins, A. B., Jr. 1988. The joys of teaching. *VCU Teaching* 1(1):13–14.

Rosenthal, R. 1973. The Pygmalion effect lives. *Psychology Today* 7(4):56–63.

Siegel, L., Adams, J. F., and Macomber, F. G. 1960. Retention of subject matter as a function of large-group instructional procedures. *Journal of Educational Psychology* 51:9–13.

Sommer, R. 1969. *Personal Space*. Englewood Cliffs, NJ: Prentice-Hall.

Steele, F. I. 1973. *Physical Settings and Organization Development*. Reading, MA: Addison-Wesley.

Steitz, J. A. 1985. Issues of adult development within the academic environment. *Lifelong Learning: An Omnibus of Practice and Research* 8:15–18, 27.

Strickland, C. G. 1975. Students' rights and the teacher's obligations in the classroom. In *Excellence in University Teaching: New Essays*, eds. T. H. Buxton and K. W. Prichard. Columbia, SC: University of South Carolina Press.

Taylor, C. (ed.). 1964. *Creativity: Progress and Potential*. New York: McGraw Hill Book Company.

Torrance, E. 1962. Developing creative thinking through school experiences. In *A Sourcebook for Creative Thinking*, eds. S. J. Parnes and H. F. Harding. New York: Charles Scribner's Sons.

Weimer, M. (ed.). 1988a. Mentors value mentoring. *Teaching Professor* 2(7):6.

Weimer, M. (ed.). 1988b. Organization: Communicating the structure. *Teaching Professor* 2(9):1–2.

Weimer, M. (ed.). 1988c. Ways and means of communicating structure. *Teaching Professor* 2(9):3.

Chapter 6

Education in the Research Laboratory

Cynthia G. Fowler and Richard H. Wilson

Research must be an integral part of professional education because every professional is required to conduct and/or use research throughout his/her career. Research, which is the application of the scientific method for observing and evaluating changes, is equally relevant for the clinician and for the investigator. The clinician uses research in assessing the validity and applicability of new diagnostic and treatment strategies described in the literature. The clinician also uses research methods during diagnosis and treatment for an individual client/patient (Perkins 1985). The investigator uses research in evaluating current knowledge in a given area, then produces research that attempts to answer innovative questions. Clinicians and investigators both must determine the aspects of research that are valid and applicable to the problems encountered in the clinic or laboratory. Nevertheless, the role of research is not fully appreciated by all members of clinical professions. Minifie (1983) reported that most speech, language, and audiology clinicians are disenchanted with the lack of clinical application of the research in their fields. Students, intent on learning clinical techniques, often regard research as irrelevant.

Applications of the scientific method are similar for the investigator and for the clinician. The steps in the scientific method include (1) observation, (2) the statement of the problem or question, (3) formulation of the hypothesis or tentative solution, (4) experimentation including data collection and analysis, and (5) derivation of conclusions and formulation of generalizations (Monte 1975). The problem may be clinical or research in nature. In clinical diagnostic sessions, the original problem is defined by the patient or referral source, but the clinician must formulate an hypothesis for the diagnosis based on observations and case history. Experimentation involves the selection and administration of appropriate tests from which data are collected and analyzed. Conclusions consist of the final diagnosis and disposition of the patient. In rehabilitative sessions, this process is repeated and the conclusions serve as a guide to continue, modify, or terminate therapy. In research, the problem arises from creative insight or from observations made from previous studies, from literature reviews, or from clinical situations. The hypothesis is derived from a review of relevant information on the topic.

The primary differences between research and clinical applications of the scientific method are the use of controls and the generalization of findings. The goal of clinical procedures, heterogeneous populations, and time constraints make the use of controls less practical in clinical situations. As a result, findings are limited to the individual patient and cannot be generalized to all patients. Identification and control of intervening variables in research protocols allow generalization of findings and consequently formulation of a theory.

Clinical fields are increasing their emphasis on the role of science and research in preparing professional clinicians whose knowledge will not become outdated. Medical institutions are increasing the research component of education to prepare medical practitioners to read and evaluate the literature critically in the interest of keeping their knowledge current (Springer and Baer 1988). Psychology and optometry, professional institutions dedicated to training practitioners, require courses in statistics and research design as well as completion of a research project (Peterson 1985).

Fleming (1980) delineated levels of research that should be taught at the baccalaureate, master's, and doctoral levels. These components are relevant to the study of communication disorders. At the baccalaureate level, students should appreciate the role of research, the steps in the scientific method, critical thinking, and research ethics. Historically, the typical audiology or speech-language pathology graduate student obtained an undergraduate major in communication disorders. With the recent technological explosion and expanded scopes of practices, many graduate programs now prefer students with undergraduate science majors that provide backgrounds in physics, mathematics, chemistry, or engineering.

At the master's level, students should be able to identify research problems within their field of interest, design a simple study, and critically evaluate research literature. Designing a study includes defining the problem, reviewing the literature, formulating appropriate methods, gathering data, analyzing the data, interpreting the results, and forming conclusions and clinical applications. Classes in research methods should include teaching research design, types of variables, sampling techniques, sources of errors, and statistics. A thesis is appropriate at this level, even if it constitutes replication of a study (Fleming 1980).

The doctoral level has always been research oriented. Although areas of concentration are individualized within a field, certain basic concepts and skills must be taught. Physiological and psychophysical bases for theories in communication sciences must be understood. A solid foundation in research tools, including advanced research design, computers, and statistics is essential. Students must be prepared to ask important questions, to test theories, and to challenge the status quo. Scientific writing skills and grantsmanship should be taught at the doctoral level (Fleming 1980). These skills cannot be developed out of a void; the basics and the orientation to science and research must be developed long before students enter the doctoral program. Clinical training and experience gained before entering the doctoral program help students to define their areas of research interest and solidify the theoretical knowledge gained at the master's level (Ludlow 1986).

TYPES OF RESEARCH LABORATORIES IN
AUDIOLOGY AND SPEECH PATHOLOGY EDUCATIONAL PROGRAMS

With the advent of computers, the differences between audiology and speech pathology laboratories have decreased. Analog equipment is generally dedicated to a specific purpose, thereby customizing laboratories both across and within specialities. Many of the functions of analog equipment have been replaced by sophisticated, inexpensive, high-speed personal computers. Now, integration of auditory and speech laboratories has resulted in more similarities than differences in instrumentation used in psychoacoustic, physiologic, and speech science laboratories.

Specialized requirements for each laboratory remain. Speech physiology laboratories require air flow gauges and radiographic equipment. Language laboratories require extensive video equipment to record and analyze data. Animal physiology laboratories require electrodes, monitoring devices, and histological equipment. Middle-ear laboratories require acoustic immittance devices.

The research function of these laboratories varies with the interests of the investigator who establishes the laboratory. Efficiency in research is achieved by an investigator who develops a cohesive line of research and maintains current knowledge of advances in computer technology. Flexibility in the laboratory is achieved easily with computer-based laboratories because modifications in software may be all that are required to set up a new study.

A relatively new concept advanced by funding agencies is the establishment of research centers that concentrate in a particular area. These are Centers of Excellence, established by the National Institutes of Health and by the Veterans Health Services and Research Administration (VA), and Science and Technology Centers, established by the National Science Foundation. The purpose of these centers is to enhance collaboration among researchers with similar interests and to encourage transfer of scientific advances to the public sector. The primary objection to these centers is that concentration of funding in relatively few centers might divert funds from individual investigators; but officials from funding agencies say that the commitment to individual researchers will continue, and that the total amount of the budget dedicated to the centers is less than 10%. The centers, however, are still in the process of development and long-term effects cannot be assessed at the present time.

It is difficult for students to use faculty laboratories because the faculty may be protective of the laboratories they have carefully established. Yet, in learning to conduct research, master's students must become familiar with all the equipment necessary to complete their projects. Doctoral students, who intend to pursue a career that includes research, must become familiar with the types of equipment they are likely to use in the future. Students, therefore, are obligated to learn safety precautions, to be aware of other projects in the laboratory, and to report immediately any equipment malfunction or alteration they cannot restore to its original condition.

THE RESEARCH LABORATORY AS A LEARNING ENVIRONMENT

Architecture of Instructional Space

Different types of laboratories require different architectural considerations. All laboratories require basic electrical, electronic, and wet facilities; secure storage space; and, as appropriate, sound-treated booths for sound isolation. Electrical circuits should be sufficient to permit multiple locations of equipment within the research space. For laboratories with mainframe computer facilities located off-site, provisions must be made for appropriate interfaces via hardwired or telephone communications. All laboratories minimally should have sink facilities with more elaborate wet facilities incorporated into physiologic laboratories. Laboratories that use chemicals require special hooded areas to eliminate fumes and a management plan for disposal of chemical wastes.

Laboratory Organization

Ideally, each audiology or speech-language project will have research laboratories available that are devoted to specific projects. Each project/laboratory unit should be under the administrative control and responsibility of the principal investigator of the project with the daily functioning of the laboratory delegated to a research assistant. In an academic environment, several additional research laboratories should be available for use by graduate students and faculty who are initiating pilot projects. In multiple purpose/use laboratories, various investigators must respect projects that are being conducted concurrently.

Laboratory Instrumentation

Instrumentation for auditory and speech-language laboratories basically revolves around computers, either the Apple Macintosh or the IBM compatible 386-based (and now 486) computer system. Computers provide speed and accuracy in the conduct of research. In general, computers are used for one or a combination of the following activities in a laboratory:

- generation and control of stimulus delivery,
- recording and storing of data,
- analysis and output of data.

In the generation of stimuli, computers are used to calculate an array of pure-tone and complex-waveform signals. Special programs are capable of generating speech signals and of controlling precisely the various parameters of a signal (e.g., duration, onset, offset, filtering, and waveform shaping). Computer-output signals, which are stored in digital form, pass through a digital-to-analog converter that changes the digital values of a waveform into corresponding voltages. While generating and transmitting a signal, computers can record psychological responses (e.g., button pushing) or physiological responses (e.g., voltage sampling) to the signals. The computer can then store and analyze the data and provide a visual representation of the data on a monitor, plotter, or printer. Although many computer functions require specialized programming, the research laboratory should have database, spreadsheet, statistical analysis, and word processing programs available for the computer.

In addition to the computer nucleus of a laboratory, other types of task-specific instruments are required in the auditory and/or speech laboratory. Electronic filters, mixers, and earphones/loudspeakers are used to shape, combine, and transduce signals. Amplifiers are used with both input (signals) and output (physiologic and electrophysiologic) functions. A variety of instruments is used to analyze signals including spectrum analyzers, counters, oscilloscopes, and multimeters. Stimuli and data are recorded on a variety of analog and digital tape recorders and compact discs. Video mixers and editors are intricate components in the language laboratory. Finally, laboratories require an assortment of tools, wire, and connectors.

Laboratory Research Subjects

One of the most sensitive issues in the laboratory is the guarantee of the rights of subjects. Ethically, every human study, funded or not, should include a subject permission form guaranteeing the rights of the subjects. These should include the subject's right to be informed of any benefits or risks involved with his/her participation and the right to withdraw at any time without penalty. A description of the methods should be explained in lay terms. Further, subjects should be guaranteed the rights of privacy and confidentiality by which their identities are not revealed; unnecessary information is not requested; and individual data are not released to unauthorized sources.

Animal subjects are guaranteed the right to humane treatment, and studies must be carefully structured to avoid waste (unnecessary killing of animals). All academic institutions and funding agencies, through the use of human and animal subjects committees, require a guarantee that the rights of all subjects will be preserved. Journals generally insist on a statement in the methods section of an article that an informed consent was obtained from human subjects or that an animal subjects committee has approved the procedure.

Instructional Considerations in the Laboratory

Laboratory demonstrations can illustrate concepts and phenomena that have been discussed in the classroom and can bridge the gap between learning about research and conducting research. Demonstrations can begin with simple examples of psychoacoustic phenomena, such as those provided on compact disc from the Acoustical Society of America, or on commercially available interactive videotapes about laboratory instruments and techniques. Once students are familiar with the phenomena and equipment, the laboratory can be set up to allow students to elicit these phenomena from their fellow students. Finally, physiological experiments can be performed to illustrate animal preparation, data recording, and electrophysiological phenomena that cannot be demonstrated through other means.

Different attitudes, expectations, and backgrounds that students bring to the laboratory can challenge instructors. Instructors must be sensitive to the fears and beliefs of students in the laboratory, especially in the case of animal experiments. The objectives of all demonstrations must be clear to the instructor and must be conveyed to the students. Ethical considerations, subject rights, and safety precautions should be explained along with the techniques and phenomena that are being demonstrated.

Laboratory documentation can be explained during demonstrations, given the necessity for students to use documentation when they begin their research projects. Records must be organized in a concise, efficient manner so that information is readily available. Although the details kept will vary with the type of study, generally valuable data on the subjects include the name or number, age, sex, physical condition, and medical history. Procedural details include the experimental variables, order of stimulus presentation, and details, results, and dates of equipment calibration. In a physiological study, the type and amount of anesthesia, and the time period for recording data are important. In a behavioral study, the listening experience of the subject and results of any qualifying tests are important. If these details are not carefully maintained, unanswerable questions will arise during data analysis, and lack of information may invalidate the study (Lipscomb 1974).

INVOLVEMENT OF STUDENTS IN THE LABORATORY

Student Attitudes Toward the Laboratory

Clinical application of research is a key strategy in fostering good research attitudes in students. The common practice of dividing audiology and speech-language pathology programs into academic portions taught by doctoral level, research-oriented personnel and clinical portions taught by master's level, clinically oriented personnel can only serve to dichotomize the roles and emphasize the separateness of clinic and research. Integration of clinical and research portions of the program can be accomplished by faculty appointments for clinical staff, joint meetings between clinic and academic staff to coordinate lessons taught at both sites, and participation of the academic staff in the clinic (Fowler and Wilson 1989). Both clinical and academic faculty must be seen as having the same ultimate goals of improving clinical skills through research and assimilation of new methods.

Several strategies can be used to improve attitudes of students toward research. These strategies include modeling, consistency, clinical application, and written assignments (Spector and Bleeks 1980). Role modeling requires involvement of the instructor, as a researcher as well as a professor and clinician, who integrates personal research or clinic material into the class. The use of the professor's own research makes research less foreign and mysterious to the student. If students see research used regularly to answer clinical questions, they will accept research as part of the ongoing clinical process.

The final strategy for improving student attitudes toward research involves written exercises. At the undergraduate or early graduate level, students can write research papers on topics of personal interest. This exercise requires that students criticize relevant literature, evaluating both strengths and weaknesses of the articles they review. Their papers should conclude with proposals for new studies, including research questions and methods, to address inadequacies in the literature. This approach allows students to use their imaginations fully to consider all aspects of a question without becoming frustrated by the realities of data collection.

For the next written exercise, master's students can complete a project or thesis, the complexity of which will vary according to each student's level of interest and career goals. The clinically oriented student can complete a project with a clinical focus, or can replicate a study. The research-oriented student can develop a more complex study that will challenge emerging research skills. The object in either case is for the student to complete a project to learn the mechanisms of research and to appreciate the difficulties involved. Having gone through the process, students will be better qualified to evaluate other studies or to pursue the next project.

Student Participation in Laboratory Learning

Projects at the undergraduate or early graduate level may be appropriately assigned to teams. The advantage to teamwork is that students can discuss with their peers different ways of approaching an issue and different methods of solving a problem. The team approach can give students support and reduce the frustration that occurs when they are confused by the progression of the experiment. Discussions among team members can bring out aspects of the problem that individuals may not have considered. Further, teamwork fosters a spirit of cooperation that makes research enjoyable. The disadvantage to team learning, of course, is that all students may not contribute equally to the project.

Following completion of a team project, each student should be assigned an individual project. Individual responsibility for a project assures that a student has experience with the entire research process. Individually, a student can explore different ideas about the topic, design, and direction of a study. The student who has complete responsibility for a project, with enough guidance to assure its successful completion, will take pride in that accomplishment. The primary disadvantage in assignment of individual projects is the amount of faculty time required for adequate supervision of all the students.

THE LABORATORY INSTRUCTOR

Roles of Researchers/Instructors

Researchers/instructors have many roles in the educational process, depending on the student's status and the relationship between the student and the researcher/instructor. At the first level, researchers must be experts in the field. To continue productive lines of research, investigators must be experts not only in the narrow aspect of the field under investigation but also in the field at large and in related fields. Only in that way can investigators develop new ideas and relate new findings to existing knowledge. The challenge to remain current applies to both research and teaching. Experts as instructors can provide students with the latest information and can provide insight into current thought.

Related to the role of instructor as expert is the role of established investigator. Recognition of an individual as an established investigator depends on that person's history of published research in peer-reviewed journals and acquisition of extra-mural funding, which requires outside reviews and competition for funding. An established investigator, therefore, has earned credibility within the field and has demonstrated an understanding of the mechanics of research. Whereas active participation in research is a necessary prerequisite for teaching research, research skills do not guarantee teaching skills.

Facilitators pave the way for research to be performed in the laboratory, and function on many levels. For students, facilitators must help to define projects and to avoid many of the pitfalls that may prevent the research from being completed. (A booklet, published by, and available from, the Council of Graduate Schools [1990], provides supervisors of research students with specific strategies to ensure that progress is being made.) Responsibilities include assuring that equipment can perform necessary functions, that equipment is functional, that the appropriate number and types of subjects are available, and that the research question is answerable.

The role of a researcher as a facilitator is not only relevant for students but also for junior faculty members. Professors with established research records have a responsibility to encourage research productivity in their younger colleagues. Assistant and associate professors can ally themselves with proven investigators to learn new research skills through collaboration. Additionally, collaboration allows junior investigators with meager laboratories to use equipment and expertise of better equipped full professors (Waller et al. 1988).

The roles of graduate schools and of individual mentors in the initial stages of a student's research career are vital. A graduate program orients students to the field, instills attitudes about professional issues, transmits expectations, and develops technical skills necessary for students to enter the profession (Creswell 1985). A prominent part of this process is the provision of mentors. Mentors typically serve as teachers, collaborators, role models, and links to other researchers in the field while students are in school. In other words, mentors provide students with knowledge and contacts that launch students' careers. Doctoral programs influence graduates' research productivity for the first six to ten years following graduation, whereas the effect of mentors lasts only about three years. Both effects gradually yield to influences of first jobs (Long 1978; Reskin 1979); but the type and setting of first jobs are typically indirectly influenced by mentors. Attitudes and values of colleagues at first jobs then exert a direct influence on the career of new investigators. Gradually, new professionals must assume responsibility for following the literature, developing independent lines of research, and acquiring research funding.

Priorities of Researchers/Instructors

The premier criterion for promotion in most academic institutions is research productivity, with teaching, clinical work, and university service distinctly secondary. Promotion from the assistant level to associate or full professor level is largely based on the number and quality of publications a faculty member has accrued. Promotion means a higher salary as well as recognition that the faculty member is contributing to the objectives of the university. Further, higher academic standings provide eligibility for administrative positions within the university (Tuckman 1976). The highest research productivity, however, generally comes from scientists who spend about one-third of their time on research, with the remainder divided among teaching, service, and administration depending on the demands of the position (Creswell 1985). Theoretically, a conflict of interest should not occur between research and teaching. The exception is that demands on a new faculty member, who must develop new courses, advise students, and provide university service, may delay establishment of a laboratory. If faculty members do not begin publishing within the first five years after graduation, then the likelihood of publishing later is greatly diminished (Creswell 1985).

Allied health professionals may not be as productive as those in other disciplines due to poor research training and basic clinical orientation. A questionnaire on the needs of allied health professionals (Waller et al. 1988) indicated that the primary skill requirements for faculty were further training in statistics and the mechanics of publishing a paper. Regardless of academic degree, the majority of respondents indicated a need for more knowledge about how to obtain funding. In an era of reduced research budgets and tighter controls over funding, this skill is among the top priorities of universities in hiring and retaining faculty. Half of the survey respondents at the bachelor's or master's levels needed further information on research design and writing a proposal. Non-tenure track individuals expressed a strong need for research skills, suggesting that people who chose a career without the intention of doing research found themselves unprepared for a position in which they either wanted to or were required to do research.

Waller and his colleagues (1988) also found that faculty from major research institutions perceived themselves as possessing fewer research gaps than did those from other types of universities, suggesting that individuals in research-oriented environments have a history of successful research experience. As individuals who have been actively involved in research, they have maintained the research skills they were taught or have developed these skills through their work. Regardless of the type of university setting, the primary need reported by respondents was information on funding mechanisms. The perceived weakness in this area may be attributed to a lack of guidance plus increasing pressures to obtain funding in the face of cuts in the budgets of funding agencies. Individuals from major research institutions also cited deficient skills in developing research designs, and individuals from other institutions cited deficient skills in submitting papers for publication. The latter insecurity involves weaknesses in a number of areas, including research design, data analysis, and writing skills, as well as a knowledge of the editorial process (Waller et al. 1988).

As allied health professionals increasingly move into academic roles, the need for research skills becomes more and more critical. Obtaining a doctoral degree would alleviate some of the needs cited by non-doctoral personnel. Additionally, universities must sponsor faculty development in research methods, encourage collaborative interaction, sabbaticals, and continuing education, and enhance the research environment through administrative support and commitment.

Laboratory Instructor as a Person

The effectiveness of instructors depends on many factors, including personality, satisfaction from teaching, and the work environment (Morton 1964). Instructors must enjoy working with students and derive benefits from working with them. Instructors must be patient in explaining concepts several times and must avoid a tone of arrogance, which will suppress questions, engender hostility, and preclude learning. Instructors who feel that time spent with students is time away from research will not be effective. A negative attitude will show; instructors will be poor role models and students will reject what is being taught.

Several personal attributes are characteristic of instructors who are successful in encouraging their students to pursue scientific careers. These professors are assertive and hold high standards for their students. These professors have broad interests, participate in administration, and relish teaching. Finally, they are respected for their research productivity (Knapp 1963). These characteristics describe professors who value research and teaching and are happy with their career choices; they attract students naturally and serve as positive role models.

A good work environment is essential to ensuring positive attitudes and research productivity of the faculty, recruitment of new faculty, and retention of existing faculty. The environmental factors investigators report as conducive to research include academic and personal freedom, opportunities for continuing education, job security, and intellectual challenges. Detrimental factors include budget instabilities; time conflicts for research, administration, and teaching; lack of money for students; lack of involvement in planning in the scientific program; poor facilities; and low salary (Taylor, Smith, and Ghiselin 1963). Some of these factors are under the control of the administration; the administration can guarantee freedoms, provide release time for productive faculty, give support and encouragement for research grants, promote the faculty, and support faculty raises and promotions. Budgetary constraints may be shared by the faculty and the administration; faculty generally are expected to procure grants to support their research and student research assistants, whereas the administration must make the environment conducive to procuring grants and completing research, and must bridge occasional gaps in research funding. Faculty, in turn, must apply for grants, produce and publish research that brings recognition to the faculty and the university, and that attracts students.

If the goal is to graduate research-oriented scholars, then instructors have only limited influence on the eventual research productivity of their students. The University of Chicago reported that only 30% of its doctoral graduates were still conducting research eight years after graduation. As students, productive graduates exhibited drive, intellectual curiosity, a measure of independence, and ability to analyze a problem and organize a research plan. Productive students had research ideas when they began graduate school and understood clearly what a research career entailed (Bloom 1964). The teaching of research skills and current knowledge in the field is all that is needed by motivated, directed, and research-oriented students.

As students, non-productive graduates did not engage in any other research projects besides their dissertation, which they generally regarded as a major hurdle. These students entered graduate school with only a vague idea of what a research career entailed and generally had no previous research experience (Bloom 1964). These students present the greatest challenge to the instructor. An inexperienced student may require extra guidance through research projects prior to the dissertation to ensure initial success that builds the confidence necessary to complete the dissertation. A mentor can be crucial in teaching students research skills and developing an awareness of the realities of a career in research and academics. Once administrative, technical, and academic hurdles are removed, however, graduates must take responsibility for their careers. Sustained intellectual curiosity and drive must be generated internally.

SUMMARY AND CONCLUSION

In summary, a professional educational program in communication sciences and disorders should include research training as an integral component rather than as a separate entity. The focus of the research training appropriately varies from undergraduate through doctoral program to meet the needs and backgrounds of students at each educational level. Educational programs can encourage the integration process by providing administrative support and faculty role models who combine clinic and research activities. Regardless of whether a person works in a research or clinical setting, each professional has a responsibility to understand, evaluate, and apply research. The integration of clinic and research by all members of the profession is necessary to insure continued growth of the individual and the field.

REFERENCES

Bloom, B. S. 1964. Report on creativity research by the examiner's office of the University of Chicago. In *Scientific Creativity: Its Recognition and Development*, eds. C. W. Taylor and F. Barron. New York: John Wiley & Sons.

Council of Graduate Schools. 1990. *Research Student and Supervisor. An Approach to Good Supervisory Practice*. Washington, DC: Author.

Creswell, J. W. 1985. *Faculty Research Performance: Lessons from the Sciences and the Social Sciences* ASHE-ERIC Higher Education Report No. 4. Washington, DC: Association for the Study of Higher Education.

Fleming, J. 1980. Teaching nursing research: Content. *Nurse Education* 5:24–26.

Fowler, C. G., and Wilson, R. H. 1989. More degrees, but no more degrees. *Audiology Today* 3:22–23.

Knapp, R. H. 1963. Demographic cultural and personality attributes of scientists. In *Scientific Creativity: Its Recognition and Development*, eds. C. W. Taylor and F. Barron. New York: John Wiley & Sons.

Lipscomb, D. M. 1974. *An Introduction to the Laboratory Study of the Ear*. Springfield, IL: Charles C Thomas.

Long, J. S. 1978. Productivity and academic position in the scientific career. *American Sociological Review* 43:889–908.

Ludlow, C. L. 1986. The research career ladder in human communication sciences and disorders. In *Speech-Language Pathology and Audiology: Issues in Management*, ed. R. M. McLauchlin. Orlando, FL: Grune & Stratton, Inc.

Minifie, F. D. 1983. Knowledge and service: Does the foundation of the profession need shoring up? *Asha* 25:29–32.

Monte, C. F. 1975. *Psychology's Scientific Endeavor*. New York: Praeger Publishers.

Morton, R. K. 1964. Personal backgrounds of effective teaching. In *College and University Teaching*, eds. H. A. Estrin and D. M. Goode. Dubuque, IA: William C. Brown Company.

Perkins, W. H. 1985. From clinical dispenser to clinical scientist. *Seminars in Speech and Language* 6:13–20.

Peterson, D. 1985. Twenty years of practitioner training in psychology. *American Psychologist* 40:441–51.

Reskin, B. F. 1979. Academic sponsorship and scientists' careers. *Sociology of Education* 52:126–46.

Spector, N. C., and Bleeks, S. L. 1980. Strategies to improve students' attitudes to research. *Nursing Outlook* 28:300–304.

Springer, J. R., and Baer, L. J. 1988. Instruction in research-related topics in U.S. and Canadian medical schools. *Journal of Medical Education* 6:591–95.

Taylor, C. W., Smith, W. R., and Ghiselin, B. 1963. The creative and other contributions of one sample of research scientists. In *Scientific Creativity: Its Recognition and Development*, eds. C. W. Taylor and F. Barron. New York: John Wiley & Sons.

Tuckman, H. P. 1976. *Publication, Teaching, and the Academic Reward Structure*. Lexington, MA: Lexington Books.

Waller, K. V., Jordan, L., Gierhart, J., Brodnik, M. P., Schiller, M. R., Flanigan, K. S., Ballinger, P. W., Grant, H. K., Bennet, D., Van Son, L. G., and Testat, E. W. 1988. Research skills and the research environment: A needs assessment of allied health faculty. *Journal of Allied Health* 17(2):101–113.

Chapter 7

Education in the Clinic

Judith A. Rassi and Margaret D. McElroy

Education in clinical professions such as audiology and speech-language pathology necessarily takes place in the clinical setting as well as in the classroom and laboratory. In the clinic, or in other environments where the profession is practiced, a student not only has the opportunity to apply previous learning, but also to gain new knowledge, new skills, and new attitudes (Purtilo 1990). The discussion in this chapter focuses on education in the clinic, as it is, and as it might be.

CLINICAL FACILITIES IN AUDIOLOGY AND SPEECH-LANGUAGE PATHOLOGY EDUCATIONAL PROGRAMS

Audiology and speech-language clinics within college and university educational programs have been the traditional sites where students have obtained their primary clinical experience. Through these on-site placements, faculty and staff have had direct influence on and control over their students' clinical learning.

Staff Composition

During the early years of educational programs, first in speech pathology, then in audiology (Pauls 1944; Hedgecock 1947; Matthews and Steer 1947; Carhart 1950), university clinics were staffed by faculty members who also served as clinical supervisors, classroom instructors, researchers, and program administrators. Over the years, with an increase in the number of programs and faculty members within those programs, with broadening knowledge and increasing research specialization, many doctoral level instructors relinquished their clinical supervisor roles to master's level clinicians who were also increasing in number.

This division of roles continues today in many programs, especially those with relatively large numbers of faculty and staff. Some programs use a combination: doctoral level persons whose primary responsibility is classroom teaching and research, and whose secondary responsibility is clinical supervision; and master's level persons whose primary responsibility is clinical supervision (Rassi 1985). Nevertheless, many professionals who are now expressing concern about the quality of educational preparation for audiologists and speech-language pathologists feel that the original model needs to be revived; that is, that doctoral level classroom instructors/researchers should be resuming the primary role as clinical supervisors (Cunningham and Windmill 1990; Hall 1990).

The reasoning of the critics is twofold: first, master's level clinicians, because of their less extensive preparation, do not have the depth and breadth of knowledge needed for quality clinical teaching in increasingly technical disciplines, especially where a blending of research and clinical processes is required; and second, doctoral level classroom instructors/researchers cannot do justice to their classroom teaching or research without current and consistent experience in the clinic. Counterpoints to these assertions are that classroom instructors/researchers who have not been directly involved in service delivery for many years are ill-equipped to supervise students in matters of contemporary clinical practice; and persons involved in clinical and supervisory work on a part-time basis do not have the same level of commitment as do those persons whose full-time job is clinical/supervisory. Each of these arguments has merit. Together, they reflect a common concern that information imparted to students be current.

Management of university speech-language-hearing clinics has become more complicated in recent years. In many places, the educational program administrator no longer serves as the clinical administrator, but rather, another faculty or staff member has been appointed to assume the responsibility. In larger programs, hearing and speech-language clinics are sometimes managed separately. Even so, these clinical managers may find that they now have less time to devote to classroom teaching, clinical supervision, or research because the clinical administrative work consumes so much of their time. This is especially likely to be the case in those clinics where there is, for example, an active, direct hearing aid dispensing program; an ongoing marketing component or quality assurance program; a computerized billing system; or contractual service agreements to initiate and maintain. In these and many other examples, the management of university clinics is not unlike that of free-standing service units or of clinical units within nonacademic institutions. The main differences, it would seem, lie in fiscal and organizational policies.

Clinical Orientation

Many universities have established at least two clinical facilities—one in a medical school or teaching hospital, the other in a nonmedical setting (Lillywhite 1961). Although the relationship between audiology and speech-language pathology and the medical and allied health professions has been somewhat tenuous, the institutions in which these liaisons have been fostered are known for the variety of enriching educational experiences they provide. Offering potential students the opportunity to learn in a university medical setting has given many programs a recruiting edge over their counterparts. That audiology and speech-language pathology are becoming more medically oriented suggests this advantage will continue and likely even increase.

Clinical facilities often differ in their emphases, depending on the interest and expertise of the clinical-supervisory staff. Philosophical and professional biases, whether held by individual clinical staff members or by the clinical education program as a whole, can influence directly the clinical approaches taken and, therefore, the kind of clinical teaching practiced. Institutional affiliations, especially those with university laboratory schools and/or university hospitals, may define a remedial-versus-diagnostic emphasis. In some instances, institutional policy or even state law may determine whether or not a particular clinical service can be offered; an obvious example is direct hearing aid dispensing.

Also having an apparent educational impact is the composition of patient populations, determined primarily by the university clinics' referral bases and secondarily by such factors as fee policies, contractual arrangements, marketing efforts, accessibility and availability of service, and types of services offered. Even the location of a university influences the composition of patient populations and ultimately a student's clinical educational experiences. Programs in urban settings, for example, may have access to a greater variety of patients than do their non-urban counterparts, but must operate within a more professionally competitive community. Those programs in more sparsely populated areas may attract patients from greater distances, yet have fewer cases representing certain types of communication disorders. Whatever the set of circumstances, a student's clinical education is shaped accordingly.

Educational Orientation

Combining clinical service and education within the structure of an academic institution has, throughout the years, been problematic. Even so, university clinics were reasonably manageable until the late 1970s and early 1980s when program administrators and clinical educators encountered difficulties of unprecedented magnitude. With diminishing institutional and research funds, with increasing pressure from university administrators to operate cost-effective clinics, and with parallel pressures on academic and research components, many CSD educational programs were faced with uncomfortable tasks, among them: reducing the size of the clinical-supervisory staff; increasing the caseload of the clinical-supervisory staff; adding clinical-supervisory responsibilities to the workload of classroom instructors/researchers; increasing clinical fees; and shortening the time allotted for diagnostic procedures and other patient services. Some educational programs survived the dramatic changes and later even expanded, while others, finding these and additional obstacles insurmountable, were eventually terminated.

Many of the surviving programs found that the kinds of changes described above had a profound impact on their clinical education endeavors. Fundamental philosophies were permanently altered: about what constitutes a viable and worthwhile program of educational preparation for professional service delivery; about the abilities of persons with dissimilar educational backgrounds and interests to provide quality clinical service and effective student supervision; and about the need to charge competitive clinical fees and market both the clinical and educational programs. In a number of ways, the upheaval was positive. At least, it forced educational programs to engage in self-evaluation. And, at most, it created changes that likely improved some programs, making them stronger.

In recent years, university and hospital pressures to increase clinical revenues and other sources of income (such as more tuition-paying students) while, at the same time, minimizing expenditures, have not abated. For those programs whose clinics are in medical schools or teaching hospitals, there is a continuing demand for more, and increasingly complicated, diagnostic services to be delivered without delay and in shorter periods of time (Rassi 1987). These developments continue to affect directly both clinical service delivery and clinical supervision.

Clinical education is expensive. Costly, yet rapidly outdated, equipment is often necessary, particularly in audiology and voice diagnostic operations. In their continuing effort to offer state-of-the-art education to students, university clinics find it especially important to have state-of-the-art equipment. Furthermore, a small faculty-to-student ratio, specifically for clinical supervision, is required for the clinical education of audiologists and speech-language pathologists. Although, according to ASHA requirements, only 25% of therapy sessions and 50% of diagnostic sessions must be supervised directly, many programs find it desirable to use one-to-one supervisor-to-student ratios, which allow 100% supervision. This has been found to be most beneficial in the supervision of students performing diagnostic and hearing aid work, and for beginning student clinicians whether they are involved in diagnostic or therapy clinical sessions. As time and personnel demands continue to change, however, maintaining this ideal ratio even for a particular subgroup of students may no longer be possible.

The time consumed by clinical teaching is also expensive in that student conference and instruction time must be added to the time spent in service delivery. This contention, of course, presupposes that a clinical supervisor actually spends extra time with students. Such is not always the case. Depending on the supervisor, and perhaps more often on the work setting, the additional time spent with students, beyond clinical session time, may be minimal. Historically thought to be happening only in service-oriented off-campus practicum settings (see Chapter 8), this situation is not uncommon in those university clinics where the time-is-money rule has taken over and where clinical supervisors are being held accountable for a set number of billable service hours. Taking the extra time necessary for conferring with students and even for allowing students to participate, knowing that they may work more slowly, presents a real dilemma for supervisors. As with supervisor-to-student ratios, the ideal time allotment may no longer be achievable in many instances, and other more workable clinical education models need to be developed.

It should be emphasized here that not all university clinics have experienced the kinds of changes noted above. Indeed, some do not provide hearing aid dispensing service; some charge low fees or no fees at all; some do not provide continuity of patient service between school terms; and some have not been subjected to administrative pressures to increase revenues or deliver more timely services. There may be as many reasons for such steadfastness as there are clinical programs falling into this category. Regardless of the reasons, it should be noted that one of the strongest criticisms of university clinics over the years has been that they are operating in "the ivory tower," providing services that do not represent what happens, or what should happen, in "the real world," and, therefore, not giving students appropriate preparatory experiences. This charge was illustrated most poignantly in the following two resolutions at the St. Paul Conference (Rees and Snope 1983):

> WHEREAS, Professional Services Board accredited clinical programs meet minimal requirements for the delivery of clinical service, and
> WHEREAS, students in university educational programs need exposure to, and practicum in, model clinical programs; therefore,
> RESOLVED, that a Professional Services Board accredited clinical service facility be a component of each educational program in speech-language pathology and audiology and further
> RESOLVED, that no graduating student shall be eligible for clinical certification unless the program from which that person graduates has an on-campus Professional Services Board accredited clinical service facility.

> WHEREAS, university-based service clinics frequently do not reflect the mode of practice common to high-quality service delivery programs in speech-language pathology and audiology; therefore,
> RESOLVED, that university-based service clinics not serve as the principal clinical practicum setting for students majoring in speech-language pathology or audiology. (p. 116)

Although both resolutions were defeated—the first, 87 to 24, and the second, 63 to 48—it should be pointed out that the majority of conferees were themselves representatives of college and university educational programs. Thus, no matter how these votes might be construed, the statements were drafted, debated, and supported by concerned professionals, many of whom were educators. When considered in the light of more recent criticisms of master's level educational programs, the resolutions convey an even stronger message.

Changes in health care delivery and higher education in the 1990s will undoubtedly continue to have an enormous impact on our educational programs. If university clinics are to endure as primary sites for students' clinical education in audiology and speech-language pathology, they must be willing to change with the times, to operate contemporary full-service clinics, and to develop innovative clinical teaching models. Not to do so would be an invitation for others to fill the void. It is encouraging that some university clinics have responded to calls for change, however painful their transformations may have been. Now, the task is not only to respond, but to initiate.

THE CLINIC AS A LEARNING ENVIRONMENT

Clinical learning and clinical teaching are corresponding, multifaceted processes, hence complex and unique. Purtilo (1990) points out that clinical education "introduces the student to the peculiarities of the work environment. The quality and quantity of teaching that take place are determined by . . . wide-ranging and unpredictable variables" (p. 10). A student's learning in the clinic can occur as a result of knowledge and skill application, modification, and refinement; interaction with patients, professionals, and environment; guided observation of a professional who is modeling or demonstrating a clinical activity; and conferring with, and following the instruction of, a professional. These, in turn, lead to other ways of learning such as problem solving, critical thinking, and self-evaluation. Learning in the clinic is effected through many different means not usually available in the classroom or even in a laboratory.

Knowledge, Skills, and Attitudes

In Purtilo's scheme of professional education components, that is, knowledge, skills, and attitudes, all three can be acquired and/or enhanced in the clinic.

Knowledge. Knowledge, particularly that which is theoretical, is perhaps best learned in the classroom; substantiation may await the clinical practicum. Conversely, because skills and attitudes, in order to be meaningful, must be built upon a solid knowledge base, clinical teachers often find it necessary to clarify for students what has been learned in the classroom or even to impart new information if the students' practicum assignments happen to precede the related coursework. Whatever the knowledge-acquisition pattern, clinical experience helps students to process and internalize information so that it becomes their own knowledge.

Skills. The skills to be learned in laboratory and clinical settings by students preparing to become health professionals are these, according to Purtilo (1990): technical skill; skill in interpersonal relationships and communication; teaching and administrative skill; and research skill. In her conceptualization, technical skill encompasses all diagnostic procedures, therapy techniques, management decisions and judgments. Also included in this category are the psychomotor skills needed by different types of clinicians, as dictated by their area of practice.

Interpersonal communication skills extend beyond those needed by students in dealing with patients and their families to relationships with other professionals, including supervisors, and supportive personnel, fellow students, and business contacts. Teaching skill is involved in the counseling and instruction given to patients and families and in the instruction of other professionals and supportive personnel, whereas administrative skill refers to organization, implementation of work, and objective peer and self-evaluations. Finally, research skill refers to hypothesis formulation and data collection either during the clinical process or as an outside project.

Medical educators, Douglas, Hosokawa, and Lawler (1988), emphasize the need for students to learn the process of clinical reasoning while engaged in patient care. Although clinical reasoning can be taught in the classroom, the clinic offers a unique learning opportunity to apply the process to an actual patient problem—ultimate decisions are consequential—while interacting with a clinical teacher. Clinical reasoning, a direct parallel to the hypothesis and data collection process in research skill, is considered by most clinical educators, regardless of discipline, to be the center of clinical learning. For teacher and learner, both process and outcome are the focus.

Attitudes. Attitudes, according to Tyler (1965), are acquired by various means. Assimilation of attitudes from the environment and development of attitudes according to the emotional effects of certain experiences are thought to be two major determinants. Acquisition of attitudes through direct intellectual processes such as studying or analyzing occurs less frequently. Therefore, although both are important, the clinic more than the classroom is seen as being conducive to attitude development and change (Purtilo 1978). Students' observation of and experience in the clinical process as well as their reactions and interactions in this environment serve as strong influences. Students' views of themselves and of others in relationship to career and profession, that is, their personal and professional attitudes, are shaped in the clinic.

Instructional Space and Equipment

The amount and kind of instructional space available in speech-language-hearing clinics vary greatly from setting to setting. In general, university clinics built for educational purposes are equipped with adjacent observation rooms where a patient's family members, clinical supervisors, and other professionals and students can observe through a one-way window and hear the proceedings of a clinical session through a communication system. There are many exceptions to this ideal, however. With program expansions, for instance, added activities and personnel often have to be accommodated within spaces that cannot be enlarged. Sound booths in audiology units frequently have small windows and sometimes these are only between the test and control areas. Other university clinics simply may not have rooms specifically designed for observation. Still others may use closed circuit television monitors which, depending on the array of equipment, allow multiple observations and may use less space.

Although perhaps not always convenient, clinical instruction and student learning can be accomplished in virtually any kind of clinical environment, with or without designated observation areas. While a clinical session is ongoing, demonstration, observation, feedback, and teaching can, and often must, take place with the clinical supervisor and student in the same room and the patient in another, or with all three in the same room. It is important to note, however, that placement of these individuals relative to one another and to their surroundings directly affects the dynamics of patient-student, student-supervisor, and patient-supervisor relationships (Rassi 1978). The amount of space within clinical rooms thus becomes a factor to consider in educational as well as clinical planning.

As already suggested, state-of-the-art equipment and materials obtained for clinical use also become educational considerations, given that students need to be familiar with current tools of the profession. If a sufficient variety is unaffordable and impractical for clinics, other means of ensuring that students are exposed to a wide array of clinical products is essential.

Clinic Structure

The entire organization of a clinic, including patient scheduling, business and administrative functions, and service delivery, can and should be adapted for instructional purposes in a university clinic. Special effort must be made to avoid the conflict between service and educational interests discussed earlier. Although compromise undoubtedly will be necessary, programs that are effective in both realms are nonetheless achievable.

Insofar as possible, at all levels of clinic administration, from staff meetings to budget preparation to quality assurance, student exposure to decision-making processes can be quite instructive. Although students' future work might not take place in a university clinic, they will be managing clinical practices of various types both inside and outside institutional settings. If a university clinic operates as a viable service facility, then its administrative and operational procedures represent an appropriate model from which these students can learn.

INVOLVEMENT OF STUDENTS IN THE CLINIC

One of the main differences between clinical and classroom learning is that the student in the clinic is responsible for demonstrating a set of skills, as well as for being knowledgeable. A second major difference between these two educational modes is the communication channel through which teaching and learning take place. In the clinic, there is one person at each end of the channel. Even if a supervisor is responsible for more than one student at a time, the supervisor typically moves from student to student, working with each on an individual basis. In the classroom, the communication channel has the instructor at one end and a group of students at the other. Although there may be out-of-class conferences between individual students and the instructor, the bulk of teaching-learning communication takes place in a group. The third major factor that distinguishes classroom and clinic learning is participation of a patient, serving as a substantial contributor, often unwittingly, to the clinical education process.

Perceptions, Expectations, and Anxiety

All three distinctions combine to make learning in the clinic a unique and unforgettable experience for students, one that has an enormous impact on their professional lives. Most students view their clinical practicum very seriously, equating it with a preview of what their future work might entail. Career directions are often established, reinforced, or rerouted as a result of students' practicum experiences. Their emotional investment is considerable.

In a study of nursing students' perceptions of clinical experience, Windsor (1987) found that, in the first stage of a three-stage development pattern, students were anxious and obsessed about task performance. Pagana (1988) studied nursing students' cognitive appraisal of stress in an initial clinical experience. Personal inadequacy was found to be their biggest fear, followed in order by fear of making errors, fear of uncertainty, fear of the clinical instructor, fear of being scared, and fear of failure. Reports by audiology students in written journal accounts of their practicum experiences and in group discussions in a supervision course taught by one of us, indicate that these same perceptions and feelings are not uncommon for student clinicians in our field.

Whether or not the stress that accompanies their practicum experiences interferes with speech-language pathology and audiology students' clinical learning and clinical performance needs to be explored. Anecdotal reports suggest that it does. Moreover, a study in counselor supervision (Ho, Hosford, and Johnson 1985) revealed that trainees' recall is adversely affected as anxiety increases during self-observation versus other-model observation, and even more so in the presence of a supervisor. Liddle (1986), looking at counselor supervision, explored the notion that in response to perceived threat, those being supervised seek to reduce their anxieties by using coping strategies that interfere with the process of learning. Whatever the learning effect, it is clear that students' anxieties need to be minimized as much as possible. One way in which this can be approached is to prepare supervisees for the supervisory process. Based on the premise that the supervisor and supervisee need to be aware of each other's expectations and perceptions about the process before they enter into it, Brasseur (1987) provides supervisees with substantial information on the supervisory process, including addressing their own perceptions about supervision and supervisor roles and their anxieties. Larson (1982) developed a Supervisory Expectations Scale that can be used to obtain information on students' expectations of their supervisors and of the supervisory experience.

Pickering (1987a), in reference to her investigative work on interpersonal communication in supervisory relationships, advises that a supervisor's expectations of a student and a student's expectations of a supervisor should be clearly stated and understood by each at the outset of a practicum assignment. On reviewing trainee expectations of supervisors in counselor education, Leddick and Dye (1987) also concluded that effective supervision features the establishment of clearly defined mutual expectations (p. 139). There are other means for reducing beginning students' general anxiety, but this initial exchange appears to be one of the most effective in alleviating students' uncertainty which, in turn, makes them less anxious about performing and more open to learning.

Periods of anxiety for students throughout a clinical practicum sequence tend to be specific to new situations, that is, new supervisors, new placements, new populations, and new procedures. The anxiety of newness apparently gives way to other student concerns. Liddle's (1986) delineation of possible perceived threats to supervisees includes evaluation anxiety, personal anxiety and issues, deficits in the supervisory relationship, and anticipated negative consequences. In their second stage of clinical development, the nursing students in Windsor's study (1987) struggled with identifying a nurse's role. It was not until the third and final stage that they became more comfortable in performing tasks, were more interested in expanding their roles and in being more independent, and identified more closely with the nurse's role. This suggests that, with time and experience, students perceive in themselves the transition from novice to practitioner in a logical progression. However, anxiety in different forms may continue to persist, hence attempts should be made to alleviate this through mutual problem solving (Liddle 1986).

Characteristic Individuality

In a study not unlike the one by Flocken (1980), Crane and Cooper (1983) examined the personality variables of female graduate students in speech-language pathology. This group profile—passive, compliant, stereotypically feminine, sensitive, anxious, highly imaginative, creative, and energetic—was found to be similar to profiles for female graduate students in education, nursing, and home economics. No comparable set of findings on audiology students is available.

Although profile data such as these suggest that there is a sameness among students, it should be noted that students bring to their clinical practicum assignments a variety of life experiences and personal characteristics. As already discussed in Chapter 5, in conjunction with classroom teaching, attitudes vary among learners. Indeed, a study of nursing students (Hodson 1985) revealed that significant behavioral differences in clinical settings were found to be related to differences in students' cognitive styles. Differences are further evident in students' interactions with clinical supervisors, patients, and others in the clinic; in their feelings about and reactions to clinical work; in their ability to learn from practice and instruction; and in their performance of clinical tasks. Individual differences, whatever they might be, are likely to be heightened more during individual clinical encounters than they are in classroom group involvements. It is this individuality that must be addressed in clinical education.

Participation in Clinical Learning

Moving from a one-to-group classroom communication configuration to a one-to-one clinic communication configuration is, for some students, a difficult transition. As previously indicated, new student clinicians are frequently anxious. This arises, in part, from being observed by a clinical supervisor while performing new tasks and being held personally accountable for actions and words—new experiences for students whose education has been confined primarily to the classroom. The patient also poses a new challenge, representing to the student yet another observer and potential critic. But the communication channel itself may be the most threatening aspect of a practicum experience. Students can no longer choose to be anonymous or silent, cannot adopt group attitudes, do not have the benefit of hearing classmates' opinions or answers, and have no classmates alongside to serve as models or standards of performance. (The latter two conditions apply only to the more typical practicum assignment of one student with one supervisor.) In short, students can no longer be passive learners.

Students who are accustomed to a traditional lecture-listen format of classroom teaching and have found comfort there may face the biggest challenge in clinical practicum with its demands for personal involvement. The risk-taking of personal disclosure becomes part of the student's responsibility for his/her own learning. Clinical students need to be active learners, who view their own work critically, who seek information from their supervisor, and who participate fully in clinical problem solving. Again, the role as supervisee needs to be clarified for groups of students as they are oriented to the clinical and supervisory processes before their first clinical practicum assignments. In Brasseur's preparation of supervisees (1987), these additional topics are covered: components of the supervisory process; joint establishment of supervision goals as well as clinical goals; prior experiences in supervision; preference for supervisor style; and baseline regarding both needs and competencies (pp. 145–47).

CLINICAL TEACHING

Traditionally, those who have educated students in a speech-language pathology and audiology clinic have been called clinical supervisors. The practice involves supervision of others, in this case, students, as they are engaged in the clinical process. Supervision in this context includes planning, observing, demonstrating, modeling, assisting, facilitating, analyzing, conferring, evaluating, and numerous other activities as delineated in the ASHA position statement on the tasks and competencies of supervision (ASHA 1985). (See Appendix C.)

Acknowledging that the word *supervision*, in its broadest sense, embraces program management as well as clinical teaching (ASHA 1978), the authors of the position statement chose to focus only on the latter, stating that clinical supervision therein "refers to the tasks and skills of clinical teaching related to the interaction between a clinician and a client" (p. 57). As further declared in the explanatory text of the position statement:

> A central premise of supervision is that effective clinical teaching involves, in a fundamental way, the development of self-analysis, self-evaluation, and problem-solving skills on the part of the individual being supervised. The success of clinical teaching rests largely on the achievement of this goal (p. 57).

Even though the words *teaching* and *instruction*, or derivatives thereof, never appear in the listing of the tasks of supervision or of the competencies for effective clinical supervision, the position statement nonetheless refers to clinical teaching as that which it defines and describes. This is significant. In the clinic, teaching is accomplished in many ways, as suggested in the list of verbs cited above and in other tasks and competencies. The avoidance of words such as telling, explaining, and advising, reflects a philosophy of clinical teaching similar to that of problem-based learning and confluent or humanistic education as they relate to classroom teaching. (See Chapter 5.)

If this position statement analysis is carried one step further, it becomes clear that didactic teaching, while not mentioned as a task or competency, is not prohibited. A competency statement such as 6.1, for example, which reads, "Ability to assist the supervisee in learning a variety of data collection procedures" (ASHA 1985, p. 59) (see Appendix C), does not suggest how such assistance should be provided. One might logically assume that traditional teaching such as telling and explaining are part of this supervisory assistance process. In some instances, they might be; in others, not. The decision is left to the discretion of supervisors. It can be seen that, regardless of the emphasis on a facilitative approach to clinical teaching, specific methodology is not stipulated. This is as it should be for a document of this kind, given that methods found to be effective for one student or group of students may not be so for others, and may not be effective even for the same student under different circumstances or at another stage in that student's clinical development.

In view of the above, traditional teaching approaches do fall within the purview of the position statement. Furthermore, the terms, *clinical instructor/instruction* and *clinical teacher/teaching* may be used interchangeably and with *clinical supervisor/supervision*, although the latter terminology prevails in audiology and speech-language pathology. It is interesting to note that *supervisor* appears to be the term of choice in counselor education, teacher education, and social work education, whereas *clinical instructor* and *clinical teacher* are used more frequently in health professions education, medical education, and nursing education, with a few exceptions and some combinations. In the latter groups, the terms, *preceptor* and *preceptorship*, are comparable to our *extern/externship* and *intern/internship*. The general term, *clinical education*, is common to all health professions, sometimes referring to that which takes place only in the clinic, other times to every phase of education pertaining to clinical subject matter, including that presented in the classroom. All of these terms, it should be noted, are used to describe similar roles and processes. Nevertheless, the terminology selected may connote different images of those who fill the role and different interpretations of what the process is (Rassi 1986). Be that as it may, supervision terms are used interchangeably with instruction and teaching terms throughout this book.

Whether clinical teaching differs from classroom teaching is another matter. If there is evidence to support Purtilo's assertion that clinical and classroom learning differ, then it seems to follow that clinical and classroom teaching ought to differ as well. In most instances, it would appear that they do. But the kind and extent of such differences may not be desirable. If, for example, classroom teaching were to involve less lecturing and more facilitating by the instructor, and if clinical teaching were to involve less supervisory explanation and more student self-discovery, classroom and clinical teaching differences would change considerably both in kind and extent. Indeed, they would be more analogous and, in the view of many researchers, more effective. Perhaps classroom and clinical teachers might benefit from working cooperatively in an attempt to find parallel and complementary instructional approaches.

THE CLINICAL INSTRUCTOR

As suggested by the foregoing discussion and documented in the ASHA position statement, the clinical instructor in audiology and speech-language pathology is called upon to perform a wide variety of tasks and needs to possess a number of competencies. Foremost in the requirements of a clinical instructor are being a competent clinician and being a competent instructor (Rassi 1978). But, even further, these must be merged skillfully into the role of competent *clinical* instructor. Just as a competent clinician is not necessarily a competent clinical instructor, neither is a competent classroom or laboratory instructor necessarily a competent clinical instructor. These principles underlie the belief that preparation for the supervisory role is important (Anderson 1981; ASHA 1985). It is fortunate that opportunities for such preparation in our field continue to increase as more information about the supervisory process becomes available.

Roles of the Clinical Instructor

As suggested by the diversity of tasks and strategies of a clinical instructor, the number of corresponding roles is equally diverse. As role labels are applied, however, it is important to heed this caveat by Brasseur (1987):

> Roles are preconceived stereotypes of supervision derived from many sources (e.g., previous experience, information obtained from various sources, theoretical approaches to supervision, personal biases, etcetera), and the complexities of the supervisory process itself make many roles available to both supervisors and supervisees (p. 145).

Still, exploring the definition and description of these roles does enhance appreciation of the many complexities. For example, of the five roles selected for discussion in Chapter 5, each is equally and similarly important for the clinical instructor: expert, master clinician/researcher, facilitator, (career) counselor, and mentor. The reasons for the importance of these roles are the same for clinical teaching as for classroom teaching.

Expert and Master Clinician Roles. Both expert and master clinician roles are indispensable to the tasks of modeling, demonstrating, and instruction. Given the rapid expansion of clinical knowledge and corresponding changes in clinical applications during recent years, staying current is as critical to the clinical instructor as to the classroom and laboratory instructor. Discrepancies in currentness (or clinical philosophy) between classroom and clinical instruction, in either direction, can confuse students and serve to diminish the quality of their overall education. Herein lie the differences between "what they teach" (classroom instructors) and "what they do" (clinical instructors)—complaints sometimes expressed by students whose instruction in the two settings comes from different individuals. Leith, McNiece, and Fusilier (1989), who analyzed this dilemma in our field, suggest several avenues of compromise when conflicts arise between clinical and classroom instructors. Resolution is clearly important not only to ensure instructional clarity but also to foster in students a healthy appreciation and respect for the connection between classroom and clinic; that is, between research and practice. We suspect that classroom-clinic discrepancies contribute, at least in part, to the research-clinic dichotomy that exists in our field today. Students whose clinical role models do not discuss or apply classroom-imparted research, for instance, may be inclined to adopt the same policy when they become practitioners.

Research in comparable areas of clinical education suggests that role modeling by clinical instructors has a considerable impact on students. Jacobson (1974) found that a group of physical therapy students identified more with their clinical instructors than with anyone else responsible for their professional education. In psychiatric education, Muslin and Thurnbald (1974) reported that students not only gained certain knowledge and understanding from a role modeling supervisor but they partially identified with that person. The instructor's clinical competence as perceived by students is essential to role modeling, according to medical educator Irby (1986), because perceived competence establishes the instructor's credibility in students' eyes. Role modeling further requires that instructors serve as exemplary professionals and as enthusiastic clinical teachers who are excited about the profession (Irby 1986). Betz (1985), a nursing educator, echoes this assertion, explaining that self-image and behavior, developed through imitation of role models, are the basis of a student's occupational role conception.

Facilitator Role. As implied earlier, a clinical instructor's role as facilitator embraces virtually all of the tasks of supervision. Indeed, the main goal of clinical teaching is facilitation of students' learning and of their becoming independent clinicians. Much of the supervision literature in speech-language pathology deals with the facilitative nature of interactions (for example, Roberts and Smith 1982; Smith and Anderson 1982; Brasseur and Anderson 1983) and interpersonal communication (for example, Pickering 1984; Pickering 1987b) in supervisory conferences.

(Career) Counselor and Mentor Roles. The job of career counselor often falls to the clinical instructor because of a student's recognition of that person as a knowledgeable clinician who is aware of job opportunities, has professional contacts, understands professional politics, and can write a letter of recommendation for a student on the basis of first-hand clinical observation. In this same vein, students often look to their clinical instructors as mentors. As discussed in Chapter 5, mentors need to be cultivated in audiology and speech-language pathology education. Until recently, mentors in most fields have been predominantly males working with male students, that is, a part of the "old boy" network, while females have had fewer mentors available for

them. Gavett (1987) points out that there has not been a mentor system in place for supervisors in our field. Unless mentors are encouraged within educational programs, the same situation will exist for many of our students as they set out to become clinicians and chart career paths. Koenigsknecht (1989), in urging supervisors to become mentors, acknowledged that "an important goal in this relationship is continued development for *both* participants—the supervisor, too, is continuously learning and adjusting. To sustain them in this demanding role, mentors need to be mentored themselves" (p. 165).

Women mentors are becoming increasingly available as more women with experience are involved in business and the professions at every level. Female-dominated professions, in particular, are just beginning to recognize the importance of mentors to professional growth and development. In nursing education, for example, there have been numerous interviews, studies, and commentaries on the topic (Darling 1985a, 1985b, 1985c, 1985d, 1985e, 1985f, 1986a, 1986b; Cahill and Kelly 1989). Based on its success in other fields, a program in which nursing students are matched with mentors who are established professionals, has been implemented at one university (Cahill and Kelly 1989). Clinical instructors in our field can take a cue from this. If students do not seek out mentors, perhaps a concerted effort is needed to foster mentor relationships.

Priorities of the Clinical Instructor

There are choices to be made by the clinical instructor, choices that, because of the likelihood of their having a direct influence on student clinicians' learning, must be weighed and given priorities. A decision as to whether clinical service takes precedence over clinical teaching, or vice versa, needs to be reached whenever these two obligations compete with one another for the supervisor's time or attention (Rassi 1978; Rassi 1987). Allowing, and even inviting, students to use workable clinical approaches other than the clinical instructor's favored ones also is a frequent challenge for a supervisor. Both of these examples involve relinquishing supervisory control.

To illustrate further, another matter of priority is the clinical teacher's willingness, along with that of the assigned student, to take personal responsibility for the student's clinical learning, rather than assume that learning gaps will be filled by other clinical or classroom instructors. This is particularly important in the case of a struggling student. In an integrated program, there must be some assurance that each of the component parts contributes its appropriate share to the clinical education of each student. A similar priority concerns the clinical teacher's willingness to put forth as much or more effort into working with beginning or intermediate students, as with advanced students. These kinds of priorities reflect a clinical teacher's attitude toward, and level of commitment to, clinical teaching and students.

The Clinical Instructor as a Person

As might be expected, personal values and personal characteristics play a role in a clinical teacher's approach to the supervisory process just as they do in a classroom instructor's approach to teaching. Because of the one-to-one relationship in clinical instruction, personal attributes may be even more consequential in this context. Blumberg, in his pioneer work on supervision of teachers (1974), discusses the importance of supervisors' learning about themselves, that is, about their own interpersonal needs, their reactions to the behavior of other people, their ability to handle conflicts, and their own competency. Self-knowledge helps supervisors to understand better their own perceptions and biases. The importance of this understanding has been substantiated by, among others, Roberts and Naremore (1983), who found speech-language pathology supervisors to be biased in supervisory decision-making behavior. In health care supervision, Munn (1982) admonishes supervisors to examine their listening skills, and Metzger (1982) recommends a "soul-searching" exercise in self-evaluation. Regardless of the field, then, the need for supervisors to understand themselves as participants in the supervisory process is considered to be paramount.

SUMMARY

Education in the clinic is key to preparation of CSD students for professional practice. Although clinical supervision by persons also involved in classroom teaching and research can enhance learning in all three areas, some kind of preparation for the supervisory process is warranted. A coming together of knowledge, skills, and attitudes in students' clinical learning is crucial to professional development. A mutual understanding between supervisor and student of each other's perceptions and expectations sets the tone for an effective supervisory working relationship. Elements of the clinical teaching-learning process are similar to those in problem-based learning and humanistic education. The roles and priorities of the clinical instructor influence education in the clinic.

REFERENCES

American Speech-Language-Hearing Association. 1978. Committee on Supervision in Speech-Language Pathology and Audiology. Current status of supervision of speech-language pathology and audiology. [Special Report]. *Asha* 20:478–86.

American Speech-Language-Hearing Association. 1985. Committee on Supervision in Speech-Language-Pathology and Audiology. Clinical supervision in speech-language pathology and audiology. A position statement. *Asha* 27(6):57–60.

Anderson, J. 1981. Training of supervisors in speech-language pathology and audiology. *Asha* 23:77–82.

Betz, C. L. 1985. Students in transition: Imitators of role models. *Journal of Nursing Education* 24(7):301–303.

Blumberg, A. 1974. *Supervisors and Teachers: A Private Cold War.* Berkeley, CA: McCutchan Publishing Corp.

Brasseur, J. A. 1987. Preparation of supervisees for the supervisory process. In *Clinical Supervision: A Coming of Age,* ed. S. S. Farmer. Proceedings of a conference held at Jekyll Island, GA. Las Cruces, NM: New Mexico State University.

Brasseur, J. A., and Anderson, J. L. 1983. Observed differences between direct, indirect, and direct/indirect videotaped supervisory conferences. *Journal of Speech and Hearing Research* 26:349–55.

Cahill, M. F., and Kelly, J. J. 1989. A mentor program for nursing majors. *Journal of Nursing Education* 28(1):40–42.

Carhart, R. 1950. Hearing aid selection by university clinics. *Journal of Speech and Hearing Disorders* 15:106–113.

Crane, S. L., and Cooper, E. B. 1983. Speech-language clinician personality variables and clinical effectiveness. *Journal of Speech and Hearing Disorders* 48: 140–45.

Cunningham, D. R., and Windmill, I. M. 1990. Faculty private practice: Implications for the future of audiology. *Audiology Today* 2(6):18–21.

Darling, L. A. W. 1985a. What do nurses want in a mentor? *Nurse Educator* 10(1):18–20.

Darling, L. A. W. 1985b. Mentor types and life cycles. *Nurse Educator* 10(2): 17–18.

Darling, L. A. W. 1985c. "So you've never had a mentor . . . Not to worry." *Nurse Educator* 10(3):18–19.

Darling, L. A. W. 1985d. Mentor matching. *Nurse Educator* 10(4):18–19.

Darling, L. A. W. 1985e. Can a non-bonder be an effective mentor? *Nurse Educator* 10(5):39–40.

Darling, L. A. W. 1985f. Mentors and mentoring. *Nurse Educator* 10(6):18–19.

Darling, L. A. W. 1986a. The case for mentor moderation. *Nurse Educator* 11(3): 27–28.

Darling, L. A. W. 1986b. Endings in mentor relationships. *Nurse Educator* 11(5): 24–25.

Douglas, K. C., Hosokawa, M. C., and Lawler, F. H. 1988. *A Practical Guide to Clinical Teaching in Medicine.* New York: Springer Publishing Company.

Flocken, J. M. 1980. Personality characteristics of communicative disorders graduate students. *Asha* 22:7–16.

Gavett, E. 1987. Career development: An issue for the master's degree supervisor. In *Supervision in Human Communication Disorders: Perspectives on a Process*, eds. M. B. Crago and M. Pickering. San Diego, CA: College-Hill Press.

Hall, J. W. 1990. Clinic practice. *Audiology Today* 2(6):17.

Hedgecock, L. D. 1947. A university hearing aid clinic. *Journal of Speech Disorders* 12:323–30.

Ho, P., Hosford, R. E., and Johnson, M. E. 1985. The effects of anxiety on recall in self versus other-model observation. *Counselor Education and Supervision* 25(1):48–55.

Hodson, K. E. 1985. Cognitive style and the behavioral differences of nursing students in the clinical setting. *Journal of Nursing Education* 24(2):58–62.

Irby, D. M. 1986. Clinical teaching and the clinical teacher. *Journal of Medical Education* 61(9):35–45.

Jacobson, B. 1974. Role modeling in physical therapy. *Physical Therapy* 54: 244–50.

Koenigsknecht, R. A. 1989. Supervision: Its place and contribution to the profession. Keynote address. In *Supervision: Innovations. A National Conference on Supervision*, ed. D. A. Shapiro. Proceedings of a conference held in Sonoma County, CA. Cullowhee, NC: Western Carolina University.

Larson, L. 1982. Perceived supervisory needs and expectations of experienced vs. inexperienced student clinicians. (Doctoral dissertation, Indiana University, 1981). *Dissertation Abstracts International* 42:4758B. (University Microfilms No. 82-11, 183)

Leddick, G. R., and Dye, H. A. 1987. Counselor supervision. Effective supervision as portrayed by trainee expectations and preferences. *Counselor Education and Supervision* 27(2):139–54.

Leith, W. R., McNiece, E. M., and Fusilier, B. B. 1989. *Handbook of Supervision: A Cognitive Behavioral System*. Austin, TX: Pro-Ed.

Liddle, B. J. 1986. Resistance in supervision: A response to perceived threat. *Counselor Education and Supervision* 26(2):117–27.

Lillywhite, H. S. 1961. Opportunities for clinical training in a medical center speech and hearing clinic. *Asha* 3:237–39.

Matthews, J., and Steer, M.D. 1947. Growth of speech correction facilities in colleges and universities in Indiana. *Journal of Speech Disorders* 12:169–72.

Metzger, N. 1982. *The Health Care Supervisor's Handbook* (2nd ed.). Baltimore: University Park Press.

Munn, H. E., Jr. 1982. The supervisor as a responsible listener. *The Health Care Supervisor* 1(1):62–71.

Muslin, H. L., and Thurnbald, J. P. 1974. Supervision as an evaluative mechanism. In *Evaluative Methods in Psychiatric Education*, eds. H. L. Muslin, R. J. Thurnbald, B. Templeton, and C. H. McGuire. Washington, DC: American Psychiatric Association.

Pagana, K. D. 1988. Stresses and threats reported by baccalaureate students in relation to an initial clinical experience. *Journal of Nursing Education* 27(9): 418–24.

Pauls, M. D. 1944. The role of the college and university hearing clinic. *Journal of Speech Disorders* 9:357–61.

Pickering, M. 1984. Interpersonal communication in speech-language pathology supervisory conferences: A qualitative study. *Journal of Speech and Hearing Disorders* 49:189–95.

Pickering, M. 1987a. Expectation and intent in the supervisory process. *The Clinical Supervisor* 5(4):43–57.

Pickering, M. 1987b. Interpersonal communication and the supervisory process: A search for Ariadne's thread. In *Supervision in Human Communication Disorders: Perspectives on a Process,* eds. M. B. Crago and M. Pickering. San Diego, CA: College-Hill Press.

Purtilo, R. 1978. *Health Professional and Patient Interaction* (2nd ed). Philadelphia: W. B. Saunders Company.

Purtilo, R. 1990. *Health Professional and Patient Interaction* (4th ed.). Philadelphia: W. B. Saunders Company.

Rassi, J. A. 1978. *Supervision in Audiology.* Baltimore: University Park Press.

Rassi, J. A. 1985. Competencies, qualifications, training: Audiology. In *Conference Proceedings of the Sixth Annual Conference on Graduate Education,* ed. J. E. Bernthal. Council of Graduate Programs in Communication Sciences and Disorders.

Rassi, J. A. 1986. What's in a name? *SUPERvision* 10(3):2–3.

Rassi, J. A. 1987. The uniqueness of audiology supervision. In *Supervision in Human Communication Disorders: Perspectives on a Process,* eds. M. B. Crago and M. Pickering. San Diego, CA: College-Hill Press.

Rees, N. S., and Snope, T. L. (eds.). 1983. *Proceedings of the 1983 National Conference on Undergraduate, Graduate, and Continuing Education* (Report No. 13). Rockville, MD: American Speech-Language-Hearing Association.

Roberts, J. E., and Naremore, R. C. 1983. An attributional model of supervisors' decision-making behavior in speech-language pathology. *Journal of Speech and Hearing Research* 26:537–49.

Roberts, J. E., and Smith, K. J. 1982. Supervisor-supervisee role differences and consistency of behavior in supervisory conferences. *Journal of Speech and Hearing Research* 25:428–34.

Smith, K. J., and Anderson, J. L. 1982. Relationship of perceived effectiveness to verbal interaction/content variables in supervisory conferences in speech-language pathology. *Journal of Speech and Hearing Research* 25:252–61.

Tyler, R. W. 1965. *Basic Principles of Curriculum and Instruction: Syllabus for Education 305.* Chicago: University of Chicago Press, Syllabus Division.

Windsor, A. 1987. Nursing students' perceptions of clinical experience. *Journal of Nursing Education* 26(4):150–54.

Chapter 8

EDUCATION IN THE FIELD

Margaret D. McElroy and Judith A. Rassi

In order to provide further opportunities for graduate students to meet or exceed the practicum clock-hour requirements of ASHA Standards for Certificates of Clinical Competence (1991) (see Appendix A) and clinical setting requirements of the ASHA Educational Standards Board (ASHA 1990b) (see Appendix B), most Communication Sciences and Disorders (CSD) educational programs arrange for additional placement of students in nonuniversity facilities. Indeed, a substantial amount of CSD students' clinical practicum experience is obtained off-campus as evidenced by the relative number of supervisors involved: of the 4717 supervisors reported to be associated with CSD programs in 1986–87, 2868 (61%) were located off-campus and 1849 (39%) were internal to the reporting institution (Cooper, Helmick, and Ripich 1987, p. 26).

FIELD PLACEMENT

Sites selected for field placement may be located anywhere, that is, near the university; within the same community, metropolitan area, geographical region, or state; or they may be in another state or country. Assignment schedules vary in duration and interval, for example: half- or full-day time blocks on a weekly basis for one school term, in conformance with a student's university class schedule and other practicum assignments; several entire workdays per week on a weekly basis for several weeks, months, or an entire school term; or full-time, that is, five workdays per week for longer time periods. The full-time arrangement is reserved usually for a culminating externship assignment which, in most programs, follows a student's completion of coursework. Also, the sites at distant locations are commonly used for the extern placements.

Purpose and Benefits

Assigning students for off-campus clinical practica or for field instruction, as this practice is called in many professions, helps a program comply with certification and accreditation standards; it also offers students specific benefits, among them: participation in a wider variety of clinical settings with variations in patient population, clinical staff composition, administrative and operational setup, and clinical and supervisory approaches; exposure to nonuniversity service operations that may have different priorities than do university clinics; development of interprofessional working relationships and involvement in interdisciplinary teamwork; application of problem-based learning skills in new environments; and, in full-time assignments, experience that more closely simulates that of a working, practicing professional.

For the university program, certain benefits accrue as well: linkage with other components of the professional community; opportunities for formal affiliation with other institutions; program visibility through the ambassadorship of students and university liaison supervisors; and continuing education and professional network exchanges. Conversely, many of these same benefits apply to the cooperating off-campus sites and their participating supervisors.

Scheduling and Timing

As suggested by the variety of scheduling patterns with and without concurrent classwork, some students are placed in off-campus sites at relatively early stages of a clinical practicum sequence, perhaps just beyond completion of the CCC and ESB standards' requirement that the first 25 clock hours be supervised by a university person. This arrangement allows several more field placements during the remaining school terms of a student's program. Other educational programs may not place students in a nonuniversity site until the final school term when a block of time has been reserved for an externship assignment. The university's timing of these placements may be related directly to the availability of field sites, to the readiness of students for more independent work in an operation outside the student-oriented university environment, or the decision may be somewhat arbitrary. In some instances, master's degree programs compressed into little more than a year's time simply may not have enough room in the curriculum to offer an externship experience, or they may offer it as an option beyond the completion of a regular program.

Student Readiness

A student's readiness for the first field placement is, with notable exceptions, likely to be related to its timing within the graduate program. That is to say, early placed students with fewer clock hours of on-campus practicum experience and less coursework completed are likely not to be as ready for an off-campus placement as are those with more preparation. In view of the supervision continuum (see Chapter

11), whereby a student is usually more dependent on close supervision at earlier stages than at later stages, this readiness-timing relationship becomes clearer. Many field supervisors, recognizing this progression, are unwilling to accept a student before the last school term of a program or the externship period.

The readiness factor is central to some of the difficulties reported by field sites in speech-language pathology and audiology. For instance, an issue of contention between university preparation programs in Colorado and the host clinics for their externs arose when the off-campus sites indicated that their investment of staff time, hence operation funds, to student supervision warranted charging the universities, or the externs, a fee (Ehrlich et al. 1983). Clinic directors maintained that, "The degree to which supervision is necessary in a professional clinic exceeds that required in a university clinic because in our clinic consumers expect and are usually purchasing professional service" (p. 26). As indicated elsewhere in this book, university programs face the same economic pressures in their own clinics, thus the difference in amount or kind of supervision provided in these two environments may no longer be so distinct. Nonetheless, the fact remains that universities are in the business of education, whereas, in most field sites, education is probably not the top priority.

The problem apparently is not unique to off-campus practicum sites for CSD educational programs because field instructors in comparable professions also state that their work load is greater when they are responsible for supervising a graduate student (Rosenfeld 1988). Reports from facilities offering clinical placements in health care professions have ranged from financial loss and decreased productivity to financial gain and increased productivity (Sheps et al. 1965; Light and Frey 1973; Halonen, Fitzgerald, and Simmon 1976; Porter and Kincaid 1977; Carney and Keim 1978; Pobojewski 1978; Moores 1979; Chung, Spelbring, and Boissoneau 1980; Garg et al. 1982; Leiken 1983; MacKinnon and Page 1986).

In view of the concerns expressed, whatever their tenor, the readiness of students becomes all the more critical in the decision to place them in off-campus sites. Further statements in the Colorado controversy are instructive in this regard. According to representatives of the clinics (Ehrlich et al. 1983):

> The credentialed staff must be responsible and present most of the time. We have seen too many omissions, too little awareness, and too many examples of inadequate judgment and limited understanding to be comfortable offering student service as professional service unless the student is very closely supervised (p. 26).

And from the universities:

> University personnel are confident that students recommended for an externship are capable of quality delivery of clinical services from the outset

of the externship, even if they may not be familiar with the specific procedures of a particular site. . . . Very close observation and supervision of
student externs is expected at the outset. Reasonably soon, however, they
(the extern supervisors) should expect to feel comfortable withdrawing
close supervision (p. 27).

This apparent discrepancy between university and field-site views
of students' ability to work independently, although a matter of perception and perhaps of philosophy as well, is nonetheless real and
something to be dealt with wherever it exists. The most important consideration, students' readiness for an off-campus placement, should be
determined individually rather than allowing all students within a particular school class to be placed at sites outside the university merely
because the students have been in the educational program for a certain period of time. Just as it cannot be assumed that all students begin
their graduate programs with the same prior educational and clinical
backgrounds, aptitude, and learning capacity, neither can it be assumed that all have had exactly the same on-campus practicum and
classroom experiences or, even if they have, that all have learned and
applied their learning in the same ways or at the same rates. Individual
readiness for the step from on-campus to off-campus practica is better
decided on the basis of clinical supervisors' evaluations of student
progress and/or results of clinical performance examinations administered at the university. As Anderson (1988) says, " . . . university supervisors must be as responsible as possible in determining the readiness of students for the off-campus experience . . . " (p. 266).

Regardless of student readiness, some universities do not have
enough variety in their own clinical population to enable students to
meet ASHA clock hour requirements in various disorder categories. In
this circumstance, it may be necessary to place students in off-campus
sites for their *initial* practicum experience with certain required populations. This often sets up a dilemma. The off-campus practicum site
may not want a student without experience in a particular area,
whereas the university needs the practicum site to provide that very
experience for the student. Compromise and understanding are obviously necessary. University programs without such resources are
clearly in a bind and, therefore, must persuade their nonuniversity colleagues to make exceptions to the requirement for advanced students
only. Reciprocal good-will gestures and supportive supervisory training on the part of university personnel can help resolve such conflicts.

Funding, Housing, and Transportation

The payment of fees to a field site may, in certain quarters, solve problems such as those cited above but, for the most part, neither univer-

sities nor students have resources set aside for this. On the other hand, some programs in communication disorders do work with graduate students to arrange full or partial funding for living costs associated with externship assignments, especially when the sites are located at a considerable distance from the university and involve long time periods. In some instances, the field site may provide a stipend or, at the least, assistance in locating reasonable housing for the student.

Because of their location, placement at some field sites may require that a student have access to a car or public transportation. In cases where the student has no car and where public transportation is not available, the university person who is arranging the practicum assignment and the student need to work together to solve the problem. Even then, there may not be a workable solution. Thus, although a desirable field site might be available for a particular student, an unsolvable transportation complication may preclude matching the student with the site.

Matching Students with Sites and Supervisors

Making off-campus placements involves the strategic matching of students with sites and supervisors. The literature on field instruction includes studies concerning matching students' personalities, specific educational and accreditation requirements, and learning styles with available clinical practicum settings and with particular field instructors who can meet a student's individual needs (Wilson 1981). Other variables that enter into placement decisions are based on information provided by the student: the availability of a car; how far a student lives from the placement; the student's self-perceived clinical strengths and weaknesses; and the student's feelings about the placement (Wilson 1981). Despite the importance attached to these factors, the literature does not support the notion that they correspond to a student's actual success in a field placement (Dailey 1970; Pfouts and Hinley 1977; Cunningham 1982).

Coordinating Placements

An extremely valuable, and often essential, member of a university CSD educational program staff is the individual who serves as coordinator of outside clinical practica, that is, a person who acts as liaison between the university and its off-campus practicum sites, contacts them initially and maintains an ongoing exchange of information, visits the facilities to determine whether or not they are appropriate as practicum sites, monitors the progress of students placed there, and keeps site supervisors informed about university policies and requirements. In many instances, this person is a university supervisor as well, and has knowledge about both the clinical and supervisory processes, which makes it possible to offer supervisory training to off-campus supervisors located within a reasonable distance. When speech-language pathology students are placed in schools, the university supervisor often works with the student's on-site supervisor as well as with the student, planning clinical and supervisory strategies and otherwise participating as a regular, integral member of the team.

In many programs the clinical practicum coordinator who serves as the university's primary liaison with field instructors serves also as the key person in the scheduling of students for their practicum assignments in the university clinics. This combination of responsibilities entrusted to the same person is particularly advantageous in that it allows for more knowledgeable scheduling, while ensuring consistency and balance in students' practicum assignments. In an ideal organizational framework, the practicum coordinator also has a thorough understanding of the academic course content and its relationship to students' clinical practicum needs. This is but one step in a program's move toward an integrated curriculum.

SETTINGS FOR FIELD INSTRUCTION

Depending on the location of a university educational program in speech-language pathology and audiology, the number and types of local and area field sites available for student practica vary. Whereas student assignment to the university clinical facilities involves working with supervisors or instructors employed by the university, assignment to outside sites may or may not involve university personnel.

Outside Placements with In-house Personnel

In recent years, the increasing number of contracts developed by university CSD departments with outside clinical facilities has allowed university supervisors to work directly with students in off-campus settings. Also, private practices conducted by university faculty or staff at nonuniversity sites afford the same kinds of field assignments. Moreover, as discussed in this book, many CSD programs operate university clinics not only in the traditional speech and hearing center but also in an affiliated medical school, medical center or teaching hospital, or in a university laboratory school. They may be staffed by personnel from another department, that is, otolaryngology or education, but these units are usually part of the university or at least closely affiliated with the university. In any such arrangements where university personnel serve as clinical instructors in an outside or affiliated facility, the clinical instruction can usually be monitored and its consistency controlled while still taking advantage of the variety in clinical experiences.

Practicum Settings

In those cases where outside sites are staffed by clinicians who are not direct employees of the university and whose primary responsibility may be service rather than education, the teaching situation may be less certain. Types of settings used as field sites are discussed in the following paragraphs.

Hospitals and Medical Centers. Clinical practicum assignments in a hospital or medical center offer CSD students a variety of experiences in working with inpatients or outpatients who may have communication disorders typically seen in a medical practice, or less common communication problems which are often accompanied by related or unrelated disease. Students assigned to an acute care unit may have the opportunity to see patients for pre-admission testing, and then to follow the patient through his/her hospitalization course (Foreman 1986). However, some patients may be released from the hospital before completion of recommended speech-language or hearing (re)habilitative services, especially because of the limitations imposed on the length of hospitalizations. In certain instances, individuals may continue to be followed for their (re)habilitative course as outpatients. Whether or not an assigned student clinician actually has the opportunity to see these patients after their release from the hospital depends greatly on developing a mutually satisfactory schedule and on the patient's ability to return to the medical center. Notwithstanding these management problems, the increased focus on ambulatory care in hospitals, another step taken to decrease the cost of medical care (Morgan 1986), has provided greater opportunities for clinicians in communication disorders, and therefore for students, to provide services within a hospital or medical center.

A medical setting offering comprehensive health care frequently finds student clinicians involved in a multidisciplinary approach to the patient's presenting problem(s), thereby broadening students' interactive as well as clinical experiences. Being involved in the daily routine of a hospital; participating in patient staffings; reviewing and contributing to the information in medical charts; and working with patients whose communication disorder is but one among many health problems represent some of the invaluable experiences available to students. In some cases, there may be opportunities for either the speech-language pathology or audiology student to observe surgery or for the audiology student to participate in intra-operative monitoring.

Veterans Administration Medical Centers (VA) traditionally have offered a broad range of experiences to clinical practicum students in audiology and speech-language pathology. In addition to seeing a variety of diagnostic and rehabilitative adult cases, students assigned to a VA facility usually have the opportunity to work with both inpatients and outpatients, use updated equipment, be involved in research projects, and interact with members of other disciplines. Also, stipends are sometimes available for students.

Rehabilitation Centers. Rehabilitation facilities usually provide students in communication disorders with a diversified population of individuals having communication problems stemming from a variety of causes. Many such facilities are residential, thereby giving added dimensions to the students' experience. There may also be opportunities to observe clients' social interactions, thus exposing students to the personal and practical aspects of a communication disorder. In these particular facilities, students may gain experience with augmentative communication systems such as communication boards and computers. Working with other disciplines is another benefit of these placements.

Nursing or Retirement Homes. A nursing home or retirement home provides experience for CSD students in working with disorders of communication that may result from strokes, accidents, illnesses, hearing impairment, or the aging process itself. Working with a primarily geriatric population affords students a special opportunity to become enlightened about the convergence of communication disorders, other health problems, aging, and all the ramifications thereof. Familiarization with the paper work associated with governmental programs such as Medicaid and Medicare and with record keeping and chart notes becomes essential in this kind of practicum setting. There are also opportunities for involvement in interdisciplinary team work and integrated patient management.

Health Maintenance Organizations (HMOs). According to many sources, the increase in health maintenance organizations (HMOs) is changing the health care system. Many individuals find HMOs attractive in terms of costs and services. However, the market for services provided by medical specialists is decreasing with the growth of HMOs, as pointed out by Foreman (1986), because HMOs focus on providers who offer services at lower costs, such as primary care physicians. Still, whether services are provided as part of a group HMO-based practice, as separate speech-language pathology and audiology units within an HMO, or as part-time consulting practices, the student can fit into the scheme in some way.

Individual or Group Medical Practice. Students in speech-language pathology and audiology who are assigned to clinical practicum in a solo or group medical practice may have different clinical experiences from those in an HMO, depending on the scope and size of the practice. Medical practices themselves vary in terms of the emphasis they place on communicative disorders. Otologists and otolaryngologists, for example, are likely to place more emphasis on these problems than are internists and pediatricians. However, more physicians are becoming aware of the importance of early identification of communication problems. Moreover, with the general population living longer, many physicians are cognizant of the vital role communication plays in the overall welfare of their patients. The availability of these kinds of settings for CSD students may be increasing, but placement decisions need to be made on the basis of the appropriateness of a clinician's available caseload, that is, on a practice-by-practice basis.

Free-Standing Units or Autonomous Private Practice. As more private practices in speech-language pathology and audiology have come into existence and their developers have become more experienced in conducting these business operations, more related opportunities have become available for students seeking real-life clinical experiences. Learning unique to these settings includes the supervisor's sharing of information about setting up a practice and about its operational aspects, thus giving students an inside perspective on a private-sector clinical practice.

Agencies. Participation in agencies, including community speech and/or hearing facilities, frequently enables students in speech-language pathology and audiology to have clinical experiences with individuals who represent a wide range of communicative disorders. Being involved in community-related activities, learning about the administrative component of an agency and, where appropriate, developing an appreciation of the role of nonprofit organizations, represent additional areas of learning for students.

Public or Private Schools. Public or private school placements offer an environment for students in speech-language pathology and audiology that is in complete contrast to a medical setting. Individuals in speech-language pathology assigned to schools work closely with the school speech-language pathologist in providing services to children with a wide range of speech, voice, language, and possible hearing problems. On the other hand, an audiology student may be assigned to work with the school's educational audiologist in conducting ongoing hearing evaluations, monitoring the amplification needs of hearing-impaired youngsters, and providing some degree of (re)habilitative services. In a school placement, the practicum student becomes familiar with forms and records used by the state department of education and the local school division—in fact, this was reported by MacLearie as early as 1947—in addition to gaining knowledge of the organizational skills necessary in working in such a setting.

Industry. An industrial setting is more appropriate as a field site for students in audiology than it is for those in speech-language pathology. In industry, the audiology student's responsibilities might include administering pre-employment baseline audiograms and conducting routine audiologic testing of employees. Providing inservice education for personnel management and employees, taking noise measurements, and administering more in-depth audiologic testing are other areas in which students in audiology might have direct involvement.

Research Settings

Research opportunities may be available in many of the same settings that offer clinical practica, including speech and hearing clinics or departments, hospitals, rehabilitation centers, community facilities, public or private schools, nursing homes or retirement centers, and private practices. Clearly, wherever the profession is practiced, research activities can be conducted. Doctoral level or research-oriented master's level students who want specific research alternatives that offer a different perspective, such as a laboratory environment, may find another university or nonuniversity laboratory appealing. In this regard, CSD educational programs might find it worthwhile to establish an exchange program with other CSD educational programs, or arrange for students to work in a nonuniversity laboratory for a designated time. Special research projects can be undertaken by students while they are learning through experience the value and efficiency of research networking and collaboration. Although such arrangements may be indicated only for certain students rather than for an entire class of students, the availability of laboratory field instruction in conjunction with an educational program appears to be warranted.

FIELD SITES AS LEARNING ENVIRONMENTS

The university individual responsible for deciding the appropriateness of specific field sites should establish guidelines regarding the facilities' professional staff, physical parameters, organizational structure, available instrumentation, service delivery, and other conditions deemed appropriate for a clinical teaching-learning experience. Indeed, facilities holding current accreditation from the Professional Services Board (PSB 1989) of the American Speech-Language-Hearing Association essentially meet all such criteria. However, PSB accreditation cannot be viewed as the single necessary criterion, given that it is not sought by all clinical facilities and, therefore, many of them may meet, or even exceed, PSB standards, regardless.

In addition, judgments about the appropriateness of a site as a teaching-learning environment must take into consideration other factors such as: the type of clinical population served relative to the program's practicum needs; the clinical modus operandi and its conduciveness to clinical teaching; the experience, both clinical and supervisory, of staff members; and the commitment of staff members to student supervision. Also, in accordance with ESB and CCC standards, all off-campus supervisors must have the appropriate CCC-SLP or CCC-A in order to supervise speech-language pathology and audiology students; that is, if the clock hours earned are to be counted toward meeting practicum requirements for the students' own certification. In selected instances, it may be desirable for a student who has already met or exceeded the minimum clock hour requirements, to observe or assist, at least during a portion of the externship assignment, non-certified individuals, for example, speech-language pathologists or audiologists (as cross professionals), teachers of the hearing-impaired, social workers, psychologists, otolaryngologists, and speech or hearing scientists. Such uncountable "enrichment" hours can complement the student's regular practicum experience.

Being personally familiar with those clinical practicum sites used routinely by an educational program is practically essential for the university coordinator who is ultimately responsible for their selection and retention. If this same individual also serves as the contact person between the educational program and the practicum site, situational changes can be monitored and accommodated as necessary. Continuity in field site planning and practicum scheduling are further assured.

STUDENT INVOLVEMENT AT FIELD SITES

The extent of students' involvement in direct service delivery at specific field sites depends, in many respects, on the composition of the client population, the prerogative exercised by the supervisor(s), and the guidelines established by the specific facility. In some circumstances, a supervisor's decision as to how much responsibility can be given to the student is related as much to these factors as it is to the student's experience with a particular disorder or population. Supervision roles relative to communication disorders work settings have been analyzed in detail by S. Farmer (1989).

Field Supervisors' Views

As indicated in the previously discussed report by Ehrlich et al. (1983), a student's readiness for certain responsibilities may be viewed differently by some field supervisors and in some field settings. The extent to which a field supervisor perceives that the facility's service delivery and accreditation reqirements may be compromised by supervision requirements apparently plays a role in this view. In a survey of Illinois audiology and speech-language pathology supervisors from university and nonuniversity settings, which was reported by Rassi et al. (1986–1987), respondents indicated, in one section, the extent of their agreement or disagreement with 11 attitude-and-concern statements. The salient findings, displayed in table I, reveal that views of the non-university supervisors in this study were not greatly different from those of university supervisors, and do not support the tenor of the Colorado report. Although the data-gathering methods were dissimilar, the contrast in findings suggests that there is a range of views, some of which are very supportive of field supervision as it currently exists.

Preparing Students for Involvement

As in any job setting, students assigned to field sites are expected to conduct themselves as professionals in dress, demeanor, and interactions with staff, clients, and peers. They should be apprised of their responsibilites in advance of their actual placement and, when possible, be given an opportunity to visit the facility and meet with their supervisor(s) before the assignment begins.

Although negative as well as positive attitudes about a specific placement are often shared among former students and those about to be assigned to a facility, it is important that new assignees begin each placement with a positive outlook. Part of a student's readiness for field placement should be his/her recognition that different client populations include persons from different socioeconomic backgrounds representing a variety of handicapping conditions, that different clinical settings vary in their accommodations and procedures, and that different supervisors have different clinical and supervisory approaches. Because it cannot be assumed that all students understand or accept these inevitabilities, the university practicum coordinator and/or other

Table I.

Attitudes and concerns of supervisors grouped according to four categories: university speech-language pathologists (SLP-U); nonuniversity speech-language pathologists (SLP Non-U); university audiologists (Aud-U); and nonuniversity audiologists (Aud Non-U); showing extent of agreement and disagreement with statements, where:

- + Agree: 67% or more agree with statement.
- − Disagree: 67% or more disagree with statement.
- = Equivocal: fewer than 67% agree and fewer than 67% disagree with statement.

Reprinted, with permission, from Rassi et al. 1986–87.

	SLP-U	SLP Non-U	Aud-U	Aud Non-U
	N = 29	N = 56	N = 16	N = 6
Before assignments are made, off-campus practicum sites should be given complete student information (e.g., previous courses and practicum assignments, outcome of student evaluations, and grades).	=	+	=	+
Off-campus practicum sites should be allowed to establish their own acceptance/rejection criteria for student placement.	+	+	+	+
Schools, hospitals, agencies, and other clinical facilities providing services in communication disorders have a responsibility to the profession to serve as off-campus practicum sites.	+	+	+	+
Quality of patient care is compromised when student supervision becomes part of a clinical operation.	−	−	−	−
Student supervision necessarily reduces the efficiency of a clinical service operation, hence costs time and money.	=	=	=	+
Off-campus practicum sites should receive monetary				

Table I—*continued.*

compensation for participating in the supervision of university students.	=	=	–	–
Off-campus practicum supervisors should receive alternate forms of compensation (e.g., tuition credits, seminar offerings, or adjunct university appointments) for participating in the supervision of university students.	+	+	+	+
A university liaison person should regularly conduct site visits at off-campus facilities where students are placed.	+	+	+	+
A contractual agreement between university and off-campus practicum facility should be completed before practicum assignment is made.	+	+	+	+
Student supervision is professionally rewarding for the supervisor.	+	+	+	+
Off-campus practicum supervisors should be given training in the supervisory process.	+	+	+	+

persons should include this kind of information when preparing students for their off-campus practicum assignments. Though specific information is sometimes better discussed individually with students, the general outline of this orientation information can be presented to them as a group. If possible, supervisors or other representatives of off-campus facilities may be brought to the university to explain their settings to students or, conversely, students may be taken in small groups to off-campus facilities for informational field trips. By whatever means, the importance of being open to new experiences and how this works to their professional and personal advantage, must be emphasized to students.

Student–Field Site Mismatching

Notwithstanding the previously mentioned matching attempts by a university coordinator in making field assignments, it is impossible to foresee all complications that might develop in conjunction with students' field placements. Just as sometimes happens in university practicum assignments, conflicts develop between students and their field supervisors, and/or other problems emerge (Rosenblum and Raphael 1987). Insofar as possible, these should be resolved at the field site by the persons involved. The university coordinator should serve as facilitator or intermediator when indicated, and should intervene or even terminate the assignment if it appears to be necessary. Taking the latter action is a last-resort option, and should be undertaken only after carefully considering all possible consequences.

Student Participation in Learning

Field-site learning, like learning in the university clinic, is influenced by the amount of the student's active participation. Students whose placements allow more hands-on involvement are likely to gain more benefit from the placement than students whose participation is restricted. Likewise, a full-time placement such as that typically arranged for an externship, affords more consistent and constant learning reinforcement than does, for example, a one-day-per-week assignment. It has been our experience that, with few exceptions, students report they "learn more" from those assignments requiring more frequent participation, for longer blocks of time.

Depending on the field setting, extra activities can help a student become involved and enhance his/her learning. In community facilities, for example, there may be occasions for students to interact with other local organizations. Involvement in their fund-raising events can be a worthwhile learning experience. Attending and presenting grand rounds and other interdisciplinary inservice presentations in medical settings is instructive. In nursing homes and retirement homes, students may be able to offer speechreading classes for patients and then participate with them in social events where they can utilize the techniques learned in class.

As in university placements, individual learning contracts may be incorporated into student field experiences, whether the clinical placement is for a school quarter, a semester, or a shorter time period. The learning contract, negotiated between student and supervisor, can be designed to allow the student to indicate the clinical areas in which he/she wishes to concentrate, the manner in which learning will be achieved, the time allotted for the learning experience, and the criteria to be used for evaluation of learning (Donald 1976; Peterson and Dyck

1986). These latter terms, of course, must conform with the university's evaluation requirements for off-campus placements. Nonetheless, an individual contractual agreement may be especially helpful in a field assignment because it provides a supervisor, who has not had the benefit of following an assigned student's clinical progress over time, with specific and current information about the student's learning needs. Conversely, it gives the student an opportunity for personal input and thus some assurance that he/she will have a role in determining the course of learning in this new, and perhaps otherwise, uncertain situation.

FIELD INSTRUCTION

The field-site instructor or supervisor plays a vital role in clinical preparation of audiology and speech-language pathology students. Individuals who contribute to the field's educational process in this capacity are not only significant teachers but usually are the first nonuniversity professional models with whom students can interact. The following discussion by Kadushin (1976) on the objective of professional training in social work seems particularly applicable to the role of off-campus, extern supervisors and of clinical-fellow supervisors in speech-language pathology and audiology. It is also a compelling statement on behalf of those who see the need in our field for more extensive clinical training over a longer period of time.

> The objective of professional training is not only to teach the knowledge, skills, and attitudes that would enable the recruit to do a competent job but also to socialize the student to the ways of the profession, to develop a professional conscience. It is the elaborate process of professional socialization, during a prolonged program of intensive training, which permits workers in all professions to operate autonomously, free of external direction and control on the basis of competence and values incorporated during training. The supervisor, is, in effect, internalized during the transformation of the lay person into a professional, and supervision does not then need to be externally imposed (Kadushin 1976, pp. 30–31).

Recruiting Supervisors

As is true in other health care fields, CSD educational programs may have difficulty recruiting field supervisors. Skolnik (1988) reports a number of possible reasons: lack of credentialed individuals who are interested; insufficient time, because of other work responsibilities; inadequate compensation (as previously discussed) or incentives offered by the educational program; lack of variety in the field site's patient population; and/or unavailable funding to support a student.

In 1981, Kahn surveyed social workers to determine their reasons for choosing to become field instructors. The three most frequently reported reasons were: the enjoyment of teaching; the learning experience related to being a field instructor; and the desire to further the profession. Some survey participants commented that supervision was one of the most interesting components of their jobs. These findings are consistent with the positive reactions of off-campus audiology and speech-language pathology supervisors to the statements displayed in table I which say that "facilities . . . have a responsibility to the profession" and "supervision is professionally rewarding . . . "

Preparing Supervisors

A number of CSD educational programs encourage their off-campus supervisors, both new and inexperienced, to participate in some form of supervisory training or preparation. In a growing number of programs, this preparation is offered by persons on the university supervisory staff in the form of group meetings, seminars, and, in some instances, coursework and/or supervision practica (ASHA 1989). The university field practicum coordinator or liaison for off-campus supervisors is usually a key person in this training effort.

As indicated in table I, supervisors in the Illinois study agreed that supervisors should receive such training. Not shown in the table is the fact that most of these same respondents indicated that the training should be provided by the universities (Rassi et al. 1986–1987). It is clearly in the university's interest to provide the training. The availability of such preparation and assistance can also be a recruitment tool.

In those educational programs where no supervisory preparation is available for off-campus people, or for that matter, for the university supervisors themselves, there should be a serious, concerted effort to make such information available to all. As discussed elsewhere in this book, there are books, articles, proceedings, and other writings available on supervision in communication disorders, along with workshops, convention sessions, conferences, and professional organizations. Continuing education opportunities in this area exist and need only to be tapped. It is up to program personnel to take advantage of these opportunities, to make them accessible for the off-campus and on-campus supervisory staff and faculty.

Administration

Agreements. The signing of formal contractual agreements between a university and a field site is sometimes required to insure that both parties are aware of their respective rights and responsibilities regarding professional liability and health insurance, coordination and evaluation of the clinical training experience, fulfillment of prerequisites for the practicum assignment, and consultation between the university coordinator and the field instructor. In those instances where neither the university nor the field site mandates this documentation, informal, oral agreements between the university practicum coordinator or the educational program director with a representative of the field site have usually sufficed. As indicated in table I, supervisors apparently favor the protection of a contractual agreement.

Compensation. Notwithstanding the previously discussed concerns about remuneration for field instruction, it is our impression that such financial compensation is not typical in CSD education. Again, as shown in table I, the majority of supervisors in this study group did not favor monetary compensation, although many were equivocal about it. All of the subgroups support alternate forms of compensation. Indeed, in both CSD and comparable disciplines, off-campus supervisors are often compensated in other ways by a university; for example, they may be awarded adjunct faculty appointments, allowed to use the university library, given discounts for the institution's bookstore, or provided opportunities to attend educational conferences (Rosenfeld 1988). In some cases, tuition credit by the university is awarded to personnel at participating sites or their individual supervisors. Some universities recognize field site instructors' contributions to the educational program through a year-end luncheon or dinner at which time a gift might also be given to each individual.

Clinical and Supervisory Processes

Clinical policies and procedures are usually well established in the field settings where students are placed. When the supervisory process is superimposed on these well-established policies and procedures, the potential for frustration and conflict exists for both clinical teacher and student, as well as for the university liaison staff person. Both the clinical and supervisory processes must be flexible and accommodating. Although service may be the field settings' priority, and clinical education the priority in a university, these priorities can be modified without being relinquished. The goal is to seek a balance between the two commitments (Nettles-Carlson et al. 1985), while being mindful of responsibilities to clients (Rassi 1978).

The supervisory process frequently needs to be adapted for a particular field setting, but the components, the sequence, and the goals can be essentially the same as those found in a university setting. When they are not, that is, when supervisory practices differ between off-campus and on-campus facilities, there are probably a variety of contributing factors. Some may be setting-specific, others may be related to individual differences in orientation to the supervisory process. All can be addressed through the preparation of students and of on- and off-campus supervisors, as discussed elsewhere.

Most, if not all, university CSD educational programs have some kind of supervision "system," that is, certain policies and rules for supervisors and students to follow: a group of forms used for goal-setting, feedback, analysis, and student or supervisor evaluation; a general framework for the scheduling and format of supervisory conferences, supervisors' meetings, and clinical conferences; and, in some programs, clinical test protocols and other guidelines for clinical decision making. That information which deals primarily with supervision can be presented to field supervisors in the form of a manual that spells out guidelines or expectations (Anderson 1988). However, those components of the system with clinical implications are not usually legitimate as university requirements for field supervisors. This unwritten rule seems to be honored by educational programs. To be sure, field sites can argue that not even supervisory requirements can be imposed on them because their time and effort devoted to the university is voluntary. To avoid potential conflict, open communication should be cultivated and contractual agreements used.

Monitoring and Analyzing Field Instruction

In addition to reviewing students' individual evaluations of a particular off-campus setting and of the supervisor(s) there, it is important for university educational programs to obtain information from other perspectives, over time, about the sites used for field instruction. Much of this task logically falls to the field practicum coordinator or university liaison person who, during site visits, telephone conferences, and supervisory training sessions, can gain valuable insight about the people and operations at field sites. Further enlightenment can come from members of the professional community who often have knowledge of the clinical reputation of persons and facilities. Because of turnover in staffs and administrations, and differing policies, the quest for updated information must be ongoing.

For purposes of monitoring and analysis, periodic meetings between the CSD program's contact person and field site instructors are extremely helpful. Face-to-face meetings are possible, of course, only for those site instructors located in fairly close proximity to the educational program. At these meetings, topics related to supervision can be discussed, as well as analysis of students' clinical performance for the current semester, and problems pertaining to specific students or situations. Telephone conferences can be arranged to maintain university contact with more distant field sites. By whatever means, regular contact between the principal parties is crucial to students' clinical experience (Hart and Falvey 1987).

Field Instructor Roles

Although the work setting and the professional orientation may differ, the audiologist or speech-language pathologist who serves as a field instructor is not unlike his/her university counterpart in the clinical education of students. However, because of the differences in setting and orientation, field-instructor roles may assume different forms or have different emphases. Some examples follow.

DeLay (1971) believes that an important part of the field instructor's role is to assist students in learning how to answer clinical questions through the utilization of resources. Indeed, field placements themselves offer a new resource from which students can draw information that will lead them to yet other resources. Another of the field instructor's roles is helping students to refine their self-evaluation skills (DeLay 1971). Because of this new and somewhat unfamiliar situation—one that challenges the student to apply skills in different and perhaps unprecedented ways—refining self-evaluation skills becomes a primary goal. Fuhrmann and Grasha (1983) charge field instructors with the responsibility of creating an atmosphere that will encourage a student's self-reliance. This is especially important, of course, in an externship scheduled in the final months of a student's graduate program just prior to graduation.

A field instructor's role as facilitator, as with any other clinical instructor, should help to build a trusting, positive relationship with the student. With this in place, an extern often seeks the field instructor's advice regarding certain aspects of the student's educational and clinical program as well as career directions and job possibilities. The field instructor's role becomes that of a mentor or career counselor which holds special meaning for the student because of the field instructor's perspective from the professional world outside the university.

Because the field instructor's association with a student typically takes place in a setting outside the university, the person who occupies the clinical teaching role may not perceive him/herself as being an educator, believing that education is confined to the university setting. This role perception, then, may determine the way in which the role is defined and carried out. When the role assumption is overlaid on a field instructor's own beliefs about clinical obligations, any unwillingness to alter well-established patterns may be difficult to change. However, change can take place with help. Field instructors can and should seek counsel from colleagues and supervisory consultants, particularly at the affiliated university. Many other available resources should also be tapped; more field supervisors need to participate in supervisors' organizations and workshops and conferences. They need to view themselves as important educators in the preparation of audiologists and speech-language pathologists. Because involvement is critical to student learning, an instructor/supervisor must have the flexibility to explore new ways of teaching (Fuhrmann and Grasha 1983), be it classroom- or clinic-related, on-campus or off-campus.

Field site instructors are critical to the clinical education of CSD students. Supervision of graduate students is a rewarding experience but, at the same time, can create problems because of the overload it causes for some site instructors (Rosenfeld 1988). Perhaps now more than ever, as the scope of practice broadens and the need for variety in practica increases, field site instruction has a vital role to play in the clinical preparation of our professions' future members. It is, therefore, essential that the rewards of teaching or supervising offset the extra work that might be involved. This is necessary to keep dedicated professionals involved in off-campus supervision and to continue attracting new professionals to it.

THE CLINICAL FELLOWSHIP

Field instruction includes the clinical fellowship in the sense that a certain amount of supervision continues, and the supervisee's clinical work usually takes place outside the university. Representing the final requirement leading to clinical certification, the fellowship typically is undertaken during the nine-month period immediately following a student's completion of the master's degree. The fellowship is a transitional experience between the preservice academic and practicum period and the independent professional years. Most clinical fellows function at a level for which consultative or upper-level collaborative supervision is most appropriate (Anderson 1988, p. 271).

Closely scrutinized and criticized over the years, the clinical fellowship has been discussed at length by, among others, those in attendence at the 1983 National Conference on Undergraduate, Graduate, and Continuing Education (Rees and Snope 1983) and by the ASHA Legislative Council (ASHA 1987). The fellowship period has survived attempts to have it abolished, but exploration for ways in which it might be improved continue. In discussions and proposals for a clinical doctorate in this field are suggestions for extensions or modifications of practica that would replace the clinical fellowship as it now exists.

As Anderson (1988) has indicated, most problems surrounding the clinical fellowship are related to matters of supervision, its quality, quantity, and availability. In a Clinical Fellowship Year (CFY) survey and subsequent convention exchange among CFY supervisors (McCready et al. 1989), a number of problems surfaced, indicating that many CFY supervisors are not well informed about the CFY itself or about supervision. The following recommendations resulted:

1. More research, publications, and presentations regarding the CFY should be done at the local, state, regional, and national level.
2. CFY supervisors should have training in the supervisory process. This can be done through formal coursework and continuing education.
3. Supervisors should be aware of, and actively participate in, supervision organizations such as CSSPA (Council of Supervisors in Speech-Language Pathology and Audiology).
4. Supervision organizations such as CSSPA should increase their efforts in information dissemination and recruitment.
5. Every supervisor and supervisee should have a copy of the (ASHA) *Membership and Certification Handbook* [1990a].
6. Every supervisor and supervisee should have a copy of ASHA's 13 tasks and 81 competencies of supervision (ASHA 1985). (McCready et al. 1989, p. 16)

Supervision of the clinical fellow, as field supervision of the practicum student, needs to be subjected to research and analysis that are unique to audiology and speech-language pathology.

SUMMARY

Placement of audiology and speech-language pathology students in off-campus or field sites for clinical practicum experience has become an integral part of clinical preparation. The university practicum coordinator is responsible for arranging field assignments and serving as a liaison with off-campus supervisors and other personnel. Students need to be prepared for field placements just as off-campus supervisors need to be prepared for the supervisory process.

REFERENCES

American Speech-Language-Hearing Association. 1985. Committee on Supervision in Speech-Language Pathology and Audiology. Clinical supervision in speech-language pathology and audiology. A position statement. *Asha* 27(6): 57–60.

American Speech-Language-Hearing Association. 1987. Legislative council report. *Asha* 29(3):38.

American Speech-Language-Hearing Association. 1989. Committee on Supervision in Speech-Language Pathology and Audiology. Preparation models for the supervisory process in speech-language pathology and audiology. *Asha* 31(3):97–106.

American Speech-Language-Hearing Association. 1990a. *ASHA Membership and Certification Handbook* (rev.). Rockville, MD: Author.

American Speech-Language-Hearing Association. 1990b. Standards for accreditation of educational programs. *Asha* 32(6/7):93–94, 100.

American Speech-Language-Hearing Association. 1991. Standards for the certificates of clinical competence. *Asha* 33(3):121–22.

Anderson, J. L. 1988. *The Supervisory Process in Speech-Language Pathology and Audiology*. Austin, TX: Pro-Ed.

Carney, M. K., and Keim, S. T., Jr. 1978. Cost to the hospital of a clinical training program. *Journal of Allied Health* 7:187–191.

Chung, Y. I., Spelbring, L. M., and Boissoneau, R. 1980. A cost-benefit analysis of fieldwork education in occupational therapy. *Inquiry* 17(3):216–29.

Cooper, E. B., Helmick, J. W., and Ripich, D. N. 1987. *1986–87 National Survey of Undergraduate and Graduate Programs*. Council of Graduate Programs in Communication Sciences and Disorders.

Cunningham, M. 1982. Admission variables and the prediction of success in an undergraduate field work program. *Journal of Social Work Education* 18(2):27–33.

Dailey, D. 1970. The validity of admissions predictions: Implications for social work education. *Journal of Social Work Education* 10(2):12–19.

DeLay, D. 1971. Preliminaries of a learning theory. In *Tough and Tender Learning*, ed. D. Nyberg. Palo Alto, CA: National Press Books.

Donald, J. G. 1976. Contracting for learning. *Learning Development* 4:2.

Ehrlich, C. H., Merten, K., Sweetman, R. H., and Arnold, C. 1983. Training issues. Graduate student externship. *Asha* 25:25–28.

Farmer, S. S. 1989. The trigonal model of communication disorders supervision. In *Supervision in Communication Disorders*, eds. S. S. Farmer and J. L. Farmer. Columbus, OH: Merrill Publishing Company.

Foreman, S. 1986. The changing medical care system: Some implications for medical education. *Journal of Medical Education* 61(9):11–21.

Fuhrmann, B. S., and Grasha, A. F. 1983. *A Practical Handbook for College Teachers*. Boston: Little, Brown and Company.

Garg, M. L., Elkhatib, M., Kleinberg, W. M., and Mulligan, J. L. 1982. Reimbursing for residency training—How many times? *Medical Care* 20(7):719–26.

Hart, G. M., and Falvey, E. 1987. Field supervision of counselors in training: A survey of the North Atlantic Region. *Counselor Education and Supervision* 26(3):204–212.

Halonen, R. J., Fitzgerald, J., and Simmon, K. 1976. Measuring the costs of clinical education in departments utilizing allied health professionals. *Journal of Allied Health* 5:5–12.

Kadushin, A. 1976. *Supervision in Social Work*. New York: Columbia University Press.

Kahn, S. L. 1981. An analysis of the relationship between social work schools and field placement agencies in their joint task of educating social workers. Doctoral dissertation, Columbia University School of Social Work.

Light, I., and Frey, D. C. 1973. Dual responsibility for allied manpower training. *Hospitals, JAHA* 47:85–90.

Leiken, A. M. 1983. Method to determine the effect of clinical education on production in a health care facility. *Physical Therapy* 63(1):56–59.

MacKinnon, J. R., and Page, G. G. 1986. An analysis and comparison of the educational costs of clinical placements for occupational therapy, physical therapy, and speech pathology and audiology students. *Journal of Allied Health* 15(3):225–38.

MacLearie, E. C. 1947. Suggestions for supervised teaching in speech correction. *Journal of Speech Disorders* 12:369–72.

McCready, V., Runyan, S. E., Farmer, S. S., Rassi, J. A., Ringwalt, S. S., and Ulrich, S. 1989. CFY supervision: A supervisors' exchange. *SUPERvision* 13(3):15–18.

Moores, B. 1979. The cost and effectiveness of nurse education. *Nursing Times* 75(16):65–72.

Morgan, W. L., Jr. 1986, September. The environment for general clinical education. *Journal of Medical Education* 61(9):47–58.

Nettles-Carlson, B., Field, M. L., Friedman, B. J., and Smith, L. S. 1985. Group faculty practice: Dreams versus reality. *Nurse Educator* 10(5):8–12.

Peterson, J. M., and Dyck, S. 1986. Systems theory facilitates student practice in self-directed learning courses. *Nurse Educator* 11(5):12–15.

Pfouts, J., and Hinley, H. C., Jr. 1977. Admission roulette: Predictive factors for success in practice. *Journal of Social Work Education* 13(3):56–62.

Pobojewski, R. T. 1978. Case study: Cost/benefit analysis of clinical education. *Journal of Allied Health* 7:192–98.

Porter, R. E., and Kincaid, C. B. 1977. Financial aspects of clinical education to facilities. *Physical Therapy* 57(8):905–909.

Professional Services Board. 1989. American Speech-Language-Hearing Association. *1989 PSB Accreditation Manual.* Rockville, MD: Author.

Rassi, J. A. 1978. *Supervision in Audiology.* Baltimore: University Park Press.

Rassi, J., Mogil, S., Bessette-Munroe, S., Murphy, B., Murphy, K., and Talbot, C. 1986–1987. Off-campus student supervision: Panel perspectives. *SUPERvision* 10(4):20–27(Summary).

Rees, N. S., and Snope, T. L. (eds.). 1983. *Proceedings of the 1983 National Conference on Undergraduate, Graduate, and Continuing Education* (Report No. 13). Rockville, MD: American Speech-Language-Hearing Association.

Rosenblum, A. F., and Raphael, F. B. 1987. Students at risk in the field practicum and implications for field teaching. *The Clinical Supervisor* 5(3):53–63.

Rosenfeld, D. J. 1988. Field instructor turnover. In *The Clinical Supervisor: Empirical Studies in Field Instruction*, ed. M. S. Raskin. New York: The Haworth Press, Inc.

Sheps, C. G., Clark, D. A., Gerdes, J. W., Halpern, E., and Hershey, N. 1965. Medical schools and hospitals: Interdependence for education and service. *Journal of Medical Education* 40(9, Pt. II):1–169.

Skolnik, L. 1988. Field instruction in the 1980s—realities, issues, and problem-solving strategies. In *The Clinical Supervisor: Empirical Studies in Field Instruction*, ed. M. S. Raskin. New York: The Haworth Press, Inc.

Wilson, S. J. 1981. *Field Instruction for Supervisors.* New York: Free Press.

SECTION III

Teaching Methods and Materials

Chapter 9

Classroom Teaching
Designing and Planning Courses

Margaret D. McElroy and Judith A. Rassi

As conscientious instructors know so well, course preparation begins long before the first day of class. This chapter is devoted to a discussion of course design and the planning of classroom teaching. In several instances, references are cited in the chapter to call readers' attention to those books considered by many educators to be definitive resources on this important topic.

COURSE DESIGN

Course design, as discussed in Chapter 3, is considered by a curriculum committee during its first deliberations on the kinds of learning experiences intended for students. Details of the design are left for the course instructor to plan.

Course Objectives

The initial step in an instructor's planning is to address the purpose of the course. Aimed at two levels, the goal is general and can be viewed as having a broad purpose, whereas the objective is more specific and exact (Westmeyer 1988). Goals can be derived from the reasons for teaching the course and the areas to be covered, whereas objectives can be met as a result of skills learned by students when the course is completed. Course content can be outlined and a list of expected skills delineated along with indicators as to how the skill or knowledge will be demonstrated.

Objectives can depict achievements the instructor wants a learner to have in order to be competent (Mager 1984) and are not unlike the competency statements referred to in Chapter 3. They should be teachable and attainable (Greive 1984), and written to describe "an instructional outcome rather than an instructional process or procedure" (Mager 1984, p. 7). Objectives can become more fully developed during actual course implementation. All subsequent course design decisions evolve from course objectives (McKeachie 1986). Westmeyer (1988) specifies three components of an adequately stated goal or objective: "the action expected of learners; the content, identification of the information expected to be learned or the skill to be developed; and statement of the level of acceptability that will let the learner move on" (p. 44). Greive (1984) recommends that no more than ten to fourteen objectives be stated and that they be "reachable" and "teachable" (p. 26).

In his publication, *Designing and Improving Courses and Curricula in Higher Education. A Systematic Approach*, Diamond (1989) gives detailed information regarding clarification of instructional objectives and assessment of outcomes. For further guidance on objectives, two classic books, developed by a committee of college and university examiners, that may be helpful to teachers representing a broad range of disciplines are: *Taxonomy of Educational Objectives. Handbook I: Cognitive Domain* (Bloom 1956); and *Taxonomy of Educational Objectives. Handbook II: Affective Domain* (Krathwohl, Bloom, and Masia 1964). Mager's book, *Preparing Instructional Objectives* (1984), also is an established model for writing course objectives.

Brinko (1991) suggests a number of goal- or objective-related questions an instructor can pose as the overall design of a course being considered. These questions are:

- What are my course goals? What do I want my students to learn primarily?
- At what level(s) do I want my students to perform?
- What class activities will help my students meet these goals and levels?
- What support will I give to my students to enhance their success in meeting these goals and levels?
- What assignments will I use to evaluate the success my students have had in meeting goals and levels?
- How much uniformity of assignments will best help my students meet these goals and levels?
- What evaluation approach will best help my students to meet these goals and levels?
- What evaluation unit for each assignment is consonant with these goals and levels?
- What type of class atmosphere will foster students' success in meeting these goals and levels?
- What kind of participation will foster students' success in meeting these goals and levels?
- What policy for class attendance will foster students' success in meeting these goals and levels?
- What pace of the course will foster students' success in meeting these goals and levels?
- What criteria will I use to determine the amount of success a student has achieved over the term?
- How will I calculate final grades for my students?
- What qualities do I expect my students to possess as they enter my class?
- What behaviors do I expect of my students while they are in class?
- What flexibility/contingencies have I planned in case my students didn't meet these expectations?
- How will I convey all of the above information to my students? (Brinko 1981, pp. 3–4)

It is helpful to students to be familiar with at least the broad-based goals for a specific course and the course requirements. This information should be given to them at the beginning of the course (Mager 1984).

Course Syllabus and Outline

The syllabus, another component of course design, comprises the course objectives, a plan of readings and activities corresponding to the dates of specific lecture topics and assignments outside the classroom, and related course information. Other items typically delineated in a syllabus are dates when assignments are due, dates of examinations or laboratory exercises, references for the course text(s) and other readings, and a list of libraries or other locations where assigned readings are available. In addition, such essential facts as course name and number; instructor's name and title; instructor's office hours; other course requirements; and the grading system should be included to establish the syllabus as the official course document. Many institutions require that course syllabi be kept on file (Greive 1984).

A second document is the course outline, which includes dates of class meetings and topics to be covered on those dates. Usually, an outline has no more than three subtopics per general topic; more detailed information can be included in lesson plans. The most typical kinds of course outlines are chronological and content or topical (Greive 1984). The chronological outline sequences classes according to some significant time element, for example, an historical or developmental sequence. The content or topical outline follows a sequence in which subject matter is presented in some kind of logical progression, for example, general-to-specific or simple-to-complex or content-related clusters.

In addition to sequencing, the pacing of course activities needs to be considered. The nature, length, and content of class assignments are incorporated into the design of a course. Regardless of the course term (for example, a compressed summer course, a school quarter or semester, or academic year in a two-part sequence), a teacher must be realistic about the time needed to cover content, projects, and other activities. Appropriate blocks of time need to be allotted for each topic, taking into account the institution's calendar, in-class discussion time, topic review, and other factors. Examination and quiz times also need to be considered in sequencing and pacing designs.

If circumstances permit, it is helpful for students to receive a preliminary schedule or outline of the dates specific topics are to be covered (Westmeyer 1988). In this way, several purposes are served. Students feel encouraged to be part of the planning before the instructor makes the schedule final. And the instructor may find that, in the students' views, time should be added or reduced for particular areas.

Moreover, a need to change the pace of the course may be revealed (McKeachie 1986). In any event, the syllabus should be made available to students the first day of class, and class time should be devoted to a discussion of the syllabus.

Another approach to describing students' responsibilities for a specific class is the use of a student manual (Diamond 1989). A manual can clarify an instructor's expectations for students' fulfillment of course requirements; enhance the proficiency of students' studying by outlining data to be addressed; decrease test anxiety by giving sample test questions; familiarize students with course details; compile a list of readings that may be difficult to find; and contain handout materials. Student manuals can be produced at a nominal cost (Diamond 1989). Copy centers offer a variety of approaches in designing such course texts comprised of entire readings, case studies, work assignments, journal articles, and lecture notes. Providing even more options, computer technology has now made possible customized textbook publishing, which includes printing information selected by a course instructor from a menu of computer databases and/or from lecture notes and other course materials. Regardless of the source, instructors must comply with copyright laws.

Planning Instruction

The type(s) of instruction to be used should be determined during course preparation. Lectures, discussion, role playing, and other approaches are all possibilities to be considered. For some courses, a combination of instructional methods is appropriate. As indicated elsewhere in this book, factors other than course objectives, such as an instructor's teaching style and even his/her personality, dictate teaching methods (McKeachie 1986).

In their book, *Teaching Techniques: A Handbook for Health Professionals,* Foley and Smilansky (1980) present seven principles of learning that they have found useful in planning instruction for health professions.

- The student should be provided opportunities to be an active rather than a passive learner.
- The student should be provided opportunities for understanding the logic underlying teaching activities.
- The student should have the opportunity to learn through a variety of educational resources.
- The student should be provided with models which serve as criteria for the expected performance.
- Until the expected level of competence is attained, students should have adequate opportunities to practice using the knowl-

edge and skills they have learned and receive feedback on their performance.
- Students should be provided with opportunities to examine ways of adapting learned knowledge and skills based upon the characteristics of a given situation.
- Overall, students should have learning experiences which are positive and satisfying rather than negative and frustrating. (Foley and Smilensky 1980, pp. 94–97)

Bases for (Re)design

In Fuhrmann and Grasha's *A Practical Handbook for College Teachers* (1983), these planning bases are recommended for consideration during design or redesign of a course: human development; creative thinking; and student and instructor skills. Each offers a distinct set of ideas upon which to design courses.

Human Development Basis. Students in communication sciences and disorders (CSD) educational programs often represent a broader age range than typical college students. Some may be new to communication disorders programs, whereas others are renewing credentials or updating their knowledge and skills. Moreover, students differ from one another on physical, cognitive, psychological, and moral levels. As individuals, they develop in a variety of ways as they are exposed to different experiences. Accordingly, teachers must be aware of various approaches to course design that accommodate these levels and promote growth.

Cognitive Development. Piaget (1947) proposed a theory that people's thinking processes change as they mature. Adults and children differ in their quantitative and qualitative thinking. Further, he theorized, people go through consistent stages that can be affected by teaching. Of interest to teachers are the stages identified by Piaget as concrete operational thinking and formal operational thinking, introduced to the reader in Chapter 2.

The formal operational stage embraces three particular thinking processes, all recognizable by teachers. First, the thinker in this category considers possibilities, thus broadening his/her ideas. Secondly, this person is capable of using "the hypothetico-deductive method to deduce from hypotheses (which may or may not be true) the logical consequence of the hypotheses as if they were true" (Fuhrmann and Grasha 1983, p. 266). Third, the thinker utilizing the formal operational stage is able to maneuver ideas, coming up with relationships that have no factual foundation. The individual who has these abilities can engage in abstract thinking.

Because not everyone achieves the formal operational stage, teachers may encounter students in their classes who pose a special teaching challenge. Students demonstrating difficulty in application, examination, synthesis, and appraisal of information probably have not attained the formal operational stage. Teachers thus need to make a special effort to foster these skills by supplementing traditional lectures with group discussions, debates, and problem-solving approaches (Fuhrmann and Grasha 1983).

Personality Development. Students' personality development is another consideration in course design. Erikson (1959, 1968) proposed that personality development occurs in a natural succession of stages, or normative crises, each of which has positive and/or negative consequences. A preponderance of positive consequences is compatible with sound personality development. The developmental implications for classroom learning are seen in students' abilities to establish an identity and in the ways in which specific courses and study formats relate to their life patterns.

Ethical Development. During the process of course design, students' ethical development should also be taken into account. Principles and responses to ethical and moral issues change over time.

Discussion of professional ethical issues as they relate to communication disorders is important in preparation of students for clinical, research, or teaching careers. Use of interactive classroom teaching methods can be especially beneficial to students as they progress in their cognitive, personality, and ethical development (Fuhrmann and Grasha 1983).

Discussion of ethical dilemmas contributes to ethical development. Because dilemmas represent circumstances in which there is no definite correct answer, students can learn to debate and defend reasons for their personal and professional choices Kohlberg (1981). At the same time, in making these arguments, students give the course instructor clues regarding the students' current stage of moral development.

Creative Thinking Basis. The proven applicability of creativity to problem solving indicates that solutions result from reflection on a number of different or alternative ideas. Attribute listing is a technique for considering alternatives. Crawford (1954) observed that new ideas derive from attributes of prevailing circumstances or, as Fuhrmann and Grasha (1983) noted, from the transposal of attributes from one circumstance to another. Crawford found that attribute listing is most effective when components of the problem are integrated to yield an innovative solution. The attribute listing process can be applied to course design, as advocated by Bergquist and Phillips (1975) in their "clock program for course design," and by Grasha (1982). Use of this method involves the following steps: listing major course attributes such as the teaching method, testing format, course materials, or time of the class; developing and elaborating on feasible alternatives to each attribute; and combining alternatives randomly, while evaluating their applicability (Fuhrmann and Grasha 1983).

Creativity is helpful not only as a mechanism for imaginative course design, but also as a thought pattern to be cultivated in students. It can be fostered through daily attempts to think of new ideas. Manipulation of thoughts, ideas, recall, facts, and information is another means for creating new ideas. Logic, not always helpful in developing ideas, can be used to refine them. Some successful inventors believe that if one states a problem, the problem can be solved more easily. Others who have been successful in creating ideas find that pausing between intense periods of thinking is just as important as the more intense periods themselves. Solutions to problems occur on occasions when "the thinker" has removed all the irrelevant factors surrounding the problem and frequently when "the thinker" takes one step at a time, not concentrating on the solution as a whole (Bertolino 1989, p. 24).

Student/Instructor Skills Basis.   Certain related categories of information are essential to course design: course objectives or goals, and the instructor and student skills needed to attain these goals; available course designs, and the instructor and student skills needed to apply each design. Readers are referred to Fuhrmann and Grasha (1983) for detailed information on a five-stage process that teachers can follow to determine the skills needed for different teaching procedures once the goals and instructor and student skills have been delineated. How to correlate the skills with different course designs is also explained.

Learning and Teaching Styles

No single teaching style or approach is entirely appropriate for all students at one time or for one student all of the time. Teachers, therefore, need to familiarize themselves with a variety of instructional methods. Many can be found in educational research reports that focus on the manner in which instructors can utilize data related to student and teacher styles.

Learning Styles.   Student learning styles stem, in part, from personality traits. Although some student personality traits have been identified, no comparative studies have been made on their relationship to student learning (Fuhrmann and Grasha 1983). On the other hand, there has been a focus on models for learning styles related primarily to "the cognitive functioning of students, the nature of the social interactions in the classroom, or the instructional preferences of students" (Fuhrmann and Grasha 1983, p. 103).

Cognitive models of learning styles stress the intellectual traits helpful to learning. As discussed in Chapter 2, two types of cognitive styles are recognized: field dependent and field independent. Insofar as professionals in the field of communication disorders must interact constantly with other individuals, they are field dependent. Field independent persons, on the other hand, are not dependent on interactions with others and tend to be more analytical. Research by Witkin, Goodenough, and Oltman (1977) suggests that recognizing these styles can be helpful in guiding students into a specific field, although neither style can be linked to satisfaction in the field selected. Teachers who are field dependent were found to have a preference for interacting with students, whereas field independent instructors seemed to lean toward a more impersonal lecture approach. Evidence has pointed to a tendency for teachers and students of the same cognitive style to like one another.

Another model of learning, this one attributed to Kolb (1976), involves four processes through which information and learning skills are acquired in an increasingly sophisticated manner: concrete experience, reflective observation, abstract conceptualization, and active experimentation. Although some persons may progress in order through these four phases of learning, others may emphasize one stage over another, depending on individual needs.

Associated with these four learning modes are four learning style clusters. The first is made up of individuals whose main aptitude for learning is abstract conceptualization and active experimentation and who are identified as *convergers*. These persons prefer specific answers and are known to act rapidly in response to a task. *Divergers*, on the other hand, tend to require concrete experience and reflective observation. Imagination is a strong trait for them, and their performance is best in creating ideas. Individuals who prefer to integrate dissimilar elements are *assimilators*. Their primary learning style is abstract conceptualization and reflective observation. *Accommodators* are risk-takers and responsive to new experiences. Their learning preference is concrete experience and active experimentation. The Kolb Learning Style Inventory is used to measure these individual learning styles (Fuhrmann and Grasha 1983; Claxton and Ralston 1978).

The Fuhrmann-Jacobs learning model (1980) is based on the place for social interactions in the learning process. This model distinguishes among three learning styles related to the classroom: the dependent style, the collaborative style, and the independent style. Although people can learn in all three styles, a particular style or circumstance may dictate a specific style.

In the Grasha-Riechmann model (1974), learning style is dependent on roles enacted by students in the classroom. How these roles are played gives clues about students' preferences for interactions with fellow students and the instructor, and about students' approaches to learning subject content. The Grasha-Riechmann model identifies six roles or learning styles that every student has in various degrees: competitive, collaborative, avoidant, participant, dependent, and independent. To measure students' use of these different roles, a two-version instrument, the Grasha-Riechmann Student Learning Style Scale, was developed. Information yielded from administering this scale can be used by instructors to adapt their instructional materials to students' learning styles. Grasha (1972) found, for example, that a more traditional lecture approach resulted in students' adoption of competitive, dependent, and avoidant styles, whereas with group or student-participation activities, students tended to demonstrate collaborative, independent, and participatory characteristics (Fuhrmann and Grasha 1983).

Teaching Styles. Fuhrmann and Grasha (1983) contend that studying teacher styles is important because of learner-instructor interactions. Studies of learning styles are more prevalent in the literature than those of teaching styles. Nevertheless, some interesting aspects of teaching styles have been noted. Axelrod (1961) sees teachers as dependent on instructive approaches, that is, giving information to, or eliciting information from, students. Adelson (1973) explored teacher concentration on self, on the course, and on the student and the student's growth. As discussed in Chapter 5, classroom teachers' roles also vary.

The Combination. An understanding of student styles and teacher styles can lead to increased classroom teaching effectiveness. Some teachers, for instance, may be interested in pairing classroom methods with individual student styles (Fuhrmann and Grasha 1983; Cross 1976). Or, conversely, intentional mismatching of teaching styles with student learning styles may be revealing. In either case, the teacher stands to be enlightened on the need to modify his or her own teaching style. The study of teaching and student learning styles can also enhance understanding of differences that exist in a teacher's relationships with some students versus those with other students. Some combinations of teacher-student styles may be more conducive to productivity than others.

Subject Matter

Good teaching requires knowledge of course content, but, according to McKeachie et al. (1986), the instructor should similarly broaden his or her knowledge for instructional effectiveness. McKeachie defines three elements of instructor knowledge: (1) sufficient familiarity with organization of course material so that concepts can be built from the simplest to the most elaborate; (2) knowledge of each class based on information being taught and the students' prior knowledge and understanding; and (3) familiarity with teaching approaches to expedite student incentive and learning.

In contemplating the types of course materials and content to incorporate into a course, an instructor should be aware that students may need to be taught how to learn and how to arrange and utilize their knowledge. In the same vein, the instructor must understand that education also involves assisting students to build confidence in themselves and their aptitudes. An instructor's role in promoting self-motivation for life-time learning is important (Editorial 1985).

Instructors should plan their courses in a highly organized fashion, taking into account the relationship of content to the aforementioned course objectives. Decisions about course content and its sequencing should be made well in advance of the beginning of a course. Armstrong (1989) favors organizational approaches to course content, for example, "the chronological approach, the thematic approach, the part-to-whole approach, and the whole-to-part approach" (pp. 78–80). Although each student brings his/her individual prior knowledge to the classroom, along with individual interests, capabilities, and expectations, an instructor must offer to all students the same course content, the same kinds of assignments, and the same methods for evaluating students' knowledge (Lowman 1984). A course designed with a broad range of goals can be helpful in addressing individuality of learners. Ericksen (1984) advocates incorporaton of such cognitive categories as factual information, performance skills, concept formulation, analysis methods, and changing values. These cognitive categories need to be adapted for each course.

Selecting Textbooks

Eble (1988) considers three major questions regarding textbooks: (1) "Which ones to use;" (2) "How to use them;" and (3) "Whether to use them at all" (p. 125). The problem of selecting appropriate texts increases almost yearly with the many texts on the market that may or may not meet an individual instructor's needs and the increased cost of texts or course materials. The cost of texts alone may dictate a teacher's decision to utilize reserve books. The first and perhaps most realistic consideration regarding text selection is whether the students are likely to read, work with, and benefit from the texts. Deciding if the instructor will augment the texts' use with other reading assignments becomes a second consideration. A third concern, related to both teacher and students, involves "learning to use the text without repeating it" (Eble 1988, p. 127). In other words, using additional materials or information during teaching rather than a text may be more effective.

One way to determine whether a text is too difficult or too easy for students is simply to ask students' opinions. Another helpful source is to consult someone who has used the text previously. Eble (1988) suggests some general guidelines in deciding about use and choice of texts: be aware of alternatives to assigned texts; experiment with ways to encourage student use of texts other than for reviews and tests; endeavor to demonstrate respect for texts while not being totally dependent on them; consider the cost and size of texts; and encourage students to obtain information beyond that available in texts (p. 129). Many publishers of textbooks offer free desk copies to university instructors.

Heye et al. (1987) describe a detailed and systematic approach to textbook selection that includes evaluation tools, evaluation criteria, methods for identifying important content areas for evaluation, procedure for selecting faculty experts to review and evaluate texts, and a data analysis method. Use of a comprehensive checksheet is another means for selecting texts (Phillips and Harman 1986). In this approach, individual evaluations are easily available to all faculty members. Questions such as these posed by Glenn and Lewis (1982) for evaluating textbooks can be incorporated into the checksheet:

1. How well does the textbook meet the goals and objectives of the course?
2. How valid is the content?
3. Does the conceptual difficulty of the text correlate with the capabilities of the students?
4. What is the readability of the text?
5. Does the text have the student practice and apply knowledge? (pp. 294–97)

In audiology and speech-language pathology, there are a number of texts geared to students, that is, with self-study guides. Examples include *Principles of Audiology. A Study Guide* by Frederick N. Martin (1984) and *ENG Workbook* by Charles W. Stockwell (1983). The *Handbook of Speech-Language Pathology and Audiology* by Norman J. Lass et al. (1989), and its companion supplement, *Study Guide for Handbook of Speech-Language Pathology and Audiology*, by Jerry L. Northern (1989), are also written for student use, although they are promoted as being good resource materials for the professional as well. These kinds of books enable students to work through the contents at their own pace.

The book, *Decision Making in Speech-Language Pathology*, by David E. Yoder and Raymond D. Kent (1988) contains algorithms that guide readers through the clinical decision-making process for various disorders. An example of an audiology textbook written in diagnostic, problem-solving format is *Auditory Disorders. A Manual for Clinical Evaluation* by Susan Jerger and James Jerger (1981). The annotated text accompanying this book augments the information presented. *Diagnostic Audiology*, edited by John T. Jacobson and Jerry L. Northern (1991), is written specifically for audiology graduate students and otolaryngology residents.

Lesson Format

Greive (1984) underscores the need to prepare lesson plans having a definite purpose, with main ideas and flexibility to accommodate current discussions. As part of an organized course design, lesson plans can be numbered and kept in a notebook. The format should include salient questions and extracts from materials that are not part of the text. Other elements of the lesson plan are definitions, remarks concerning the purposes of the course, learner activities, and teacher projects. Because a lesson plan is not constricted by institutional directive but rather is the individual expression of an instructor's work, creativity can prevail. Ideally, a lesson plan should be formatted for each class meeting.

Library Resources

A major objective in the educational process is to assist students to develop self-directed, lifelong learning skills (Saunders, Northup, and Mennin 1985). Providing students with a course bibliography, references, and/or annotated reading lists prompts them to seek information outside course texts and the classroom. This can be built into a course design. The ability to use library information to its greatest advantage can be cultivated in students through meaningful, directed course assignments, which make use of various indices, textbooks, references, audiovisual materials, and computerized access to informational networks.

The library, an important part of every student's educational program, helps students learn how to learn. In particular, the library is an essential component of a program with a problem-based curriculum. Using information gained through library resources, a student can develop a personal library or filing system that will be useful in both present and future work.

Homework and Work Assignments

Working on course assignments outside the classroom may be as meaningful to students as in-class learning experiences—perhaps more so. Therefore, homework and other class-related work assignments should be carefully planned and monitored by instructors. Instructors can help students improve study approaches by providing guidelines or offering constructive suggestions. Many students need to be encouraged by their instructor to improve study practices. Instructors should seek ideas that help students learn material more readily (Weimer 1987).

Writing a paper, long or short, on a pertinent course topic is a typical class assignment given to students in higher education. Sorrell (1989) describes effective ways for instructors to review student writing in a reasonable time. In evaluating student papers, teachers should focus on the clarity of content; how the information is organized; and how well the content addresses the needs of the person reading it. Instructors are advised to comment on at least a single strength of each paper and to give ideas for enhancing other areas. Instructors' goals should be to guide students in improving the re-draft. Offering criteria that must be met in writing papers is also beneficial to students (Wolfe and Reising 1983). In turn, these criteria will provide means for instructors to be constructive, uniform, and consistent in evaluating students' papers.

Wolfe and Reising devised a rating form (1983) to be used in evaluating student papers. In Sorrell's (1989) adapted version of this format, the "composition rating" form delineates three main areas: general (ideas, organization, appropriateness for audience); mechanical (grammar, sentence structure, punctuation, spelling); and a grading scale. Incorporated into the latter are low, middle, and high rankings for rating the composition (Sorrell 1989, p. 25).

It is often helpful for a student to discuss in advance with the instructor the outline for a paper. This approach helps the student develop ideas and generate appropriate information for the paper. Peer review can also be helpful to the writer (Sorrell 1989). Such an approach can result in cooperative learning among peers. With these approaches, instructors can view evaluating a paper as a teaching strategy (Sorrell 1989).

Workbooks can also be used in the learning process. They are utilized more frequently in laboratory teaching, but are common to other learning situations as well. There are two kinds of workbooks: practice books that contain content-associated problems to be solved, and guides to course study. Although practice books are available through publishers, guide books may or may not be accessible commercially; therefore, in some instances, instructors may have to develop an appropriate course workbook (Westmeyer 1988).

Workbooks are suitable for courses in which: content is topical rather than sequential; content is conducive to assignments that students can do actively; activities can be explained in print; pacing of the course allows students' workbook progress to match progress in class; physical space is adequate for individual and team work; the workbook can be duplicated; and students have the necessary motivation to work independently (Westmeyer 1988). Included in the workbook should be stated goals for the course, objectives for each goal, and a detailed description of activities, particularly those in the workbook, as they relate to the objectives.

Handout materials, like workbooks, may be distributed to students for homework purposes. Used also to augment information provided in a class lecture (de Tornyay and Thompson 1987), they help students to organize class notes and further serve as a reminder to students of information addressed in lecture. The use of handout materials ensures that all students have at least some of the same material.

Learning Contracts

Learning contracts between teacher and student, in the traditional sense, are implied rather than exact. In this sense, teacher and student may have definite expectations of one another and themselves, but, because of the lack of explicitness, misunderstandings, presumptions, and frustrations can result (de Tornyay and Thompson 1987). As it relates to elements of course design, the learning contract is defined as a written, signed agreement between instructor and student(s). It is exact in its identification of the expectations of all parties involved. Its emphasis on learning and not grading includes established learning objectives, resource materials, and procedures for evaluating learning (de Tornyay and Thompson 1987).

Among the basic principles identified with learning contracts (de Tornyay and Thompson 1987) are: individual students' learning styles, varied backgrounds, and distinct needs; the ability of adult students to be self-directed, creative in finding learning alternatives, and responsible for their own learning; and acknowledgement by all parties that learning constitutes a lifelong process. The independence inherent in a learning contract teaches students control over learning that will extend over their lifetime.

A number of authors have specified components important to a learning contract (Clark 1981, p. 588; Moran 1980, p. 82; Reilly and Oermann 1985, p. 132). These elements can vary according to individuals and schools, but the nucleus of learning contracts comprises objectives, activities to be performed, materials and procedures to be used, and an evaluation of results (de Tornyay and Thompson 1987). The contract develops from these key elements and additional structural factors. A time frame is also included in the contract. All individuals involved in a learning contract must sign the contract or a letter of agreement and be given a copy of the contract following the signing process (de Tornyay and Thompson 1987).

SELECTING AND PLANNING INSTRUCTIONAL DESIGN

Instructional theory should focus on the most effective techniques of learning, that is, it should relate to the identification of instruction that will optimize learning, recall, and transmission (Gagne and Dick 1983). As stressed in Chapter 5, one important instructional design factor that contributes to effectiveness is the learning environment (McCord 1985). Indeed, Jason and Westberg (1982) maintain that "the instructional setting can shape the instructional experience" (p. 84).

In the steps he considers necessary for learning, Gagne (1977) cites the following characteristics of effective instruction: obtaining attention; familiarizing the learner with the objective; inciting recall of required learning; introducing stimulus material; giving guidance for learning; evoking performance; giving feedback regarding performance correctness; evaluating performance; and enhancing memory and transmittance. Although a number of instructional models exist, research is lacking for most as they relate to higher education. One exception is the Ausubel Model of Advance Organizers (1960) which serves as a model for use in assessing classroom learning and the clinical application of that learning. Used by Ouellette (1986) with nursing students, the model emphasizes individualized student learning, accounting for different learning styles and backgrounds.

In his practical book, *Teaching Tips. A Guidebook for the Beginning College Teacher*, McKeachie (1986) provides a list of instructional methods along with possible goals for each. Regardless of the teaching approaches an instructor might select, he stresses, accompanying goals should be formulated. McNergney (1988) points out that instructional planning facilitates the following: monitoring students' progress; making the instructor feel organized; determining the successful and unsuccesful aspects of a specific teaching approach; and obtaining feedback from observers. A final factor in planning is self-confidence, which teachers must have (Hanning 1984).

Lecturing

Probably the oldest instructional method used in teaching larger groups is the lecture (de Tornyay and Thompson 1987). To be effective, the lecture should be used:

- For the development of general interest at the introduction to the main topic of the course.
- To provide additional information on a topic that is explored in detail with other teaching methods.
- To present information on a topic that is not readily available. (Grieve 1984 [paraphrased], p. 40)

Advantages of the lecture as an instructional approach include efficiency in communicating content information, minor additional preparation, relative inexpensiveness; suitability for large and small classes, and effectiveness in transmitting cognitive materials (Grieve 1984). While this instructional approach allows eye contact and can hold students' attention, the instructor must remember that attention to a lecture decreases dramatically after approximately 20 to 30 minutes, necessitating periodic breaks for listeners (Eble 1988). Currently a widely used approach in college teaching, the lecture allows an instructor to convey a considerable amount of material within a brief time (Greive 1984; Foley and Smilansky 1980). The lecture's disadvantages include its lack of variation in activity, the need for instructor and students to be familiar with the same vocabulary, and the importance of a dynamic presentation/delivery to maintain students' interest (Grieve 1984).

Eble (1988) considers the following points of advice crucial to effective lecturing:

- Fit the material to the time at your disposal.
- Seek concise ways to present and illustrate content.
- Begin each class by stimulating the interest of the audience.
- Develop an ability to improvise and to sustain an improvisational quality even in a carefully structured presentation.
- Provide the audience with frequent breathing spaces and opportunities for questions.
- Provide an ending for every lecture but maintain a continuity with what has gone before and what lies ahead.
- Develop and use a range of voice, gestures, and physical movement that is appropriate to your style, to the material, and to the occasion and that reinforces content, fixes attention, and stimulates the audience.
- Be guided by the living audience and the most pressing need of striking up discourse with as many class members as possible. (pp. 80-81)

Greive (1984) suggests a number of ways in which lecturing might be improved. Teachers, he says, should be sure they have adequate references, appropriate stories, and other such materials to augment the lecture. The lecturer's physical appearance should be satisfactory, and the lecturer should feel confident about his/her presentation. Providing cues for class participants about key points of the lecture and summarizing important lecture points can enhance and reinforce learning. Furnishing an outline of the lecture to students can be an effective teaching tool. Vocabulary used by the lecturer should be familiar to students. The lecturer can use a blackboard or other visual aids to supplement his/her presentation. Time should be allocated for student reactions, inquiries, and discussion.

Lecturing skills can be improved in many ways, and useful ideas can be found in these references: Westmeyer (1988) provides guidelines on lecture delivery; Palmer (1983) suggests videotaping a lecture and then asking a colleague in faculty development to criticize the video; Foley and Smilansky (1980) discuss audiovisual aids; and Foley and Smilansky offer helpful ideas on lecture techniques.

Direct Instruction

Instructional effectiveness can be heightened by tutoring or individual teaching. The one-to-one relationship between teacher and student can be particularly helpful to a student in acquiring skills. The biggest problem related to tutoring is the time required for working with students on an individual basis. Adhering to established office hours, working with students in small groups, or announcing particular times that specific topics will be discussed are possible ways that a teacher might address the time factor (Eble 1988).

Demonstration Methods

The demonstration instructional approach is very effective in teaching skills, especially since this approach involves both auditory and visual modes. Other advantages are: it is motivational; it fosters variety in classroom activities; and it can gain attention and be used for both group and individual learning situations (Greive 1984).

Demonstration does necessitate preparation. Simulation of the activity prior to actual presentation is helpful in foreseeing problems that may occur. The instructor can even caution students about specific problems and can solicit students' assistance in addressing the problems. Students should be made aware of demonstration objectives (Greive 1984).

Discussion Methods

Following lectures and textbooks, discussion is probably the most frequently used instructional method in higher education (Kozma, Belle, and Williams 1978). Discussion facilitates active student participation, and students' knowledge of material, techniques, and competence can be explored through the discussion format. Discussion can provide the instructor with information regarding the need for further clarification of a topic, and give students opportunities to respond to questions in the presence of peers. Another advantage of discussion is that it fosters a closer working association among students and instructor (Humphreys and Wickersham 1987). In particular, discussion can assist students in the application of theoretical concepts to practice in the clinic (Foley and Smilansky 1980).

McKeachie (1986) offers a number of suggestions for effective discussions. In one approach, a discussion period is held following a presentation. To facilitate discussion, he recommends that chairs be placed in a circle, issues for discussion listed in a location visible to each individual, and a time limit set to give everyone a chance to speak. Another discussion method that can be used following a presentation calls for the instructor to be the facilitator and the group to formulate issues to be addressed. A panel presentation can also include discussion. In this approach, a panel member gives a presentation and then questions are posed by other panel members and the class. Discussions can also be held in conjunction with role-playing activities (Fuhrmann and Grasha 1983; Brinko 1987a, 1987b). Lowman (1984) suggests that discussions of ten to fifteen minutes per class session are usually the most beneficial.

An inherent problem in the discussion approach is that some students may refrain from participating in the discussion. To remedy this, the instructor can try different tactics: using a smile to encourage participation by infrequent contributors; calling students by name to facilitate involvement by those who are more reticent; employing subtle body language or more direct means of discouraging participation by an individual who monopolizes discussion; balancing personality conflicts that develop during discussion; and interjecting instruction throughout the discussion by stating objectives, providing summaries, encouraging listening, and influencing the discussion design (Brinko 1987a, 1987b).

Seminars

In the seminar instructional approach, the student is the expert on a specific topic that he/she researches and then presents to the class. Audience members are also involved, asking questions of the presenter.

Eble (1988) believes that each participant should offer information on the presentation topic. The seminar can be effective if the content of the course consists of only one main topic or if the content can be divided into two or three main topics. The instructor's roles are confined to assigning topics, guiding research, and serving as a participant (Westmeyer 1988). In addition, the instructor should be careful to monitor discussion to maintain focus on the main topic (McCord 1985). Instructors should be cautious in carrying out the responsibilities associated with the seminar approach. Sykes (1988) believes that many teachers leave too much responsibility for the seminar to students and fail to structure the seminar as a true learning experience.

Teacher-Centered versus Learner-Centered Instruction

In teacher-centered learning, instructors are completely responsible for students' learning. The point of this approach is that students have no responsibility for structuring the learning situation. Teacher-centered learning is advantageous for instructors whose responsibilities permit only limited time to devote to teaching. Teachers can utilize lectures, seminars, and reading assignments. On the other hand, this format does not take into account differences in students' abilities, deficiencies, or understanding of new knowledge. Teachers must stay current in all areas of information being conveyed to students (Barrows and Tamblyn 1980).

In learner-centered instruction, students determine the material they should know. Instructors offer guidance in the beginning, after which students soon assume responsiblility for all aspects of learning. Students, therefore, become motivated and actively involved, making decisions related to their overall education. Disadvantages of this learning format include problems associated with the availability of resource materials, individualization of evaluation or testing procedures, a possible lack of maturity on students' parts, and different levels of facilitative and evaluative skills on the teachers' parts (Barrows and Tamblyn 1980).

Individualized Instruction

Individualized instruction has been used more frequently as differences among students have become more evident. As discussed elsewhere, the student population in CSD education, like that in other academic programs, has become increasingly diverse in age and, seemingly, in learning pace as well. Learning styles differ. "Learning style refers to the unique ways in which a person perceives, interacts, and responds to the various elements in a learning situation" (de Tornyay and Thompson 1987, p. 182). The best learning style for each student, then, is the individual student's favored method of gaining and processing information from instruction.

Learning independently should be considered a necessity if students are expected to view learning as a lifelong process, according to McKeachie (1986). He describes two forms of independent study—individual projects and small-group independent study. Independent study projects usually entail research and synthesis of data completed by one or more student. Individual and group meetings with the instructor vary according to the needs of the individuals involved and the nature of the study being undertaken.

Another form of individualized instruction is illustrated in a personalized system of instruction (PSI) developed by Keller (1968). Five major points differentiate this instruction method from other forms of teaching. Keller's "course is (1) mastery oriented, (2) student proctored, and (3) a self-paced course that uses (4) printed study guides to direct the student's learning, and (5) occasional lectures to stimulate and motivate the students" (McCord 1985, p. 110). This procedure enables students to assimilate information and to be tested at their own pace. Writing is emphasized to effect meaningful communication between teacher and student. Before going to the next unit, students must learn the preceding unit. To motivate students, lectures and illustrations are provided at the students' request. Students who did well in the course previously may be designated course proctors.

Grouping for Instructional Purposes

Team learning was developed as an instructional plan to address problems associated with teaching large classes. Students attending large classes may be passive and disinterested because of class size. Team learning allows active participation in the learning process (Michaelsen 1983). The most effective team learning appears to depend on having team members with different viewpoints and with the ability to complete activities. Instructors assign students to specific groups on the basis of individual backgrounds and needs. Because the teacher is not the focal point in team learning (Michaelsen 1983), a group assistant may be needed to develop and maintain cohesiveness in the group.

As students assume more responsibility for their own learning in the team approach, the sequence of instructional activity often differs from that in more traditional classroom teaching. Some of the logistics of group learning are the distribution and collection of materials, pacing of activities, obtaining a room of adequate size for group work, and recognizing group efforts as legitimate relative to grading (Michaelsen 1983).

Fuhrmann and Grasha (1983) point out four important requirements for effective classroom group activity: "meeting members' needs; providing norms that encourage and support interactions (teachers' conduct determines the norms of involvement); selecting an appropriate leadership style (group maturity is a factor); and designing group structures" (pp. 148–54). Specific actions should be taken to solicit comments and inquiries and to facilitate interactions among group members. Presentations can be followed, for example, by question and answer periods, discussions, group-generated agendas, panel presentations, or role-playing activities. The instructor needs to be aware that the teaching method should be compatible with the goals for the class session, the students' level of maturity, and the instructor's personal style.

A number of institutions employ a small-group tutorial in conjunction with problem-based learning. In the educational setting, the instructor is a critical factor in the success of this approach. The purpose of the tutorial group is to foster "self-directed learning, clinical reasoning and problem-solving, communication skills, self and peer evaluation, and support" (Lucero, Jackson, and Galey 1985, p. 46). Use of this approach may necessitate a change in the attitudes of some faculty members, because it focuses on student learning rather than content teaching. With this method, students learn to synthesize and apply information, resolve problems, and have meaningful interactions. The most important element in a problem-based learning program is the quality and preparation of tutors. Workshops for training tutors are encouraged (Lucero, Jackson, and Galey 1985). The majority of participants' time is devoted to independent work, away from the tutorial; from six to ten hours a week are spent in the framework of the tutorial itself. Both independent work and group discussions have been found to benefit students in selecting helpful resources (Lucero, Jackson, and Galey 1985).

Small Group Teaching in Medicine and Nursing. A working understanding of group learning is important to all instructors, especially those engaged in health care professions. Conveying this appreciation of the process to students in helping professions can also increase students' sensitivity to others and their understanding of themselves. Diekelmann and West (1981), among others, provide guidelines for implementation of this teaching approach in health care professional education. Among those in nursing education, Fontes (1987) reports positive results of a group-work teaching strategy in which students' active participation in learning was encouraged.

Boardwork

Greive (1984) emphasizes the positive effects of using chalkboard or porcelain board and encourages use of a board by the instructor as a device to motivate students and as an aid to learning. But he cautions that there are fundamental principles and purposes for board use. One should write on the board from the right side of the room to the left side for a right–hander and the opposite for a left–hander, thereby preventing the instructor's body from obstructing students' views of the written material; use the board for listings so that the instructor can periodically re-establish eye contact with the class; write material on the board that is important to remember, such as definitions, thus allowing the teacher to pause while looking at the students and stimulating questions or comments; put on the board procedures or objectives for a task; and write assignments and short quizzes on the blackboard (p. 44).

Care should be taken that writing on the board can be read from all parts of the room. Although instructors can talk while giving attention to the board, they should remember to increase the volume of their voices slightly and turn toward the class occasionally (Greive 1984). Instructors should be aware also if there is a hearing-impaired or other handicapped student who may need visual clues. Board use by the students can also be encouraged, depending on the teaching format being used.

Gaming and Simulation

In recent years, gaming has become increasingly important as an educational approach. Games, in this context, involve some form of contest or accomplishment associated with a learning goal. Their purpose in many cases is to imitate or simulate an actual problem. Regardless of the circumstances, the person planning the activity should define the teaching objectives and designate those elements that relate to the objectives (McKeachie 1986). A primary benefit of games is that they require active participation by students. Both games and simulation can be components of lectures or a teaching method in themselves (Mitchell 1982).

Many disciplines employ educational gaming. In a research study conducted by Cessario (1987), for example, a board game was found to help motivate nursing students. Hartsock and Lange (1987) developed a trivia game to expand and strengthen learning in pediatrics. Students assisted in its planning and implementation through researching and writing questions to be used in the game, designing the game board, and deciding the manner in which the game would be played. Students felt that this project served as a motivation to learning. It helped them prepare for exams and for patient care. The authors viewed the games as an instructional method to complement more traditional teaching approaches.

Simulation has specific application to the field of communication disorders because of the clinical component. This instructional approach can serve as a teaching and evaluation tool by providing experience in clinical areas where students may have fewer opportunities to develop particular skills (de Tornyay and Thompson 1987). Simulation allows presentation of real situations without danger to clients, provides repeated experience for students, gives students opportunity for feedback, and expands students' proficiency for clinical application of knowledge. In addition, students are given the opportunity to apply what they have learned, engage in critical thinking, and gain self-confidence (Boss 1985). Appropriate in both the classroom and the laboratory, simulated activities are time-efficient (Whitis 1985). In their representation of reality, simulation games permit students or learners to perceive the framework of some component of the actual world (Kozma, Belle, and Williams 1978), while promoting group learning, entertainment, and relaxation. Futhermore, simulations require students to be accountable for their own learning (Boss 1985) and require the instructor's direct involvement (Lange 1981). Duke (1986) has reviewed and compiled games and simulations adaptable to nursing education, many of which also are applicable to communication disorders education.

Written simulations, also directly applicable to our field, can be designed to present students with clinical problems related to patient management. Through this activity both the instructor and learners can become more aware of clinical decisions that need to be addressed in a clinical setting. At specific junctures in the written simulation, for instance, the teacher-writer offers decision options which, in turn, increase the teacher's awareness of the option best suited to a situation or perhaps the realization that there is no best decision (Jason and Westberg 1982).

Another form of simulation designed as a prelude to clinical practicum, and discussed further in Chapter 11, is the simulated patient. In this arrangement, an ordinary person, an actor, or a patient with medical problems is trained to depict a real patient. If the training is carefully done, a skilled clinician will have difficulty differentiating this person from a real patient. An advantage of this simulation is that "the patient" can provide information to the learner regarding the learner's interpersonal abilities or professional bearing (Barrows 1985; Norman et al. 1985).

Role Playing

Role playing, another activity that encourages learning and student involvement, is most effective when used as a course component or as a method to augment course presentations. Role playing does not involve rules and competition as do simulation games. Among the many possible types of role playing situations are: explanations of problems with no single correct answer; student characterizations of actual or imagined individuals; and instructor characterizations of actual or imagined individuals (Fuhrmann and Grasha 1983).

Debriefing, an important element of role playing, allows examination and interpretation of conduct (Kozma, Belle, and Williams 1978). The presented problem, rather than the role player, should be evaluated. In addition, de Tornyay and Thompson (1987) point out the helpfulness of videotaping the simulated activity for purposes of accurate recall on the observers' parts. Westmeyer (1988) advises that learners be assigned roles but that a person not be coerced to assume a role he/she does not want to assume; that the individual playing a role not have the personality of the person he/she is playing; that goals be limited; and that role playing be confined to short time periods, no longer than five to ten minutes. McKeachie (1986) recommends that instructors avoid presenting problem situations that might resemble those experienced by students in the class.

Group and Individual Projects

Although teachers acknowledge the merit of group projects, many do not assign them because of concern that projects do not fit easily into an instructional mode. Nevertheless, if group projects are planned, instructors are well advised to follow these guidelines: assign tasks that are specific to a particular group; limit the number of students in a group to no more than seven; specify definite time periods for project work; and state a definite objective(s) for use of the group's findings (Weimer 1988b). Projects can be instructionally advantageous by leading students to learning experiences outside the classroom. Moreover, if properly designed, projects can be directed toward the interests of individual students.

Margolius and Duffy (1989) used a student-project teaching approach to promote creativity in patient care by nursing students. These authors' reflections on the educational value of this effort are captured in the following words, which seem especially relevant to the concerns of CSD educators:

> How do we encourage students to think beyond traditional boundaries and learned limitations? How do we help students to feel autonomous in a profession in need of autonomy? Perhaps the answer is simply to free our minds from previously established constraints and, in discrete but planned stages, provide educational opportunities to creatively promote a clear balance between the science and art of nursing (p. 32).

If, as Torrance (1975) asserts, students are versed in conventional approaches to patient care but recognize when these methods are not adequate, then instructors' fostering of students' creativity through project assignments is a worthwhile educational pursuit.

Guided Design. While learning, students need to combine data, ideas, and rationale with new information so that they can make decisions related to problems with which they will be confronted. Guided design, a classroom teaching process developed to assist engineering students in acquiring decision-making skills (Wales and Stager 1977), uses a structured problem-solving approach that enables students to learn not only the substance of course content but also how to explain problems, formulate solution options, and choose responses (de Tornyay and Thompson 1987). This approach to the study of course material and its application to professional tasks focuses on student projects rather than on subject matter given by the instructor to the student in a more traditional manner.

Activities for a guided-design course are arranged around a number of organized projects that students work on during class. Open-ended problems are presented instead of more conventional course material. Problem designs require students to manipulate the subject material they are learning, while the instructor's prepared printed data direct the decision-making process for groups of four to eight individuals. This teaching method allows students to be active participants in their learning, while, at the same time, they are given prompt evaluations of their cognitive abilities (de Tornyay and Thompson 1987).

Learning Modules

A method of individualized, self-contained learning that has become more prevalent in recent years is the learning module, referred to in Chapter 3. This individualized instruction mode centers on a single topic with explicit objectives. A crucial component of learning modules is independent study, which enables the student to determine the time and place for learning. The actual design of a module dictates the individualization of the learning setting. Whatever the design, the module should be integrated in terms of objectives, procedures, and assessment (de Tornyay and Thompson 1987).

The components of a learning module typically include a table of contents to specify sections and pages; an introduction concerning the module's purpose, the value of material to be studied, and the manner in which one can move through the module; a listing of prerequisites and suggested resources; detailed learning objectives for the module; a pretest that reflects the learning objectives; a listing of resources to assist in attaining the objectives; learning activities for use in mastering the objectives; progress self-checks to give the student prompt feedback about his/her progress; a posttest to ascertain if the student has met the learning objectives of a particular module; and, usually, a request for the students' impressions concerning the module (de Tornyay and Thompson 1987).

As an integrated learning system, the module can be put into use for any subject in any setting. In addition, its flexibility allows application for part of a course, a whole course, or an entire curriculum. It is also useful for remedial teaching or review of information previously learned. Although there are many advantages to using a learning module, instructors should be aware of potential disadvantages. These include a student's inability to manage self-study; failure of students to take responsibility for their own learning; difficulty in maintaining updated information for the module; and insufficient learning resources (de Tornyay and Thompson 1987).

Problem-Based Learning

The Principle and the Process.   Learning in the field of CSD, as in medicine, involves the acquisition of basic science knowledge and clinical skill. Medical educators report that there is minimal evidence, however, that students' actual knowledge corresponds to their clinical competence (Wingard and Williamson 1973). It is therefore incumbent upon educators, whether in medicine or in CSD, we believe, to emphasize the clinical application of knowledge.

Subject-based learning can be designed for a group, an individual, or it can be self-paced. This approach can be teacher- or student-centered but, because the learning of a particular subject is emphasized, memorization of information is required, and learners are typically not exposed to problem situations. The advantages of this method are that the subject determines the boundary points of student learning, resource materials are readily available, and instructors feel assured in identifying material for students to learn. Moreover, subject-based learning has proven effective, and the assessment of students' recall poses no problem. On the other hand, learners in this mode are not being required to integrate newly learned information with that in other subject areas. In the absence of such integration, the transfer to clinical application is unlikely to occur.

Problem-based learning derives from striving to solve a problem. It focuses on a problem related to a patient, to health delivery, or to research. Acquiring a unified body of material associated with the problem and applying skills of problem solving are the two educational objectives. Problem-based learning is compatible with student-centered learning as well as with teacher-centered learning. In the latter, teachers designate the problem, the topics of study, and the resources pertinent to the problem (Barrows and Tamblyn 1980).

The advantages of problem-based learning for students are evident. Working with a problem allows for the integration of information, ideas, and aptitudes that can be utilized with current and future problems. Skills in clinical reasoning and problem solving emerge. However, students must discipline themselves to work with difficult problems that may defy their skills development. In addition, concentration on clinical assessment and management may be detrimental to the acquisition of facts and of in-depth knowledge in the basic sciences and, further, may constitute an inefficient learning approach. Barrows and Tamblyn (1980), in their book, provide ways to lessen these possible consequences.

Adopting the Approach. Problem-based learning can be embedded in the curriculum in various ways. Depending on content, laboratory and classroom courses can provide appropriate opportunities for assigning problem-solving exercises, or an elective course in problem-based/self-directed learning might be offered. Because instructors must be familiar with this teaching-learning mode before they engage in it, faculty workshops and resource development sessions are necessary. Studies have shown that the time required for teachers to serve as facilitators of a problem-based learning class is approximately six hours a week. Both faculty and administrative support are, therefore, essential. In addition, students' schedules must be sufficiently flexible to accommodate meeting times for implementation of their self-study plans (Barrows and Tamblyn 1980).

Identifying Problems for Study. As a first step in determining the problems to be addressed in a problem-based learning format, faculty members representing a specific curriculum area can list the course information and skills they consider essential for students to learn (Barrows and Tamblyn 1980). Next, instructors select patient problems that correlate with the first list. In another approach, which can be used to transform an existing course into a problem-based format, instructors generate a list of problems related to course topics, then select those with related clinical features. At the same time, instructors should be certain that the selected problems will direct students into separate major subject areas of the course (Barrows 1985; Barrows and Tamblyn 1980).

Constructing Problem-Based Learning Units. The design of problem-based learning units should include patient simulations that will require students to develop clinical reasoning skills and to engage in self-directed study. These units should also foster self-assessment skills while allowing instructors to evaluate students' performance in reasoning, knowledge, clinical application, and self-study efficiency (Barrows and Tamblyn 1980).

Just as in real life, any simulation should not provide all the data required to solve the problem (Elstein et al. 1972). In that instructional media are an important component of the problem-based learning approach, they should be carefully selected (Barrows and Tamblyn 1980).

The basic organization of a problem-based learning unit, according to Barrows and Tamblyn (1980) involves:

- Identification of the objectives of the session
- Interaction with the patient problem
- Identification of self-study questions raised by work with the problem
- Self-directed study
- Application of acquired information back to the problem
- Review and synthesis of what has been learned
- Evaluation (p. 71)

Ongoing evaluation of a unit's instructional value is extremely important. Both positive and negative information about a unit should be weighed by the instructor, particularly during any experimental phase of this approach (Barrows and Tamblyn 1980).

Clinical Reasoning. An awareness of the problem-based learning process as it involves clinical reasoning relative to patient problems facilitates self-directed study and further clinical reasoning (Barrows and Tamblyn 1980). A group of four or five students, an instructor, and a simulated patient can be combined to illustrate the clinical reasoning skills associated with problem-based learning. It is essential that the group have definite objectives for the specific learning experience, that the group recognize there are no right or wrong answers associated with this learning approach, and that group members work in a cooperative spirit.

The simulated patient is interviewed by students, the findings are discussed during frequent breaks to assess components of the reasoning process as it develops, brainstorming about possible hypotheses is pursued, and the entire process is evaluated. Self-directed learning occurs when students become aware of areas in which they may be deficient (Barrows and Tamblyn 1980). Other formats can be used to facilitate clinical reasoning. A patient's or client's actual problem, for example, can be introduced to individuals who are studying the clinical process.

Clinical reasoning is the cognitive process involved in assessment and management of medical problems. Barrows and Tamblyn (1980) describe a model having five steps for teaching clinical reasoning to physicians and students in the health care professions. At each step, the thinker must employ clinical reasoning in order to move on to the next one.

Step 1—Perception or observations by the physician or clinician of a number of patient cues

Step 2—Generation by the physician or clinician of two to five hypotheses as possible reasons for the patient's problem based on the physician's or clinician's past experiences

Step 3—Refinement of early hypotheses by use of possible patient interviews or evaluations and utilization of scan questions or specific data gathering

Step 4—Accumulation of data as patient contact continues

Step 5—Decision is made by clinician that no further data are available; notes are made of significant data (pp. 22–30)

Critical Thinking. Fundamental to clinical reasoning is the ability to think, and teachers have a responsibility in each course they teach to cultivate students' thinking. Making sound clinical judgments and being proficient in decision making, both essential skills for all professionals in health-related fields, can be fostered through critical thinking. According to Paul (1989), "When students are adept at thinking critically, they are adept at gathering, analyzing, synthesizing, and assessing information . . ." (p. 2). Indeed, each of these abilities is vitally important to the clinical process. As stated by Malek (1986), "stimulation of the thinking process becomes the essence of clinical instruction" (p. 20). Specific suggestions for fostering critical thinking in the classroom have been cited by Meyers (1986):

- Begin each class with a problem or controversy
- Use silence to encourage reflection
- Arrange classroom space to encourage interaction
- Wherever possible, extend class time
- Create a hospitable environment (pp. 61–67)

The instructor must establish an atmosphere conducive to the kind of interactions that facilitate critical thinking; that is, where imaginations are stimulated and new ideas encouraged (Demetrulias and Shaw 1985). McMillan's *Enhancing College Students' Critical Thinking: A Selected Annotated Bibliography of Resources* (1985) is a helpful resource for instructors who recognize the need to improve their skills in teaching critical thinking.

Clinical Problem Solving. The combination of clinical reasoning and critical thinking logically culminates in clinical problem solving, another thinking process to be nurtured in the classroom as well as in the clinic. In either setting, students can be involved in data collection, evaluating and assembling findings, developing management plans, and assessing results (Foley and Smilansky 1980). Again, as participants in this process, classroom instructors, like clinical instructors, are responsible for creating environments that encourage student problem solving and provide instructive feedback. The use of carefully formulated and sequential questions related to clinical experience is one means of facilitating problem solving (Foley and Smilansky 1980). In addition to simulated experiences in the classroom, an instructor can also use computer applications, case presentations, and role playing to teach clinical problem solving.

Boyd and Diekelmann (1981) have devised a model, based on cognitive behaviors, for teaching problem solving to students in primary care medical education. Described as "a comprehensive system that accounts for the major cognitive processes" (p. 72), their model emphasizes differentiating, structuring, integrating, abstracting, and generalizing. Nehring, Durham, and Macek (1986) describe an adaptation of Pridham, Hansen, and Conrad's Paradigm of Problem Solving (PPS) for teaching interpersonal problem solving in primary care settings. Both approaches could be adapted for use in speech-language pathology and audiology education. Also, in our field are available resources (e.g., Slosson Educational Publications 1988, 1989) on cognitive skills testing that can be useful to individuals in learning or teaching problem solving.

Presentation of Patient Problems.   In problem-based learning, problems must be accessible to students for study, while their presentation should contribute to development of clinical reasoning skills. More traditional presentations available to students in the medical profession have been real-life patients and written case histories or studies. Although real patients definitely motivate students in the learning process, their use has disadvantages: appropriate patients are not available consistently; patient variables can be a matter of contention; and students in training may not be sensitive to the patient (Barrows and Tamblyn 1980). Written case histories may contain the necessary information about a particular patient and his or her medical problems, but students do not have the benefits of interview, examination, and personal interactions.

In many case-study teaching formats, the student cannot exercise clinical reasoning unless there is an opportunity at specific stages to make decisions prior to reading the next segment of the case. However, in an investigation (Johnson and Purvis 1987) of case studies used with nursing students, faculty and students responded positively to the approach, reporting that decisions could be made in "controlled situations"

(p. 119). Moreover, the students believed they gained insight into problems they might not have encountered in a laboratory setting. Analytical skills that students used to make clinical decisions also improved.

Medical educators have discovered additional ways to circumvent some of the difficulties encountered with typical presentation formats. Variations of both traditional and non-traditional approaches include: having patients available on demand; using printed case histories; employing simulated patients; delineating patient management problems (PMP) or sequential management problems (SMP) that present a picture of the patient to the student, giving options from which to select for subsequent inquiry; adopting the P4, a card format allowing students to choose among actions that would be usable with real patients, or using computer formats (Barrows and Tamblyn 1980).

Implications for Education.   Problem-based learning allows elements of clinical reasoning to be discerned by instructors and students. For educational purposes, clinical-reasoning components can be arranged into the following distinctive behaviors for evaluation and learning (Barrows and Tamblyn 1980): "information perception and interpretation; hypothesis generation; inquiry strategy and clinical skills; problem formulation; and diagnostic and/or therapeutic decisions" (pp. 39–55).

CONSIDERING TEACHING STRATEGIES

Following selection and planning of course and instructional design, instructors need to consider specific ways in which teaching strategies will be applied. Some of the key underlying factors are discussed in this section.

Determining Set

The word *set* denotes a response pattern that influences a person to examine a problem in a pre-established way. (This is addressed again in Chapter 11 in a discussion of clinical observation.) Hyman (1964) defines *set* in this context as an attitude of intellect and arrangement of facts. Those facts eliciting set in the learner are referred to, in learning psychology, as set induction. The idea of set induction suggests that actions pre-existing a learning activity will affect the consequence of that action. The motivation to learn is related to set induction. Arousal, expectancy, and incentives, three concepts determined by De Cecco and Crawford (1974) to be associated with motivation, can be helpful to teachers in motivating students to learn. More detailed information about the relationship of these factors to the learning process can be found in de Tornyay and Thompson (1987).

Bearing in mind that these are matters of influence, instructors might incorporate some of the following strategies into the first class meeting to relieve students' initial anxiety about the course and, not incidentally, to influence students' set. Information about the instructor can be handed to students along with the syllabus, then explained. Students can be asked to share thoughts they associate with the main words from the title of the course, or their expectations about the course. In the same vein, the instructor can recall some of his/her own reflections when he/she took the course as a student (Weimer 1988b). A positive, stimulating experience on the first day of class can help to shape a student's motivation for the duration of the course.

Explaining and Clarifying

Explaining and clarifying are integral components of teaching, and clear communication is essential to effective teaching. If messages communicated in either direction do not include definitions and descriptions understood by both the instructor and students, the information may be confusing or meaningless. Models, examples, analogies, illustrations, comparisons, anecdotes, and other such devices are often required so that the information conveyed by an instructor to students is more easily conceptualized and understood.

The explanation of technical, scientific information, such as typical material in speech-language pathology and audiology courses, often requires considerable forethought on the part of the instructor. Indeed, students' understanding of difficult concepts may depend directly on an instructor's ability to translate phenomena into understandable language. Although textbooks and other printed information, along with computerized graphic illustrations, may serve the purpose of clarification, it is the instructor's responsibility to ensure that course content is understood.

Applying Reinforcement

Reinforcement is a potent strategy in teaching. Reinforcers—"anything that strengthens behavior and increases the probability of its occurrence" (de Tornyay and Thompson 1987, p. 3)—may include recognition, tangible rewards, learning activities, school responsibilities, status indicators, verbal and written incentives, and personal activities (Tosti and Addison 1979). Only those reinforcers actually related to learning performance will motivate students to learn (de Tornyay and Thompson 1987).

Questioning and Listening

Asking questions, an important instructional strategy, can be used to ascertain whether students have comprehended basic information, to assist students in understanding relationships between concepts, and to enable students and the teacher to investigate ideas jointly (de Tornyay and Thompson 1987). Questions have been categorized and investigated in many different ways. In a simple, three-way classification according to instructional purpose, these types of questions emerge—factual, clarifying, and higher-order. Factual questions, relying on memory or description, involve the recall of previously obtained information. Clarifying questions require more than recall, seeking additional information or asking for justification of the response (de Tornyay and Thompson 1987; Far Western Laboratory for Educational Research and Development 1969). Higher-order questions are more complicated. To answer these, students must generalize, reason, or categorize (de Tornyay and Thompson 1987), deduce, synthesize, or hypothesize, thereby leading to critical thinking.

In using questioning as a classroom teaching strategy, the instructor should "set the focus" (de Tornyay and Thompson 1987) to confirm the subject to be addressed and to keep students' attention on the topic. Greive (1984) emphasizes that teachers should frame questions using discrete vocabulary levels and timing. He points out some of the advantages in employing questions as an impetus for class discussion: "stimulation of thought; arousing curiosity; stimulating interest; development of student confidence in expressing himself/herself; determination of student progress in the class; reinforcement of previous points; and evaluation of the preparation of the student" (p. 42). Greive has found that directing questions to the class as a whole and then "readdressing" the question to a member of the class is helpful in giving students sufficient preparation time to think through their responses.

Whether an instructor is listening to a student's response or to a student's volunteered opinion, comment, or observation, the instructor must be an interested and attentive listener, showing respect for the speaker and the message. Gordon (1974) calls this "active listening" and considers it to be crucial to successful class discussion. As in question-asking, an instructor's timing is a factor in listening, in this case allowing the student time not only to formulate ideas and statements but also to expand on them, and giving other students the opportunity to engage in discussion.

Mackey and Appleman (1988) and Wenk and Menges (1985) are helpful references on the use of questions in teaching.

Attaining Closure

When the objectives of a course have been met, the instructor is responsible for effecting closure. The reciprocal to set induction, this final phase bridges new knowledge to knowledge learned in the past. Three strategies that help students achieve closure are suggested by Allen and Ryan (1969): reviewing and summarizing topics; applying new information to examples in order to assist students in organizing recently acquired information; and expanding new information to unfamiliar circumstances to aid in the students' transfer of knowledge. It is appropriate to have orderly closure on a unit or course of study before proceeding to a new topic (de Tornyay and Thompson 1987).

LABORATORY INSTRUCTION
AS AN ADJUNCT TO CLASSROOM TEACHING

Courses may require laboratory meetings for the demonstration and learning of specific skills such as those needed in clinical procedures, research experiments, observation, and data collection, or of multistep problem solving, practice exercises, and the like. These meetings, usually described as "labs," may occur during regularly scheduled class periods or in extra sessions, either in a classroom or other appropriate location such as the clinic or scientific laboratory. Scheduling labs in conjunction with a course gives students additional time and opportunity to become active participants in their own learning, to ask questions, and to interact with classmates as well as the instructor. Often, the instructor or aides serve as facilitators, allowing students to work as independently as possible.

The Clinical Lab

The lab supplement to classroom teaching can serve as a bridging activity between coursework and clinical practicum. In learning to administer diagnostic tests for both speech-language pathology and audiology, for example, students can practice the procedures in laboratory activities, testing classmates or other persons. Videotaping practice sessions, followed by self-, peer-, and instructor critiques can be conducted via lab assignments. As appropriate software becomes increasingly available, self-practice through computer programs can now be carried out with a whole new array of lab teaching activities. Clearly, educational lab opportunities will continue to increase with new technological developments. Educators have an obligation to keep current in this area just as they do with classroom teaching. Lab activities can be as varied and enriching as is an instructor's ability to be creative.

Teaching labs ought to play a prominent role in audiology and speech-language pathology education, given the discontinuity that so often occurs between classroom study of clinical matters and actual practice in the clinic. It is not uncommon for students to be inadequately prepared for their initial practicum assignments, thus causing them undue anxiety and requiring more teaching and modeling by clinical supervisors. Preclinical practice labs can remedy many of these clinic-classroom "gap" problems. A number of approaches, combining laboratory and clinical teaching strategies, are suggested in Chapter 11. However, it should be noted that lab teaching activities are just as important as classroom teaching. The lab teacher, either solely, or in combination with the clinical supervisor, must provide bridging activities that link theory with practice.

Health professions education literature offers a number of examples on the use of teaching labs, also reported in the clinical discussions in this book. For instance, a preclinical laboratory experience, named "Mock Hospital" (Cowan and Wiens 1986), enabled nursing students to gain extensive prepracticum supervised experience in different phases of patient care. In this two-step lab program, each student learned to perform specific skills on peers and, then, after demonstrating competence in these areas, each student participated in the Mock Hospital that had community volunteers acting as patients. Results of this experiment indicated that student nurses' anxiety regarding patient care decreased and their competence in interacting with patients increased. Moreover, videotaping lab activities enabled nursing students to evaluate their own clinical performances. Patient input also proved to be valuable to subsequent discussion of the clinical situations.

The Research Lab

The connection between classroom teaching and related instruction in the scientific laboratory is obvious. (See Chapter 10 for a detailed discussion.) In some instances, this kind of lab instruction is akin to workbook instruction in that both may have a guide format (Westmeyer 1988). The course textbook may include a laboratory guide or the instructor can prepare a guide. On the whole, laboratory instruction motivates students. Westmeyer (1988) emphasizes the need for closely related lab instruction and course content. In addition, students should be advised of the manner in which their laboratory activities will be judged.

Skill Lessons

As in most health care professions, educational preparation in audiology and speech-language pathology involves teaching and learning specific skills necessary to the profession. Indeed, students' psychomotor or hands-on skills (Foley and Smilansky 1980) are principal elements of practical examinations to determine the performance levels of graduates in many of these fields. Results of skill assessments, in turn, can serve as a guide for future educational program planning.

Although all classroom, lab, and clinical instructors should contribute to students' orderly acquisition of psychomotor skills, it is the lab instructor who is usually responsible for basic skill development. In carrying out this task, the instructor should give students an overview of the objectives, methods for learning the skill, and procedures for evaluating performance (Foley and Smilansky 1980). Richardson (1969) has described psychomotor skills "as manipulative skills that require the learner to perceive and coordinate sensory stimuli to complete purposeful movements" (de Tornyay and Thompson 1987, p. 60).

In the psychomotor domain, instructor demonstration of a specific skill, either live or videotaped, is followed by a student's learning through guided practice. Skill mastery is often not achieved until the student has had numerous practice opportunities, hence this final step may not occur during the learning phase, but after.

Other skills, appropriately taught first in a practice lab environment, are the interpersonal, interviewing, and counseling skills needed by health professionals, including speech-language pathologists and audiologists. Here, the continuity from classroom to lab to clinic is crucial and, thus, is a major consideration for curriculum planners as well as clinical instructors. These cooperative endeavors are discussed in the curriculum and clinical chapters of this book. The important point here is that lab instruction is a vital link in teaching these skills, and in many CSD programs, this link appears to be missing or inadequate. (See articles cited in Chapter 3.)

Other fields provide information on teaching these skills through practice. Sklare, Portes, and Splete (1985), for example, provide guidelines for teaching effective questioning in counseling with application in our field. Block and Coulehan (1987) describe the use of a module, mentioned earlier in this chapter, as a lab tool for teaching students skills in detecting the main problem of an interview. This instructional strategy makes students aware that the origin of the problem may be the client, the interviewer, or both individuals. In addition, the module helps students recognize that obtaining accurate information is the primary purpose of a patient interview.

Maintaining Clinical Focus

Insofar as the application of classroom theory to the clinical setting is problematic, Volcek and Nelson (1986) state that maintaining a clinical focus is the key to relating theory in the classroom to practical application. The two authors delineate the following main purposes of clinical focus: "to identify student objectives for the clinical experiences; to unify the approach by faculty members applying classroom theory in the clinical setting; to direct the selection of learning experiences; and to promote self-directed learning by the student" (p. 34). Presumably, lab activities are instrumental in achieving these ends. In addition to being beneficial to the student, the maintenance of clinical focus in clinically related courses promotes a cooperative spirit and working relationship between teaching faculty and clinical faculty.

Duban and Kaufman (1985) endorse a clinical skills course as a means of transition between theoretical concepts and practical applications. This kind of course, they say, reinforces the relationship of basic sciences to the students' clinical reasoning processes and the clients' clinical evaluations. Students are given opportunities to become more aware of the clients' needs through role playing and other classroom and lab activities. Finally, this bridging effort offers an opportunity for collaboration between classroom and clinical faculties.

Many instructors in audiology and speech-language pathology do teach clinically related courses, but whether these courses include teaching of skills through classroom or lab activities is less certain. In a study of course design in ESB-accredited educational programs within our field, Rassi and McElroy (1989) found that 34 of the 49 examined courses reportedly had clinical content. Twenty-nine required projects or homework assignments, 16 required clinical observations, and 10 required laboratory participation in conjunction with the course. Among the 21 special course features reported were the use of guest lecturers, including patients as well as professionals; taking a field trip; role playing; administering tests; and collecting clinical data. Although these findings are somewhat encouraging, they may not be representative of all clinical courses in the field.

PLANNING ASSESSMENT OF STUDENTS' LEARNING

Assessment of students' learning takes various forms. Tests should be given for purposes of learning, motivation, and measurement. Eble

(1988) also stresses the importance of giving students feedback on their test performances and considering novelty in test design. References on the design of tests include Copperud (1979), Ebel and Frisbie (1986), Gronlund (1982), and Walsh (1985). The use of tests in education has been addressed by Levy (1984).

Jason and Westberg (1982) studied ways in which medical school faculty members evaluate students. Fundamental differences between responses of basic science teachers and clinical teachers were found. (Clinical teachers involved in medical education typically do their teaching in classrooms as well as in clinics.) Basic science teachers appear to stress conventional, prompt results, such as the type yielded by national board exams, whereas clinical teachers emphasize the need for "more long-term, career-linked outcomes" (p. 108). A marked contrast between basic science instructors and clinical teachers was also shown on a number of other study items. Multiple-choice questions, essay questions, and laboratory student observations, for instance, are used more often by basic science teachers. Clinical instructors, on the other hand, more frequently rely on observations of students in patient-care settings, on written simulations, feedback from students, oral exams, and contributions to class discussion. In discussing the results of their study, the investigators commented that students' critical thinking abilities cannot be facilitated effectively by most multiple-choice examinations. Jason and Westberg (1982) state that students' contributions in class are important indicators of their level of understanding; of the degree of keenness in their thinking; of their capability in applying knowledge to problem solving; and of their overall competence.

Evaluating students' knowledge through the use of examinations administered by nationally recognized testing agencies or boards such as the National Board of Medical Examiners for medical students and the National Teacher Examinations (NTE) Programs of the Educational Testing Service for speech-language pathologists and audiologists constitutes a distinctly different approach from university examinations. Designed for purposes of certifying or licensing individuals for professional practice, these comprehensive tests provide a set of scores and a basis for equating schools or programs. This type of testing typically stresses the importance of factual information at the possible sacrifice of evaluating necessary elements of clinical performance. It, therefore, has limitations. Nevertheless, examinations of this nature provide information for the public, for governmental facilities, and for accrediting agencies about the common knowledge base of members of a particular profession. Whether or not professional competence can be measured or predicted by these examinations is debatable and, thus, the subject of controversy and the object of research.

Selecting Types of Tests and Examinations

Classroom instructors have a wide array of tests from which to choose, ranging from group tests to individual tests in a variety of formats. Each yields different kinds of information and/or serves different purposes. A selected number are described here.

Practical and Performance Examinations. Practical examinations or performance tests (Corley 1981; McGuire 1983), particularly applicable to the clinical professions, can be administered in several ways. Some are analyzed in Chapter 11 relative to their application by a supervisor in a clinical setting. From the classroom instructor's perspective, these and other approaches can also be used. Oral simulations, for instance, can be conducted with the instructor and student in a simulated setting where the student is asked by the instructor to respond to a set of questions and/or perform a series of fact finding activities. Immediate oral feedback and/or delayed written feedback can be given. Oral simulations can be used to require the student to solve real or hypothetical patient management problems in which a number of options exist. Role playing, another form of oral simulation, is extremely versatile in that it can be used not only to demonstrate, model, or teach, but also to evaluate a student's interpersonal clinical skills.

Because all types of oral examinations employ an approach that requires the student to give oral responses to specific questions or problems, they are most appropriately used for assessing problem-solving abilities and clinical reasoning skills. This format can be stressful (Muzzin and Hart 1985). Notwithstanding its anxiety-producing nature, the opposite effect can be achieved, as shown in a study conducted by Rassi (1988), where audiology students reported an increase in self-confidence following an interactive practical examination. Furthermore, as a result of this examination, students reported learning about their specific competencies and achievement levels which, in turn, led to perceptions of increased self-evaluation skill.

Written simulations include a problem-solving process that allows exploration of a specific order of questions and data to lead students to draw conclusions about diagnosis and management. Again, answers can be given orally, allowing an exchange of ideas between the examiner and student, and/or students can be required to perform certain tasks, making this another type of performance examination.

Written Examinations. Each instructor can construct examinations to suit individual learning needs of students and instructional objectives of a particular course, so there are probably as many variations in written exams as there are instructors. Those exams used frequently enough to compose a test category are mentioned below. Examinations are discussed in more detail in Chapter 10.

Projective testing techniques are those involving tasks or problems that require constructive thought on the part of the student, and can be presented in written and oral form. Essay examinations, the oldest written examination format and commonly used in the university classroom, are subjective in nature and, therefore, unreliable for scoring purposes. However, these exams, if constructed properly, require the recollection of information, organization of thoughts, and effective expression—useful information in evaluating students' abilities to synthesize information and make judgments (Greive 1984; Douglas, Hosokawa, and Lawler 1988). Open-ended examinations also include questions that give students opportunities to use their own ideas in addition to those generated by the course.

Recall tests are used infrequently at the college or university level, but there are some advantages to this test format including the simplicity of its construction and grading; the allowance for questions covering broad or diverse content; and the requirement of definitive recall by students (Greive 1984). Short-answer tests, designed to examine recall of factual information, can be constructed in two different formats: one contains questions or statements that require, respectively, a brief response or sentence completion; the other asks for the association or matching of two words or phrases (Douglas, Hosokawa, and Lawler 1988).

True-false tests, although a matter of concern regarding objectivity and validity, have proven to be useful in specific situations, for example: when a number and variety of questions need to be asked; when time and simplicity are factors; when only two answers are possible; and when the instructor wishes to give an easily scorable test (Greive 1984; Douglas, Hosokawa, and Lawler 1988). Objective, multiple-choice tests, popular among many educators in higher education, are difficult to construct but easy to score and demand reasoned thinking by students. Verbal reasoning tests are examinations that require students to arrive at a conclusion through deduction or induction.

External or open-book examinations, usually comprehensive in nature, allow students to obtain information from outside sources, but demand resourcefulness, selectiveness, organization, integration, and other such skills that need to be cultivated. A library search can be evaluative as well as instructive. Student-generated questions from which the instructor selects items can be incorporated into examinations. Experiential tests can be administered following a lab demonstration by asking questions about specific concepts related to the experience. Computer-managed testing—a broad category—includes all of the aforementioned testing formats and myriad others, the number and variety of which are limited only by the ingenuity of instructors.

Evaluating Problem-Based Learning. The Clinical Reasoning Test Module (CRTM), as described by Barrows (1985), is a problem-based learning tool used to evaluate objectively a student's clinical reasoning. The evaluation is based on an unfamiliar problem or a simulated patient task presented in a series of workbooks. A challenge to their reasoning ability, the exam requires students to make initial hypotheses, pursue the inquiry strategies, determine more feasible hypotheses, recommend suitable diagnostic tests, and then make a final hypothesis based on the test results. The exam has a scoring system and can be administered even by clerical staff. Another feature of the CRTM is its ability to assess students' self-directed study. In a notebook, students summarize the information they have learned and evaluate their accomplishments. Should the instructor feel that further information is needed, multiple-choice questions or modified essay questions can be administered following the students' completion of the CRTM (Barrows 1985).

Among the multiple-assessment methods used in evaluating problem-based learning is the use of clinical stations (Harden et al. 1975). These can be self-assessment units with a simulated patient and videotape player located in a clinical examination room. Patient problems presented for solution allow students to evaluate their own problem-solving abilities by making videotaped comparisons of their performances (Barrow and Tamblyn 1980).

Other Assessment Methods. In addition to examinations, other methods for gathering data and assessing outcomes can be used. Several are mentioned here because they can also be used in conjunction with the laboratory sections. For instance, anecdotal reports can be used to study and report student behaviors. As pointed out in the clinical chapter, however, great care must be exercised to make this kind of data collection objective. Rating scales, whether numerical or descriptive, allow a more exact method for recording behavioral changes, though they still rely on an evaluator's subjective judgment. Checklists requiring yes-no or present-absent judgments are useful in determining whether skills have been acquired. Self-assessments in which students note their own progress are also applicable to the class-lab situation (Fuhrmann and Grasha 1983).

Jason and Westberg (1982) have pointedly reminded educators that tests or examinations represent only one component of evaluation. Indeed, they refer to an objective test as "an event, which may or may not be part of a fully formulated, ongoing process" (p. 166).

Constructing Tests and Examinations

Valid test construction, regardless of format, is not an easy task. Anderson's (1972) review of exams from a research perspective revealed that they generally do not adhere to a major measurement principle, that is, defining what is to be measured. Even the obvious measurement objective—to assess knowledge about course content—can be interpreted differently from one instructor to another. Carmichael and Caldwell (1988) note that testing should be planned at the same time an instructor is outlining a course. In other words, tests should evolve from lesson plans.

In his classic work, Bloom (1956) advises instructors to design tests that evaluate the learning effects or results deemed important. He classifies learning outcomes in the following sequential order: knowledge, comprehension, application, analysis and synthesis, and evaluation. Accordingly, Fuhrmann and Grasha (1983) suggest that teachers follow these guidelines in selecting examination content:

- Determine the factors of the content to be measured, perhaps looking at Bloom's classifications relative to course information.
- Plan a chart or outline for exams on the basis of desired learning results.
- Inform students of the learning results that have met the class objectives.

Items requiring students to engage in intuitive thinking during test taking are recommended by Blomquist (1985) for inclusion in evaluations administered to nursing students. Layton (1985) suggests that item analysis be undertaken after test administration in order to determine if any test elements need to be revised.

Oral Examinations. Construction of oral examinations is based on their purpose and varies according to type. If the exam is not a practical or performance one, but rather an oral version of what could be a written essay examination, the design does not necessarily need to be different. Its advantage over a comparable written exam is that the instructor has the opportunity to ask students for elaboration or clarification of answers.

Design of those oral exams that are practical in nature may focus on integration of theory and application by presenting questions and situations requiring students to diagnose, formulate a treatment plan, solve a clinical or research problem, or explain operational procedures. If the exam is consistent and uniform, exact phrasing of questions is strictly followed by the instructor or other test administrator. If, on the other hand, it is to be interactive and consequently more subjective, such as allowing dialogue between the tester and student, standardization is precluded. Such an exam cannot be planned entirely in advance because much of the questioning is contingent upon students' answers. When an oral examination is performance-based, items are obviously task-oriented, requiring the student to demonstrate a clinical or research procedure. Performance tests also can be standardized or individualized.

As already indicated, oral examinations can pose problems in reliability and validity. An examiner's personal prejudices and biases can affect phrasing of questions and interpretation of answers. If examiners who give oral examinations were trained, say Barrows and Tamblyn (1980), some of the problems associated with this evaluation tool might be controlled better, and this has been borne out in supervision research.

Essay Examinations. Essay examinations should be clearly written, answerable within the allotted time, and challenging to the student. As suggested earlier, they should require answers that depend on thinking processes rather than just memory (Fuhrmann and Grasha 1983). Furthermore, this type of test should demand organization and creativity on the part of students (Barrows and Tamblyn 1980).

Within the realm of essay exam construction is the modified essay question, described by Knox (1980) as "an account of a series of events in the evolution of a case study, narrated as they occur" (p. 20), and designed specifically to test students' problem-solving abilities that foster the problem-based learning approach. In this combined oral-written format, explicit questions are asked by the instructor at regular intervals, requiring brief written responses. As used in medical education, a real patient is the basis for this form of exam. Diagnostic and management problems usually make up the content. Although this test form needs more research, Neufeld (1985) sees it as a workable procedure for evaluating clinical competence.

Multiple-Choice Tests. Fuhrmann and Grasha (1983) suggest that these guidelines be followed in devising multiple-choice questions: take more than one sitting to write the questions; write the stem first, the correct response second, and distractors last; and use index cards to write the questions. Cherry (1989) reported that, in a workshop on creating tests (sponsored by the Northwest Regional Educational Laboratory), suggestions about formulating multiple-choice items include avoiding double negatives and making certain that only one response is correct. Greive (1984) recommends that the following points be considered in formulating multiple-choice questions: have four possible responses; exclude implausible answers; do not use "none of the above" and "all of the above"; be consistent regarding punctuation and other elements; do not use qualifiers such as "usually" and "always";

write questions in a positive format; and have all statements similar in length. A more extensive checklist for assessing multiple-choice tests from a different perspective has been compiled by Ory (1983).

Barrows and Tamblyn (1980) stress that the multiple-choice format presents difficulty in assessing problem-based learning and clinical reasoning. Likewise, Neufeld and Norman (1985) indicate that its validity as a test for clinical competence in medicine is limited to the "clinically relevant knowledge" element. They say that this particular test's best features are its efficiency in grading and providing direct feedback to students and teachers, and its suitability for educational research.

Problem-Based Evaluations. In deciding the individual skills or behaviors to be assessed in problem-based learning, an instructor should look at the competencies previously identified as instructional objectives. By definition, the problem-based learning approach requires that both clinical reasoning skills and technical skills be assessed (Barrows and Tamblyn 1980). Interpersonal skills are included in both of these areas.

Because evaluation is considered an essential component of the overall learning process, students should be given verifiable feedback concerning their progress, and specific learning needs should be identified. Because the objective of self-directed learning is to make learning an integral part of a student's professional life, it is important that students be able to use the evaluation instruments. Evaluation design for problem-based learning should incorporate a self-assessment component, giving students insight into their own knowledge and helping them differentiate the "when and how" (Barrows 1985) of using skills they have learned. Similarly, the instructor can look at students' skills in assessing themselves by posing specific, related questions to determine student's aptitude for generalizing and synthesizing information during problem-solving (Barrows and Tamblyn 1980).

Grading Coursework

The use of grades in the educational system has been well established, although grades are not necessarily good predictors of performance in later life (Eison 1980). From a different perspective, grades serve as motivating forces for students.

Grading Criteria and Calculation. Classroom instructors should establish a solid basis for grading. In the interest of instructor accountability, criteria for grading should be specific, logical, and defensible. Greive (1984) suggests the following guidelines in grading format:

- Communicate to students early in the course the grading criteria to be used, allowing time for student response.

- In addition to test scores, use other grading criteria such as class participation and projects.
- Do not use irrelevant factors such as tardiness and class absence as grading criteria.
- Give careful weighting to criteria established for grading.
- Use students' own achievement of course objectives (criterion-referenced) for determining grades rather than comparing their performances with those of other students (normative-referenced).

Fuhrmann and Grasha (1983) and McKeachie (1986) also recommend that instructors be cautious in using normative-referenced grading, that is, grading on the curve, because of problems with the normal distribution of ability. In addition, Weimer (1988c) emphasizes that grading on the curve can create strong competition among students. Lowman (1984) urges instructors not to force grades to fit quotas or theoretical expectations.

An instructor will find it helpful to develop an evaluation plan in the form of a chart or worksheet, indicating the weighted percentage assigned to various factors and points for each factor such as completion of outside assignments and laboratory work. Whether or not students' participation in class should be graded is a topic of controversy (Weimer 1988a). In group learning situations, it is advisable to have a grading system that recognizes group performance. Students' responsiveness to other students should be taken into account also (Bouton and Garth 1983).

Carter (1977) stresses that objectivity, reliability, mastery of content, and flexibility are necessary elements of all grading systems. The conventional mode of averaging test scores, according to Fuhrmann and Grasha (1983), may result in imprecise assessments of some students. They suggest that classroom instructors consider other possibilities to supplement conventional grades, such as contract grading, student-assigned grades, students grading each other, and descriptive feedback. Eble (1988) advocates giving a number of grades during a course, believing that students can benefit from varied kinds of evaluation carried out frequently. He stresses the use of regular feedback as a means of guiding the instructor and students in identifying students' needs.

Essay examinations are more difficult to grade than many other forms of tests because of their subjectivity. McKeachie (1986) offers these guidelines to instructors in grading essays:

- Read all or several of the examinations in a preliminary fashion to establish some notion of the general level of performance.
- Write models of excellent, good, adequate, and poor papers to which you can refer to refresh your memory of the standards by

which you are grading. This technique is particularly useful if an assistant is helping to grade or if grading is carried out over a period of time.
- Establish a set of grading criteria.
- Give a global grade—not several subgrades which are summed. Your overall impression is likely to be more reliable than the sum of grades on such elements as content, organization, originality, etcetera.
- Read essay exams without knowledge of the writer.
- Do your grading in teams (if you use an assistant). (pp. 102–103)

Giving Feedback on Performance. Giving students feedback lets them know their course standing. Educators seem to agree that frequent feedback is important. Accordingly, Fuhrmann and Grasha (1983) compiled a list of ten basic feedback principles, displayed with an accompanying rating scale of 1 to 7, where 1 means "never," 3 means "hardly ever," 5 means "fairly often," and 7 means "always." This rating scale can be self-administered by instructors. Fuhrmann and Grasha (1983) recommend that items with a rating of 4 or below constitute areas the course instructor may wish to refine.

1. _____ I try to give feedback to students based on how well their performance met the objectives and standards of the course.
2. _____ I try to be as specific as I can when giving feedback.
3. _____ I try to give feedback as soon as possible.
4. _____ I try not to be evaluative when giving feedback.
5. _____ I try to give positive feedback frequently.
6. _____ I try to give feedback only when I am sure a student wants it.
7. _____ I ask students what behaviors they would like feedback on.
8. _____ I check my feedback to make sure that it was heard.
9. _____ I give feedback to the person who should get it.
10. _____ I personally model giving and receiving feedback in my own behavior. (pp. 179–82)

In situations involving feedback to members of groups in team-learning classes, conflicts can develop more readily than in settings involving individual students. Members of team-learning classes are supportive of one another and may be more likely to disagree with an instructor. When disagreements occur in conjunction with test performance, the instructor can address the problem by offering "an ideal" answer to the test question or discuss the matter within the group. Usually, a confrontation can be avoided (McKeachie 1986).

SUMMARY AND CONCLUSION

Designing and planning courses is a multistep process requiring a number of decisions. Course design entails writing objectives, preparing a syllabus, and planning instruction. Learning and teaching styles should be considered along with selection of textbooks and planning of lesson formats. Classroom instructors have a wide range of instructional modes and teaching strategies from which to choose. Whatever is used, it is important that clinical reasoning, critical thinking, and/or clinical problem solving be among the primary instructional objectives in appropriate CSD courses.

REFERENCES

Adelson, J. 1973. *The University Teacher as Artist*. San Francisco: Jossey-Bass.

Allen, D., and Ryan, K. 1969. *Microteaching*. Menlo Park, CA: Addison-Wesley.

Anderson, R. C. 1972. How to construct achievement tests to assess comprehension. *Review of Educational Research* 42:145–70.

Armstrong, D. G. 1989. *Developing and Documenting the Curriculum*. Boston: Allyn & Bacon, Inc.

Ausubel, D. P. 1960. The use of advance organizers in learning and retention of meaningful verbal material. *Journal of Educational Psychology* 51:267–72.

Axelrod, J. 1961. The teacher as model. *The American Scholar* 30:395–401.

Barrows, H. S. 1985. *How to Design a Problem-Based Curriculum for the Preclinical Years*. New York: Springer Publishing Company.

Barrows, H. S., and Tamblyn, R. M. 1980. *Problem Based Learning. An Approach to Medical Education*. New York: Springer Publishing Company.

Bergquist, W. H., and Phillips, S. R. 1975. *A Handbook for Faculty Development*. Washington, DC: Council for the Advancement of Small Colleges.

Bertolino, C. E. 1989. Secrets of creativity. *Chicago Life, Spring*, p. 24.

Block, M. R., and Coulehan, J. L. 1987. Teaching the difficult interview in a required course on medical interviewing. *Journal of Medical Education* 62(1):35–40.

Bloom, B. S. (ed.). 1956. *Taxonomy of Educational Objectives. Handbook I: Cognitive Domain*. New York: Longman, Inc.

Blomquist, K. B. 1985. Evaluation of students. *Nurse Educator* 10(6):8–11.

Boss, L. A. S. 1985. Teaching for clinical competence. *Nurse Educator* 10(4):8–12.

Bouton, C., and Garth, R. Y. (eds.). 1983. *New Directions for Teaching and Learning: Learning in Groups* (no. 14). San Francisco: Jossey-Bass.

Boyd, R. D., and Diekelmann, N. L. 1981. Problem solving with students. In *Approaches to Teaching Primary Health Care*, eds. H. J. Knopke and N. L. Diekelmann. St. Louis: C. V. Mosby Company.

Brinko, K. T. 1987a. Getting it going: How to initiate a discussion. Unpublished manuscript. Appalachian State University, Boone, NC.

Brinko, K. T. 1987b. Keeping it going: How to facilitate a discussion. Unpublished manuscript. Appalachian State University, Boone, NC.

Brinko, K. T. 1991. Visioning your course: Questions to ask you as you design your course. *Teaching Professor* 5(2):3–4.

Carmichael, H., and Caldwell, M. 1988. Evaluation. In *Guide to Classroom Teaching*, ed. R. McNergney. Boston: Allyn & Bacon, Inc.

Carter, K. R. 1977. Student criteria grading: An attempt to reduce some common grading problems. *Teaching of Psychology* 4:59–62.

Cessario, L. 1987. Utilization of board gaming for conceptual models of nursing. *Journal of Nursing Education* 26(4):167–69.

Cherry, S. 1989. Writing a good test part science, part art. *Chicago Tribune, School Guide*, pp. 2, 6.

Clark, T. F. 1981. Individualizing education. In *The Modern American College*, ed. A. W. Chickering. San Francisco: Jossey-Bass.

Claxton, C. S., and Ralston, Y. 1978. *Learning Styles: Their Impact on Teaching and Administration*. AAHE-ERIC/Higher Education Research Report No. 10. Washington, DC: Association for Higher Education.

Copperud, C. 1979. *The Test Design Handbook*. Englewood Cliffs, NJ: Educational Technology Publications.

Corley, J. B. 1981. Simulation principles and techniques in the evaluation of student performance. In *Approaches to Teaching Primary Health Care*, eds. H. J. Knopke and N. L. Diekelman. St. Louis: C. V. Mosby Company.

Cowan, D., and Wiens, V. 1986. Mock hospital: A preclinical laboratory experience. *Nurse Educator* 11(5):30–32.

Crawford, R. P. 1954. *Techniques of Creative Thinking*. New York: Hawthorne Books.

Cross, K. P. 1976. *Accent on Learning*. San Francisco: Jossey-Bass.

De Cecco, J. P., and Crawford, W. R. 1974. *The Psychology of Learning and Instruction* (2nd ed.). Englewood Cliffs, NJ: Prentice-Hall.

de Tornyay, R., and Thompson, M. A. 1987. *Strategies for Teaching Nursing* (3rd ed.). New York: John Wiley & Sons.

Demetrulias, D. M., and Shaw, R. J. 1985. Encouraging divergent thinking. *Nurse Educator* 10(6):12–17.

Diamond, R. M. 1989. *Designing and Improving Courses and Curricula in Higher Education. A Systematic Approach*. San Francisco: Jossey-Bass.

Diekelmann, N. L., and West, D. A. 1981. Primary health care education: A group process approach. In *Approaches to Teaching Primary Health Care*, eds. H. J. Knopke and N. L. Diekelmann. St. Louis: C. V. Mosby Company.

Douglas, K. C., Hosokawa, M. C., and Lawler, F. H. 1988. *A Practical Guide to Clinical Teaching in Medicine*. New York: Springer Publishing company.

Duban, S., and Kaufman, A. 1985. Clinical skills: Enhancing basic science learning. In *Implementing Problem-Based Medical Education. Lessons from Successful Innovation*, ed. Kaufman. New York: Springer Publishing Company.

Duke, E. S. 1986. A taxonomy of games and simulations for nursing education. *Journal of Nursing Education* 25(5):197–206.

Ebel, R. L., and Frisbie, D. A. 1986. *Essentials in Educational Measurement* (4h ed.). Englewood Cliffs, NJ: Prentice-Hall.

Eble, K. E. 1988. *The Craft of Teaching* (2nd ed.). San Francisco: Jossey-Bass.

Editorial. 1985. Editorily speaking. *Journal of Chemical Education* 62(10):821.

Eison, J. 1980. Grades: What do they tell? *Teaching-Learning Issues* 10(43):3–26.

Elstein, A. S., Kagan, N., Shulman, L. S. Jason, H. and Loupe, M. J. 1972. Methods and theory in the study of medical inquiry. *Journal of Medical Education* 47(2):85–92.

Ericksen, S. C. 1984. *The Essence of Good Teaching*. San Francisco: Jossey-Bass.

Erikson, E. H. 1959. Identity and the life cycle. *Psychological Issues* 1(1):25–30.

Erikson, E. H. 1968. *Identity, Youth and Crisis*. New York: Norton.

Far Western Laboratory for Educational Research and Development. 1969.

Handbook for Minicourse III: Effective Questioning in a Classroom Discussion. Unpublished manuscript. Berkeley, CA.

Foley, R. P., and Smilansky, J. 1980. *Teaching Techniques: A Handbook for Health Professionals.* New York: McGraw Hill Book Company.

Fontes, H. C. 1987. Small group work: A strategy to promote active learning. *Journal of Nursing Education* 26(5):212–14.

Fuhrmann, B. S., and Grasha, A. F. 1983. *A Practical Handbook for College Teachers.* Boston: Little, Brown and Company.

Fuhrmann, B. S., and Jacobs, R. 1980. *The Learning Interactions Inventory.* Richmond, VA: Ronne Jacobs Associates.

Gagne, R. M. 1977. *The Conditions of Learning.* New York: Holt, Rinehart & Winston.

Gagne, R. M., and Dick, W. 1983. Instructional psychology. In *Annual Review of Psychology*, eds. M. R. Rosenzweig and L. W. Porter. Palo Alto, CA: Annual Reviews.

Glenn, A. D., and Lewis, V. J. 1982. Analyzing the textbook to improve student reading and learning. *Reading World* 21:294–97.

Gordon, T. 1974. *T.E.T.: Teacher Effectiveness Training.* New York: Peter H. Wyden, Publisher.

Grasha, A. F. 1972. Observations on relating teaching goals to student response styles and classroom methods. *American Psychologist* 27:144–47.

Grasha, A. F. 1982. *Practical Applications of Psychology.* Cambridge, MA: Winthrop.

Greive, D. 1984. *A Handbook for Adjunct and Part-Time Faculty.* Cleveland: Info-Tec, Inc.

Gronlund, N. E. 1982. *Constructing Achievement Tests* (3rd ed.). Englewood Cliffs, NJ: Prentice-Hall.

Hanning, R. W. 1984. The classroom as theater of self: Some observations for beginning teachers. *Association of Depts. of English Bulletin* Spring.

Harden, R. McG., Stevenson, M., Downie, W. W., and Wilson, G. M. 1975. Assessment of clinical competence in using objective structured examination. *British Medical Journal* 1(2):447–51.

Hartsock, J. M., and Lange, R. H. 1987. Trivia games: Stimulating student learning. *Nurse Educator* 12(1):24–27.

Heye, M. L., Jordan, L. E., Harden, J. T., and Edwards, M. J. 1987. A textbook selection process. *Nurse Educator* 12(1):14–18.

Humphreys, W. L., and Wickersham, B. (eds.). 1987. *A Handbook of Resources for New Instructors at UTK (University of TN at Knoxville).* Knoxville, TN: University of Tennessee, Learning Research Center. (ERIC Document Reproduction Service No. ED 289 440.)

Hyman, R. 1964. Creativity and the prepared mind: The role of information and induced attitudes. In *Widening Horizons in Creativity*, ed. C. W. Taylor. New York: John Wiley & Sons.

Jacobson, J. T., and Northern, J. L. (eds.). 1991. *Diagnostic Audiology.* Austin, TX: Pro-Ed.

Jason, H., and Westberg, J. 1982. *Teachers and Teaching in U. S. Medical Schools.* Norwalk, CT: Appleton-Century-Crofts.

Jerger, S., and Jerger, J. 1981. *Auditory Disorders. A Manual for Clinical Evaluation.* Boston, MA: Little, Brown and Co.

Johnson, J., and Purvis, J. 1987. Case studies: An alternative learning/teaching method in nursing. *Journal of Nursing Education* 26(3):118–20.

Keller, F. S. 1968. "Goodbye, teacher . . . " *Journal of Applied Behavior Analysis* 1(1):79–89.

Knox, J. D. E. 1980. How to use modified essay questions. *Medical Teacher* 2:20–24.

Kohlberg, L. 1981. *The Philosophy of Moral Development: Essays in Moral Development*. New York: Harper & Row, Publishers.

Kolb, D. A. 1976. *The Learning Style Inventory: Technical Manual and Self-Scoring Test and Interpretation Booklet*. Boston: McBer and Company.

Kozma, R. B., Belle, L. W., and Williams, G. W. 1978. *Instructional Techniques in Higher Education*. Englewood Cliffs, NJ: Educational Technology Publications, Inc.

Krathwohl, D. R., Bloom, B. S., and Masia, B. B. 1964. *Taxonomy of Educational Objectives. Handbook II: Affective Domain*. New York: David McKay Company.

Lass, N. J., McReynolds, L. V., Northern, J. L., and Yoder, D. E. (eds.). 1989. *Handbook of Speech-Language Pathology and Audiology*. Philadelphia: B. C. Decker, Inc.

Lange, C. M. 1981. Constructing simulations. In *Approaches to Teaching Primary Health Care*, eds. H. J. Knopke and N. L. Diekelmann. St. Louis: C. V. Mosby Company.

Layton, J. M. 1985. Item analysis for teacher-made tests. *Nurse Educator* 10(4):27–30.

Levy, P. 1984. *Tests in Education: A Book of Critical Reviews*. London: Academic Press.

Lowman, J. 1984. *Mastering the Techniques of Teaching*. San Francisco: Jossey-Bass.

Lucero, S. M., Jackson, R., and Galey, W. R. 1985. Tutorial groups in problem-based learning. In *Implementing Problem-Based Medical Education. Lessons from Successful Innovations*, ed. A. Kaufman. New York: Springer Publishing Company.

Mackey, J., and Appleman, D. 1988. Questioning skill. In *Guide to Classroom Teaching*, ed. R. McNergney. Boston: Allyn & Bacon, Inc.

Mager, R. F. 1984. *Preparing Instructional Objectives* (rev. 2nd ed.). Belmont, CA: David S. Lake Publishers.

Malek, C. J. 1986. A model for teaching critical thinking. *Nurse Educator* 11(6):20–23.

Margolius, F. R., and Duffy, M. M. 1989. Promoting creativity: The use of student projects. *Nurse Educator* 14(2):32–35.

Martin, F. N. 1984. *Principles of Audiology. A Study Guide*. Austin, TX: Pro-Ed.

McCord, M. T. 1985. Methods and theories of instruction. In *Higher Education: Handbook of Theory and Research, Vol. 1*, ed. J. C. Smart. New York: Agathon Press, Inc.

McGuire, C. H. 1983. Evaluation of student and practitioner competence. In *Handbook of Health Professions Education*, eds. C. H. McGuire, R. P. Foley, A. Gorr, R. W. Richards, & Associates. San Francisco: Jossey-Bass.

McKeachie, W. J. 1986. *Teaching Tips: A Guidebook for the Beginning College Teacher* (8th ed.). Lexington, MA: D. C. Heath and Company.

McKeachie, W. J., Pintrich, P. R., Lin, Y., and Smith, D. A. F. 1986. *Teaching and Learning in the College Classroom. A Review of the Research Literature*. Ann Arbor, MI: National Center for Research to Improve Postsecondary Teaching and Learning, University of Michigan.

McMillan, J. H. 1985. *Enhancing College Students' Critical Thinking: A Selected Annotated Bibliography of Resources*. Richmond, VA: Center for Educational Development and Faculty Resources. Virginia Commonwealth University.

McNergney, R. 1988. Planning. In *Guide to Classroom Teaching*, ed. R. McNergney. Boston: Allyn & Bacon, Inc.

Meyers, C. 1986. *Teaching Students to Think Critically*. San Francisco: Jossey-Bass.

Michaelsen, L. K. 1983. Team learning in large classes. In *Learning in Groups*, eds. C. Bouton and R. Y. Garth. San Francisco: Jossey-Bass.

Mitchell, P. D. 1982. Simulation and gaming in higher education. In *New Directions for Teaching and Learning: Expanding Learning through New Communication Technologies* (no. 9), ed. C. K. Knapper. San Francisco: Jossey-Bass.

Moran, V. 1980. Facilitating self-directed learning. The role of the staff development director. In *Self-Directed Learning in Nursing*, ed. S. S. Cooper. Wakefield, MA: Nursing Resources.

Muzzin, L. J., and Hart, L. 1985. Oral examinations. In *Assessing Clinical Competence*, eds. V. R. Neufield and G. R. Norman. New York: Springer Publishing Company.

Nehring, W. M., Durham, J. D., and Macek, M. M. 1986. Effective teaching: A problem-solving paradigm. *Nurse Educator* 11(3):23–26.

Neufeld, V. R. 1985. Written examinations. In *Assessing Clinical Competence*, eds. V. R. Neufield and G. R. Norman. New York: Springer Publishing Company.

Neufeld, V. R., and Norman, G. R. (eds.). *Assessing Clinical Competence*. New York: Springer Publishing Company.

Norman, G. R., Barrows, H. S., Gliva, G., and Woodward, C. 1985. Simulated patients. In *Assessing Clinical Competence*, eds. V. R. Neufield and G. R. Norman. New York: Springer Publishing Compay.

Northern, J. L. (ed.). 1989. *Study Guide for Handbook of Speech-Language Pathology and Audiology*. Philadelphia: B. C. Decker, Inc.

Ory, J. C. 1983. *Improving Your Test Questions*. Measurement and Evaluation Division, Office of Instructional and Management Services, University of Illinois at Urbana-Champaign.

Ouellette, F. 1986. Facilitating classroom learning: The Ausubel Model. *Nurse Educator* 11(6):16–19.

Paul, R. W. 1989. *The Ninth Annual & Seventh International Conference on Critical Thinking & Educational Reform* (Brochure). Rohnert Park, CA: Center for Critical Thinking & Moral Critique.

Palmer, S. E. 1983. The art of lecturing: A few simple ideas can help teachers improve their skills. *Chronicle of Higher Education* 26:19–20.

Phillips, C., and Harman, E. 1986. Criteria for selecting textbooks. *Nurse Educator* 11(2):31–34.

Piaget, J. 1947. *The Psychology of Intelligence*. New York: Harcourt, Brace, and World.

Rassi, J. A. 1988. Student evaluation of an audiology practicum examination and of self-achievement. *SUPERvision* 12(2):32–38(Summary).

Rassi, J. A., and McElroy, M. D. 1989. Analysis of course design, organization, and content in ESB-accredited programs. Miniseminar presented at the annual convention of the American Speech-Language-Hearing Association, St. Louis, November.

Reilly, D. E., and Oermann, M. H. 1985. *The Clinical Field: Its Use in Nursing Education*. Norwalk, CT: Appleton-Century-Crofts.

Riechmann, S., and Grasha, A. 1974. A rational approach to developing and assessing the construct validity of a student learning style scale instrument. *Journal of Psychology* 87:213–23.

Richardson, A. 1969. *Mental Imagery*. New York: Springer.

Saunders, K., Northup, D. E., and Mennin, S.P. 1985. The library in a problem-based curriculum. In *Implementing Problem-Based Medical Education. Lessons from Successful Innovations*, ed. A. Kaufman. New York: Springer Publishing Company.

Sklare, G., Portes, P., and Splete, H. 1985. Training model. Developing questioning effectiveness in counseling. *Counselor Education and Supervision* 25(1):12–20.

Slosson Educational Publications. 1988. *1988 Catalog*. East Aurora, NY: Author.

Slosson Educational Publications. 1989. *1989 Catalog*. East Aurora, NY: Author.

Sorrell, J. M. 1989. Responding to student writing. *Nurse Educator* 14(2):24–26.

Stockwell, C. W. 1983. *ENG Workbook*. Austin, TX: Pro-Ed.

Sykes, C. J. 1988. *ProfScam: Professors and the Demise of Higher Education*. Washington, DC: Regnery Gateway.

Torrance, E. P. 1975. Creativity research in education: Still alive. In *Perspectives in Creativity*, eds. I. Taylor and J. Getzels. Chicago: Aldine Publishing.

Tosti, D. T., and Addison, R. 1979. A taxonomy of educational reinforcement. *Educational Technology* 14(9):24–25.

Volcek, M. K., and Nelson, A. E. 1986. Clinical focus: Bridging theory and practice. *Nurse Educator* 11(3):34–37.

Wales, C. E., and Stager, R. A. 1977. *Guided Design*. Morgantown, WV: Center for Guided Design, West Virginia University.

Walsh, W. B. 1985. *Tests and Assessment*. Englewood Cliffs, NJ: Prentice-Hall.

Weimer, M. (ed.). 1987. Teaching aids. Study skills. *Teaching Professor* 1(9):5.

Weimer, M. (ed.). 1988a. Forum follow-up. Participation: To grade or not to grade. *Teaching Professor* 2(1):3–4.

Weimer, M. (ed.). 1988b. Teaching aids. Making group projects work. *Teaching Professor* 2(3):8.

Weimer, M. (ed.). 1988c. Grading on the curve: Some thoughts. *Teaching Professor* 2(5):3–4.

Wenk, V. A., and Menges, R. J. 1985. Using classroom questions appropriately. *Nurse Educator* 10(2):19–24.

Westmeyer, P. 1988. *Effective Teaching in Adult and Higher Education*. Springfield, IL: Charles C Thomas.

Whitis, G. 1985. Simulation in teaching clinical nursing. *Journal of Nursing Education* 24(4):161–63.

Wingard, J. R., and Williamson, J. W. 1973. Grades as predictors of physician's career performance: An evaluative literature review. *Journal of Medical Education* 48(4):311–32.

Witkin, H. A. 1977. Cognitive styles in the educational setting. *New York University Education Quarterly* 8:14–20.

Witkin, H. A., Goodenough, D. R., and Oltman, P. K. 1977. Role of field-dependent and field-independent cognitive styles in academic evolution: A longitudinal study. *Journal of Educational Psychology* 69:197–211.

Wolfe, D., and Reising, R. 1983. *Writing for Learning in the Content Areas*. Portland, ME: J. Weston Walch.

Yoder, D. E., and Kent, R. D. 1988. *Decision Making in Speech-Language Pathology*. St. Louis: C. V. Mosby/B. C. Decker.

Chapter 10

Research Laboratory Teaching
Preparing Lessons and Planning Instruction

Cynthia G. Fowler and Janet S. Leonards

Laboratory teaching is appropriate when practice and hands-on experience are essential to learning (Kozma, Belle, and Williams 1978). Research laboratory experience in communication sciences covers a wide range of activities and objectives. The general objectives of laboratory courses are to promote inquiry, develop performance skills, and provide practical experience with experimental concepts. Specific objectives are to familiarize students with laboratory equipment, provide an introduction to reading and designing research studies, guide preliminary small-scale or group research projects, and instruct individual students in the conduct of research projects. Students must think and solve problems during a laboratory session, not simply learn techniques.

A real limitation in teaching research is the attitude of clinically oriented students who see research as irrelevant. To overcome this attitude, a research instructor must serve as a role model; an instructor must believe in the value of research and personally conduct it. Further, a research instructor must understand clinical issues and use examples from research in the context of the clinical interests of students (Overfield and Duffy 1984).

PREPARING LABORATORY LESSONS

Lesson Objectives

Laboratory lesson objectives must be clearly delineated and tailored to the laboratory situation. Objectives that focus on the development of skills, research methods and tools, and observation, demonstration, or manipulation of materials are appropriate. A common complaint from students is that laboratory objectives are vague, independent of classroom activities, and irrelevant to career goals (Weimer 1988). These complaints can be assuaged if laboratory objectives are determined carefully.

As in any small-group instructional setting, it is crucial to discuss with students their backgrounds and expectations for the laboratory class. Specific objectives of each class can then be tailored to the needs, backgrounds, and attitudes of the students (Kozma, Belle, and Williams 1978). Despite the importance of this step, Jason and Westberg (1982) indicate that instructors rarely begin an instruction session by investigating students' backgrounds.

Subject Matter

The subject matter in a laboratory class varies with objectives of the laboratory. If the objective is to teach students how to conduct or read research, the component parts of the project and the critical thinking behind each step must be taught. The first classes should be devoted to identification of a research question. Students who have been thinking about their clinical and classroom experiences should be able to ask a few questions that have not been adequately answered by the textbooks or instructors. The laboratory instructor and other classmates can then discuss different ways of phrasing questions to devise experimental hypotheses.

The second step is to determine the current status of knowledge on the subject. Strategies and resources to locate current information on a topic are emphasized. Students must learn to conduct computerized library searches based on key words, topics, authors, or citations. Students should learn to use cumulative indices such as *Index Medicus, Psychological Abstracts, Dissertation Abstracts,* and *References to Contemporary Papers on Acoustics.* They should review journal indices, current issues of journals, and recent textbooks and chapters for information and references. Abstracts of convention programs and copies of relevant papers may be helpful. Finally, students should consult professors, fellow students, or other authorities in the field for current information.

A literature review, based on current information, should build a case for the study, including the history and rationale. Students must learn to phrase the purpose carefully to link the literature review to methods, and to orient readers to the direction of the study. Phrasing of the purpose determines the type and framework of the study that follows.

Once the purpose is clarified, students must choose appropriate methods. Each possible research design has inherent weaknesses as well as strengths that must be considered. Students must determine critical characteristics of subjects and choose the best way to measure those characteristics. One of the most difficult decisions is the choice of an appropriate number of subjects, which depends on research design and statistical analysis. Appropriate equipment for the study must be chosen with an understanding of its characteristics and any limitations that may affect the results. Choice of test materials is also crucial; any inherent flaws in test materials will affect the outcome of the study.

For procedures, students must identify appropriate dependent and independent variables, and critical mechanics of data collection. Finally, the method of data analysis must be determined. Students must understand the rationale for procedural details that will be included eventually in the methods section of a research paper.

Once data are collected, students must learn to present the results in a clear, concise written form using appropriate statistics, tables, graphs, and illustrations. The narrative portion of the results section can link data displays and guide the reader through the data. Generally, the results should follow an orderly progression, such as general to specific, and subsections should be arranged in parallel fashion for consistency.

In the discussion section, students must learn to compare and contrast results with relevant studies in the literature. Similar findings may confirm results of the study; conflicting results may suggest previously unknown methodological variables or challenge accepted ideas. Results can be discussed in terms of prevalent theories or can be used to propose new theories. Implications of the study indicate possible applications and any relevance the study has beyond the subject group that was studied.

The conclusions section may be the most difficult part for a student to write. The entire paper must be distilled by stating simply and succinctly what the author expects readers to have gleaned from the paper. The extent to which the initial question was answered should be addressed.

A critical investigator should be able to identify aspects of the study that could have been done in another way, or the existence of certain variables that may have influenced the outcome. A student's ability to critique personal work is an indication of the student's objectivity and self-assessment abilities, qualities that are important in a scientist. One frustrating aspect of research, especially for an inexperienced investigator, is identification of problems during the study or data analysis. Although circumventing these problems may not be possible during the study, the investigator must be aware of the limitations they impose on results and conclusions. The investigator can use the experience to prepare for the next study. Students can become aware of this process in the simplest study they conduct, and will appreciate thereafter the difficulties and limitations inherent in any study they read. A discussion of research problems experienced by other student investigators can be invaluable to the entire class.

Textbook/Workbook/Manual Content

Textbooks that provide basic tools for understanding and conducting research in communication disorders are available, primarily in the fields of audiology and speech-language pathology, psychology, and education. These textbooks (e.g., Ventry and Schiavetti 1986) provide an overview of the types of research designs used in these fields and the strengths and weaknesses inherent in each design. Data collection and analysis are described briefly. Adequate data analysis and statistical design require independent classes. These texts also provide step-by-step approaches to preparation of a research article, and serve as guides for students who will be primary consumers, as well as producers, of research.

Lesson Formats

Lesson formats in a research laboratory are necessarily loosely structured within the framework of objectives. As long as students are asking pertinent questions, the instructor will find that following their lead is more important than rigidly adhering to a structured plan. A strict format may lead to a cookbook approach; students may be pushed through prescribed steps rather than allowed to explore and learn on their own. The emphasis of laboratory instruction is placed more appropriately on the process of learning than on the actual content that is taught (McKeachie 1986). An instructor must be sufficiently flexible to meet challenges presented by individual students.

Although lesson formats for laboratory meetings should be informal, structured activities must be assigned and completed between class meetings. These assignments should guide students in learning problem-solving skills, and, therefore, should follow the steps in conducting a research project. For the first assignment, an instructor may select a topic and have students do a computer search for relevant literature. For the second assignment, students may critique two to three articles identified through the computer search. A helpful 12-step checklist compiled by Lehman and Mehrens (1971) can help students critique an article. If the same article is assigned to all students, the class can compare opinions of the article. For the third assignment, students can identify relevant variables for a research project and discuss measurement techniques; for the fourth assignment, they can present ways in which variables might be measured better, i.e., overcome previous methodological limitations noted in articles. Subsequent classes can be devoted to discussing assignments and building on the foundation that completion of assignments has established.

Pacing and Sequencing Learning Activities

A laboratory course should follow an introduction-to-research class that provides students with the knowledge to critique a study, and a statistics class. Computer programming and applications classes are becoming increasingly necessary, because laboratories are relying on computers to generate stimuli, control experiments, collect and analyze data, generate graphics, and serve as word processors to complete manuscripts.

After students have a theoretical background, the laboratory class will permit them to apply theory to design and implement their own studies. Students can choose questions that require simple research designs and have a high probability of completion. Even a simple study will allow students to understand research, and alert them to the necessity of precise record keeping, effects of uncontrollable or unexpected variables, and problems that can arise in scheduling subjects or maintaining equipment.

Guidance from the laboratory instructor is crucial during development of the study; the instructor must make sure that students choose topics within their capabilities and time commitments. The nature of the laboratory class requires that instructors know the capabilities of their students and monitor progress accordingly. Advanced students can be encouraged to move quickly through their laboratory projects, whereas beginning students can be guided slowly through each step to assure understanding of underlying concepts. In all cases, the instructor must order lessons appropriately to ensure that each lesson builds on the foundation established by the previous one.

A laboratory work schedule should initially provide each student access to the research instructor or a laboratory assistant who can assure that the student does not become frustrated early in the project. Later in the course, the student should exhibit a degree of independence so that the constant presence of an adviser is not necessary.

SELECTING AND PLANNING INSTRUCTIONAL DESIGN

Lecture

Lecture classes are appropriate for the efficient transfer of facts, theories, and philosophies, imparting general background knowledge, statistics, and research design. These lectures should be taught or coordinated by the same instructor who teaches the laboratory practicum to ensure that the information is compatible and concurrent. For students to have an understanding of the entire process of research, lectures are insufficient; laboratory experience and active participation by students in a research project are required.

Demonstration

Demonstrations can illustrate concepts that cannot be described adequately in lectures, such as auditory and speech phenomena and use of equipment. Demonstrations may be based on commercially available or locally prepared audiotapes, videotapes, and compact discs. More complex demonstrations involve setting up the laboratory to create the phenomena. Although demonstrations are efficient ways to present background material to groups of students, demonstrations cannot replace hands-on experience in manipulating the equipment or creating the auditory or speech phenomena of interest.

Discussion

Discussion sections encourage students to think actively about research and its application to clinical and basic science questions. Students should bring questions that have arisen in their clinics or readings to the discussion session so that class members and the instructor can frame the questions into hypotheses, compare possible research designs, and discuss variables that might influence the outcome. Exercises such as these allow students to relate research to their own experiences and become personally involved in research.

Student groups can discuss literature in journal groups. Students identify in an article the definition of a problem, the methods used, and the results. They should summarize the authors' conclusions and present their own conclusions. This exercise gives students an appreciation for well-designed studies, warns them of possible pitfalls, and prepares them for designing their own studies (O'Grady and Haukenes 1978). Students are encouraged to overcome the perception that all published studies are valid. If the instructor offers personal work for student discussion, a good example in objectivity is set for the students.

Seminars

Seminars are valuable for exposing students to a wide variety of research topics. Seminars can be given by local professionals who are actively engaged in research and willing to use their own work as examples of problem solving in both the research laboratory and clinic. Experts from outside the university can provide insights from examples of types of research and research applications not being carried out at the university (Leach and Champion 1989).

Seminars can also be used as forums for students presenting their own work to a group of interested peers and faculty. This prepares students for presenting papers at meetings, and helps them gain experience in speaking in front of groups, presenting and defending their research, and evaluating the research of others.

Individualized Instruction

Laboratory research is particularly suited for individualized instruction, especially for students with a background in research. Individualized instruction allows students to advance at their own pace, to delve into aspects of research especially interesting to them, and to spend time strengthening areas in which they need extra help. Although individualized instruction is the most costly teaching method in terms of faculty time and laboratory space and equipment, it is the most appropriate teaching method for advanced students and for students who display an above-average interest in research.

Grouping for Instructional Purposes

Group conferences are relatively effective for teaching research to naïve students. The purposes of conferences are to (1) provide faculty access for small groups of students with similar research backgrounds, (2) use faculty time efficiently, and (3) allow students to discuss research ideas and problems with a limited peer group (Pardue and Sisson 1986). If these sessions are held weekly, they can facilitate student-faculty interaction, and can lead to quick resolutions of problems that arise during the course of students' experiments. Students are also encouraged to ask questions they might not consider important enough to warrant individual conferences.

Group conferences also have disadvantages. Primary problems involve students who monopolize the conference and students who are intimidated by perceived superior knowledge of other students and, therefore, do not participate during sessions (Pardue and Sisson 1986). An instructor with experience in group leadership can circumvent these problems and facilitate full participation by all students.

Project Method

The best way to learn to conduct research is to do research. Student participation in research can be accomplished either through group or individual research projects. Although students should choose their projects, an instructor should provide a list of potential topics to facilitate students' choices. Topics in line with each student's expected career goals will be more acceptable and successful in reaching educational goals than topics that are perceived as irrelevant (Overfield and Duffy 1984).

Although, ideally, students should be free to choose any topic, in reality the laboratory instructor will have ongoing research and well-defined research interests. A student project not within the realm of interest of the professor may require a longer time commitment than is practical in developing the topic and in acquiring or setting up appropriate equipment. If funding is an issue, funds for a new project may not be available, whereas funds for an ongoing line of research may be covered by existing grant money. Further, time is a consideration; if the project is part of a course, the course will be over before the experiment is begun; if the study is a thesis, the student will have graduation deadlines. These limitations are part of any research project and students should be fully aware of them. A practical compromise can be reached if students and professor discuss availability of equipment and the nature of ongoing research prior to selecting a topic.

Problem-Based Teaching

Problem solving requires first, specific knowledge in the field, and second, general problem-solving skills (Mayer 1983, p. 347). If the knowledge base is weak, then problem-solving skills are useless. Problem-solving skills develop from experience and imitation of problem-solving abilities of others. The entire scope of the problem must be understood, including the givens, goals, and obstacles (Mayer 1983). The goal is to find a comprehensive solution that encompasses all aspects of the problem.

Common strategies for problem solving exist. First, the problem must be clarified with identification of relevant and irrelevant facts. Second, similarities between the current problem and past problems are explored for clues to possible solutions. Third, innovative approaches and unconventional solutions are considered. Fourth, comprehensive solutions are sought, rather than individual, unrelated solutions directed at each aspect of the problem. Fifth, thinking processes of successful problem-solvers are explored for ideas about new approaches to the problem. Sixth, a discussion of the problem with others might provide new insights or viewpoints that have not been considered. Once the solution is determined, a critical re-evaluation of the solution may determine its accuracy and its application to other situations. By putting the problem and its solution into a general context, an investigator adds to the existing problem-solving strategies, and facilitates making analogies to new problems (Mayer 1983).

Skill Lessons

Skill lessons are practical and must be individually tailored to the needs of each student. For example, students in audiology or speech-language pathology must know specifics about calibration, acoustics, electronics, and computers; physiology students must know about animal care, surgical techniques, and effects of drugs; psychoacoustics students must understand advanced statistical methods and signal processing. Speech students may need to know radiographic techniques and speech digitization; language students may need to know video equipment. All students must be familiar with any equipment's safety precautions.

Once an instructor determines the types of skills that are necessary, a brief orientation or demonstration of equipment is required. This introduction can be accomplished by lecture, audiotape, or videotape. Complex skills can be broken down into component parts and taught in steps. After an introduction to the equipment, students are allowed to handle the equipment by performing increasingly difficult operations. A specific set of instructions or tasks is then given and students pursue that set independently of the instructor. Minimal instructor guidelines will encourage students to work out problems themselves. An instructor, however, must oversee the work to prevent errors that will be harder to eliminate once they have become established as habits (Kozma, Belle, and Williams 1978).

SELECTING AND PLANNING TEACHING STRATEGIES

Creating Set

A learning set is a set of instructional objectives written in terms of learning outcomes. Performance of any task requires previous mastery of a group of learning sets arranged in a hierarchy. Each learning set is based on other subordinate learning sets, which must be mastered and recalled before achieving higher sets. Instructional objectives in the laboratory must be constructed with an understanding of the hierarchy of learning sets leading to an understanding of research processes. This hierarchy of learning sets is defined by asking what students must know to perform each specific task required in the laboratory exercise. If students are missing some subordinate learning sets, these sets must be taught before the students can accomplish the expected task (Wittrock 1968).

Instructional objectives should be stated as desired learning outcomes in terms of student performance. Too often instructional objectives are phrased in terms of the learning process (e.g., learns terminology), the course content (e.g., studies research methodology), or teacher performance (e.g., teaches how to caculate t-tests) rather than in terms of student performance (e.g., identifies the various types of research designs, computes t-scores) (Gronlund 1985). Learning outcomes are best stated in specific terms, using verbs such as *defines, identifies, infers,* and *relates.* Specific terms clarify what students must do to demonstrate their understanding. Writing clear and specific instructional objectives is not easy. Readers who are not well versed in writing such objectives can consult the following sources for ideas, examples, and explanations: Mager (1962); Johnson and Johnson (1970); Popham and Baker (1970).

Employing Reinforcement

Providing feedback to students is critical in directing their research performance. Students need to know what is expected, and whether or not they are meeting expectations. Students learn better from constructive criticism, i.e., instruction on ways to improve performance, rather than from negative feedback (Kozma, Belle, and Williams 1978).

Unless progress is monitored regularly, students will not make the expected progress toward established objectives. One common instructor strategy is to tell students to seek him or her for advice as needed. Jason and Westberg (1982) indicate, however, that students who are most in need of help are least likely to ask. Frequent monitoring can be assured by assigning and grading weekly assignments; if a student has difficulty with the assignment, the problem can be discovered and addressed before the student falls too far behind the class.

Questioning, Listening, Observing

Open-ended questions require students to reason and allow the instructor to evaluate students' problem-solving skills (Weimer 1988; Foley and Smilansky 1980). If questions are presented in a logical sequence with hints from related problems within students' experiences, they will learn the process of reasoning through a problem. Students often discover that they have the knowledge and skills to solve problems that they initially considered completely new. They need to be shown the way to determine an answer based on a restructuring of their current knowledge through associations with similar situations. A sequence of open-ended questions, each building on information from the answer to a previous question and each directed to a different student, will engage the entire class in the reasoning effort.

Achieving Closure

Closure occurs when students make the knowledge they have acquired their own; that is, when students internalize knowledge. Only then can they use their newly acquired knowledge as a theoretical background for learning advanced concepts and as a practical background for solving future problems (Wittrock 1968). Concepts learned through understanding or discovery are internalized and transferred more easily to other situations than concepts learned by memory (Mayer 1983, p. 42).

Closure is facilitated if an instructor emphasizes the clinical or theoretical relevance of facts. Not only is learning easier when facts are placed in a practical framework, but facts are also more easily recalled when they are related to previously encountered situations. Students are encouraged to form many associations for facts rather than isolate the facts in their original contexts. Indeed, educators recommend spending less teaching time on isolated facts and more time on forming associations and interrelations among the facts (Small 1988).

PLANNING THE ASSESSMENT OF STUDENTS' KNOWLEDGE AND/OR EVALUATION OF STUDENTS' PERFORMANCE

The primary goal of any evaluation of student knowledge or performance is to obtain a reliable and valid assessment. Achieving this goal requires that a series of decisions be made about the evaluation process prior to the development of any assessment tool. These decisions include determining the purpose of the evaluation, the specifics of the test, the appropriate item types, and the way relevant test items are to be prepared (Gronlund and Linn 1990).

Purpose of the Evaluation

One of the critical steps in creating a test or assessment tool is to make the test compatible with the purpose of assessment. An instructor must decide whether the purpose of evaluation is to determine the relative ranking of students, or to determine if students have mastered a certain set of skills or knowledge.

The first instance, that of determining relative ranking (i.e., who has learned the material best), assumes that there will be students who are more proficient than others, that the degree of proficiency among students will approximate a normal distribution, and that the degree of proficiency is important. Tests based on these assumptions are called "norm-referenced" tests and the goal of such testing is to differentiate among, or rank, students. Norm-referenced tests are most appropriate measures to use when making summary statements about students, such as final grades (and, frequently, midterm grades). Norm-referenced tests can also be used to determine the levels of prerequisite skills the students have. These tests typically contain items with a moderate range of difficulty to identify fine distinctions among students in the amount of knowledge learned.

The second instance, that of determining if a student has mastered a certain set of skills, assumes that above a certain cut-off score, all students are proficient. Tests designed to fit this purpose are called "criterion-referenced" tests and are the most appropriate measures for making statements from weekly quizzes or laboratory exercises that inform students of their current levels of understanding. Criterion-referenced tests typically contain items that are relatively easy, as it is assumed that the objectives tested have been met by a majority of students.

For a research course in communication disorders, both norm-referenced and criterion-referenced assessments may be appropriate. For example, as weekly homework assignments function primarily as aids to the learning process, their construction might be criterion-referenced. If a student scores 75% or better on an assignment, credit can be given for that assignment. In general, the aggregate score for such homework assignments typically constitutes between 15% and 25% of the total grade for a semester. Final tests, or papers, however, are better designed as norm-referenced measures, because these assessments tap a student's mastery of the problem solving, synthesis, evaluation, and performance aspects of conducting research.

Developing Test Specifications

The primary goal in any assessment is to be confident that the assessment process is fair, that the test provides an accurate estimate of a student's ability and that the test measures what it set out to measure. The psychometric concepts of validity and reliability underlie good assessment processes.

Validity refers to how well a test measures what it purports to measure. In achievement-based situations, a valid test is one in which the learning objectives are appropriately measured, i.e., the relevant content is tested at desired levels of cognitive skills. For example, in a research class in communication disorders, definitions and terms are best tested at the knowledge level, whereas identification of the most serious threat to validity in a research design is best tested at an evaluative or judgment level. Readers unfamiliar with various taxonomies of cognitive skill levels are referred to Bloom (1956), Gerlach and Sullivan (1967), and Ebel (1979).

An excellent way to ensure "content validity" is to prepare a table of specifications that links relevant content with its corresponding cognitive skill level. Inherent in any learning objective is both the general area of content to be tested and the corresponding cognitive skill level. For example, the learning objective "identifies basic terms" designates a cognitive skill level (identification or comprehension) as well as a general content area (basic terms). The first step, therefore, in preparing the table is identification of pertinent learning objectives. The second step is grouping learning objectives according to cognitive skill level (e.g., knowledge, application, or synthesis). The third step is outlining specific content areas and designating proportion of test items or assessment procedures to be spent on each content area. For further information on construction of a table of specifications, see Mehrens and Lehman (1984), Cunningham (1986), and Gronlund and Linn (1990).

A table of specifications can be created for each test or assessment procedure to be given during a course; or a global table of specifications can be created covering all objectives to be taught that semester. An example of an abbreviated table of specifications for a final test in a research laboratory course in communication disorders is shown in table I.

Once a test specification table has been constructed, steps are taken to ensure test reliability. Reliability refers to the consistency or trustworthiness of a test. The interested reader is referred to texts on

Table I. Abbreviated table of specifications for a test on research laboratory techniques, showing the percentage of items by content and cognitive skill level and giving examples of a task to test that objective

| Content Area | Instructional Objective | | |
	Analysis 30%	Synthesis 40%	Evaluation 30%
Designing a study 40%	Identifies appropriate variables 12%	Proposes a plan for an experiment 16%	Judges consistency of written material 12%
Conducting a study 30%	Identifies appropriate assessment techniques 9%	Devises new methods to assess relevant variables 12%	Explains why new/revised techniques are warranted 9%
Evaluating a study 30%	Recognizes unstated assumptions 9%	Writes a well-organized report on a study 12%	Judges adequacy with which data support conclusions 9%

measurement procedures (see Ebel 1979; Mehrens and Lehman 1984) for cogent discussions on determining the reliability of a test. Several factors that influence the reliability of a test are under immediate control of the instructor. The following rules can enhance the reliability of a test/assessment procedure.

The longer the test is, the greater its reliability. Longer tests generally allow for a greater sampling of students' knowledge. A typical rule of thumb is to have three items per learning objective, especially in objective tests.

Objectively scored test items produce greater test reliability. Tests composed of objectively scored test items eliminate rater bias. If one must use subjectively scored essay items, the reliability can be increased by having multiple graders, grading tests without knowledge of student identity, grading one item across all papers, and providing specifics on what is to be included in the answer (termed restricted essay items).

The more homogeneous the item content is, the greater the test reliability will be. Tests composed of items that are homogeneous in content (e.g., all items are related to methods of conducting research) typically have greater reliability than tests that cover more than one broad content area (e.g., a combination of research-based and clinically based items).

The more heterogeneous the student performance is, the greater the test reliability will be. The amount of variability in test scores (i.e., heterogeneous group performance) directly contributes to the statistical calculation of reliability. Heterogeneous group performance occurs when the group itself is heterogeneous in ability for the area being tested, and when the test measures fine distinctions in ability.

In contrast to norm-referenced tests, criterion-referenced tests, which are constructed so that the majority of items are easy for the majority of students, measure minimal variability among students. Traditional methods of establishing reliability do not apply. Instead, the reliability of criterion-referenced tests is established by calculating the percent of students classified as masters or nonmasters (APA 1985).

In addition to validity and reliability, other issues of test specification include whether the test is to be completed by an individual or by student groups, whether the test will be open- or closed-book, and whether the test will primarily be a speeded or a power test. These three issues are discussed below.

Individually Completed versus Group-Completed Assessment. At the graduate level, group-completed assessments, in which the grade for an assignment is given to all members of a group, can be appropriate for homework and other assignments that inform a student of his/her progression in a course. Group or cooperative exercises can have a positive effect on academic achievement, especially with low-achieving students (Ames 1981). These students benefit from an exchange of ideas with other members of the group and from observations of the ways other students approach and solve problems. If the purpose of evaluation, however, is to rank students on how well they, individually, learned the course material, such as performance on a final exam or term paper, then individually completed assessments are most appropriate.

Open- versus Closed-Book Assessments. Open-book assessments are those in which students are free to use references to complete the test. Closed-book assessments are those in which access to references is not allowed. In general, when the objectives of a course are at the lower cognitive skills levels, e.g., recall or recognition of facts, then closed-book exams and assessments are preferred. If, however, the objectives of the course are at the upper end of the cognitive skill hierarchy, such as analysis, synthesis, and evaluation, then open-book exams may be appropriate.

In a research course in communication disorders, open-book assessments may be preferred. Given that the general goals of the course are to promote critical inquiry and problem solving while developing research skills, it may be more realistic to determine if a student can demonstrate these skills with access to references rather than without them. After all, professional researchers make frequent use of references when designing, conducting, and analyzing studies.

Speeded versus Power Testing. Speeded tests are designed to measure how many items an individual can answer correctly within a certain time. Time, therefore, is used as a basis for differentiating among the better and poorer students. For speeded tests, the assumption is that the better students answer items faster and will answer more items in a given time. Better students, therefore, will have "access" to all test items, whereas poorer students will not.

In contrast, power tests are designed to measure how many items an individual can answer correctly. Items on the test are arranged in order of difficulty with the assumption that better students will be able to answer the most difficult items correctly. Both types of students should have sufficient time to attempt to answer all items. True power or true speeded tests are rare. Speeded tests usually contain some items of varying difficulty and power tests usually have a time limit. For a graduate-level, laboratory research course, the assessment procedures should lean toward power testing to assess clarity of thinking and problem solving rather than the speed with which students make decisions.

Appropriate Item Types

Appropriate items must be matched to the learning objectives of the course. This matching involves analyzing the cognitive skill specified in a learning objective and then constructing an item that taps that level of skill for specified content. Item types typically are categorized as either objective or essay. Objective items are characterized by dichotomous scoring: an answer is either entirely correct or entirely wrong. In addition, objective items are structured tasks that limit the type of response a student can make. Within the objective category are selection-type items where the student "selects" the correct response, such as true-false, matching, multiple-choice; and supply-type items in which the student "supplies" the correct answer, such as a short answer consisting of one to four words. Most objective items are written to test lower level cognitive skills, such as recall, recognition, and identification.

Essay items are characterized by multipoint scoring (a range of possible scores): an answer can be entirely correct, partially correct, or entirely wrong. In addition, essay items are loosely structured tasks with limited responses. Essays can be restricted, varying from two sentences to a page, or extended, varying from four to five pages with the content limited only by the scope of the item. Essay items are used to tap higher levels of cognitive skills, such as analysis, synthesis, and evaluation.

Preparing Relevant Test Items

Preparing relevant test items is neither easy nor quick. Objective tests are lengthy to write, but quick to score. Writing objective tests requires time because of the large number of items required and because constructing plausible distractors is difficult. Essay tests, by contrast, are quick to write, but lengthy to score. Combining test items with an interpretive exercise is an excellent way to use objective and essay items to test higher-level cognitive skills. An interpretive exercise is one in which a set of test items is based on a common set of data, such as tables, charts, paragraphs, and graphs. Further information on guidelines and examples for interpretive exercises is available in publications such as Wesman (1971), ETS (1973), and Nitko (1983).

Advantages of interpretive exercises include: the amount of factual information given can be controlled; all students are presented with the same task; and a variety of learning outcomes can be measured, such as identifying relationships, evaluating conclusions, and interpreting findings. One problem with objective items linked to an interpretive exercise is that a student may not remember specific facts, and, therefore, will not be able to demonstrate higher-order learning. Items based on an interpretive exercise, however, can provide facts, and can test whether or not a principle is understood.

The primary disadvantage of interpretive exercises is the difficulty of construction. Modifying the material appropriately takes time, resources, and creativity. A second disadvantage is that an interpretive exercise does not tap a student's global problem-solving skills, or sense of integration. For this level of learning, extended response essay questions are required.

Interpretive exercises are typically combined with objective items or with restricted-response essay questions. When objective items are used, the learning outcomes are based on a student's ability to select correct answers that test cause and effect relationships, validity of conclusions, and limitations of data. In contrast, when interpretive exercises are used with restricted-response essay questions, the learning outcomes are based on a student's ability to explain, rather than identify, cause and effect relationships, to formulate valid conclusions, and to describe the limitations of data.

Table II.   Means and standard deviations (in parentheses) for the latencies and amplitudes of wave V(L + R) and peak A and the amplitude ratio of peak A: wave V(L + R) for the four stimulus conditions

	1000 Hz	4000 Hz
Wave V(L + R)		
Latency, ms		
80 dB pe SPL	7.46(0.35)	6.89(0.45)
100 dB pe SPL	6.71(0.25)	6.24(0.24)
Amplitude, uV		
80 dB pe SPL	0.31(0.14)	0.32(0.12)
100 dB pe SPL	0.86(0.31)	0.57(0.18)
Peak A		
Latency, ms		
80 dB pe SPL	7.84(0.40)	7.25(0.39)
100 dB pe SPL	6.98(0.26)	6.49(0.22)
Amplitude, uV		
80 dB pe SPL	0.11(0.07)	0.11(0.04)
100 dB pe SPL	0.22(0.08)	0.15(0.05)
Ratios of A:V(L + R)		
80 dB pe SPL	0.25(0.26)	0.18(0.18)
100 dB pe SPL	0.28(0.08)	0.19(0.14)

Note: Values are conservative estimates because data were only used from subjects in whom the binaural interaction component was present in all four stimulus conditions.

The questions below illustrate an example of an interpretive exercise, first with objective items, and then with a restricted-essay question. According to Gronlund and Linn (1990), the set of objective items shown here tests whether a student can recognize warranted from unwarranted generalizations. Making such distinctions tests learning outcomes at the evaluation level. The common set of data in this example is presented in table II. These data are taken from a study on the Binaural Interaction Component of the Auditory Brainstem Response (Fowler and Leonards 1985).

Directions: Use the data in the preceding table to respond to the following statements. For each statement, use the following key to mark your answer.

Circle: S   if the statement is SUPPORTED by the data.
                R   if the statement is REFUTED by the data.
                N   if the statement is NEITHER supported nor refuted by the data.

1.   S   R   N   Wave V(L + R) latency was latest in the 4KHz, 100 dB SPL stimulus condition.

2.   S   R   N   Wave V(L + R) amplitude was largest in the 1KHz, 100 dB SPL stimulus condition.

3.   S   R   N   There were frequency- and intensity-dependent differences in the wave V(L + R) latencies.

4.   S   R   N   Peak A amplitude was equivalent for the following stimulus conditions: 1KHz, 80 dB SPL; 4KHz, 100 dB SPL; and 4KHz, 80 dB SPL.

The next example uses a restricted-essay question to test a student's ability to explain and appraise the relevance of data. As with the previous set of items, this item is testing a learning outcome at the evaluation level.

Directions: Using the data in the preceding table, answer the following question in no more than one page.

Explain what is meant by the note, "Values are conservative estimates because data were only used from subjects in whom the binaural interaction component was present in all four stimulus conditions." Determine whether or not the inclusion of the note is relevant to data interpretation: justify your position.

When the learning outcome requires students to produce, organize, or integrate information, then extended-response essay questions, research papers, or technical reports are required. Writing extended-response essay questions requires skill and questions should be linked to specific learning outcomes. Using verbs such as *compare, relate, justify, summarize, classify, create, apply, analyze, synthesize,* and *evaluate* requires students to demonstrate higher-level cognitive skills. Moreover, these actions are used in specific learning objectives and link questions to learning objectives. They also clarify what is expected of the students. Additional guidelines in writing extended-response essay questions include: setting an approximate time limit for each question, then erring by overestimating the time needed to answer the question; and avoiding the use of optional questions.

CONCLUSION

In conclusion, laboratory classes present both advantages and disadvantages to the educational curriculum. The main disadvantages are that the classes are time-consuming and expensive, requiring low student-faculty ratios as well as dedicated space and equipment. The main advantages are that laboratory classes present both challenges and opportunities for creativity on the parts of the instructor and students. The instructor must be flexible, inquisitive, and knowledgeable to adapt to varying student backgrounds and interests and to take advantage of direct student-faculty interactions. A student must be motivated, challenged, and stimulated by the instructor. The student, in turn, must participate actively in the laboratory and willingly experiment with new techniques and skills. Despite difficulties and limitations, laboratory classes contribute substantially to the development of a student into an active and independent learner and problem-solver.

REFERENCES

American Psychological Association. 1985. *Standards for Educational and Psychological Testing.* Washington, DC: Author.
Ames, C. 1981. Competitive versus cooperative reward structures: The influ-

ence of individual and group performance factors on achievement attribu-tions and affect. *American Educational Research Journal* 73:411–18.

Bloom, B. S. (ed.). 1956. *Taxonomy of Educational Objectives. Handbook I: The Cognitive Domain.* New York: Longman, Inc.

Cunningham, G. K. 1986. *Educational and Psychological Measurement.* New York: Macmillan Publishing Company.

Ebel, R. L. 1979. *Essentials of Educational Measurement* (3rd ed.). Englewood Cliffs, NJ: Prentice-Hall.

Educational Testing Service. 1973. *Multiple Choice Questions: A Close Look.* Princeton, NJ: Author.

Foley, R. P., and Smilansky, J. 1980. *Teaching Techniques: A Handbook for Health Professionals.* New York: McGraw Hill Book Company.

Fowler, C. G., and Leonards, J. S. 1985. Frequency dependence of the binaural interaction component of the auditory brainstem potential. *Audiology* 24: 420–29.

Gerlach, V. S., and Sullivan, H. J. 1967. *Constructing Statements of Outcomes.* Inglewood, CA: Southwest Laboratory for Educational Research and Development.

Gronlund, N. E. 1985. *Measurement and Evaluation in Teaching* (5th ed.). New York: Macmillan Publishing Company.

Gronlund, N. E., and Linn, R. L. 1990. *Measurement and Evaluation in Teaching* (6th ed.). New York: Macmillan Publishing Company.

Jason, H., and Westberg, J. 1982. *Teachers and Teaching in U. S. Medical Schools.* Norwalk, CT: Appleton-Century-Crofts.

Johnson, S. R., and Johnson, R. B. 1970. *Developing Individualized Instructional Material.* New York: Westinghouse Learning Corporation.

Kozma, R. B., Belle, L. W., and Williams, G. W. 1978. *Instructional Techniques in Higher Education.* Englewood Cliffs, NJ: Educational Technology Publications, Inc.

Leach, A., and Champion, V. 1989. Research teaching strategies. *Nurse Educator* 14(1):5.

Lehman, I. J., and Mehrens, W. A. 1971. *Educational Research Reading in Focus.* New York: Holt, Rinehart & Winston, Inc.

Mager, R. F. 1962. *Preparing Objectives for Programmed Instruction.* San Francisco: Fearon Publishers.

Mayer, R. E. 1983. *Thinking, Problem Solving, Cognition.* New York: W. H. Freeman and Company.

McKeachie, W. J. 1986. *Teaching Tips: A Guidebook for the Beginning College Teacher* (8th ed.). Lexington, MA: D. C. Heath & Co.

Mehrens, W. A., and Lehman, I. J. 1984. *Measurement and Evaluation in Education and Psychology.* (3rd ed.). New York: Holt, Rinehart & Winston, Inc.

Nitko, A. J. 1983. *Educational Test and Measurement: An Introduction.* New York: Harcourt Brace Jovanovich.

O'Grady, D. J., and Haukenes, E. 1978. Teaching research methods to under-graduates in nursing—learning by doing. *Journal of Nursing Education* 17(8): 48–52.

Overfield, T., and Duffy, M. E. 1984. Research on teaching in the baccalaureate nursing curriculum. *Journal of Advanced Nursing* 9:189–96.

Pardue, S. F., and Sisson, R. A. 1986. Group conferences as a student advise-ment teaching strategy. *Nurse Educator* 11(2):12, 22.

Popham, W. J., and Baker, E. L. 1970. *Planning an Instructional Sequence.* Englewood Cliffs, NJ: Prentice-Hall.

Small, P. A., Jr. 1988. Consequences for medical education of problem-solving in science and medicine. *Journal of Medical Education* 63(11):848–53.

Ventry, I. M., and Schiavetti, N. 1986. *Evaluating Research in Speech Pathology and Audiology* (2nd ed.). New York: Macmillan Publishing Company.

Weimer, M. (ed.). 1988. Forum: Laboratory instruction. *Teaching Professor* 2(9):4.

Wesman, A. G. 1971. Writing the test item. In *Educational Measurement* (2nd ed.), ed. R. L. Thorndike. Washington, DC: American Council on Education.

Wittrock, M. C. 1968. Three conceptualized approaches to research on transfer of training. In *Learning Research and School Subjects*, eds. R. M. Gagne and W. J. Gephart. Itasca, NY: F. E. Peacock, Inc.

Chapter 11

Clinical Teaching
Delineating Competencies and Planning Strategies

Judith A. Rassi and Margaret D. McElroy

Compared with the lack of available material for classroom and laboratory instruction in audiology and speech-language pathology, clinical supervision information, in the form of convention presentations, conferences, workshops, books, journal articles, and coursework, has burgeoned over the years. A doctoral program at Indiana University (Anderson 1981), dedicated to the preparation of researcher-scholars in the supervisory process, has, along with individual dissertations on supervision from other speech-language pathology and audiology programs, provided the field with a research base and a corpus of researchers. These persons, in turn, are leading others in the study of supervision. ASHA has lent its support to the supervision movement by the establishment of a Committee on Supervision in Speech-Language Pathology and Audiology and by the adoption of an official position statement on the tasks of supervision and the competencies needed by supervisors to perform these tasks (ASHA 1985). The National Student Speech Language Hearing Association (NSSLHA) has given supervision a forum in a number of its publications, including the clinical series edition on self-supervision (Casey, Smith, and Ulrich 1988). A national professional organization (the Council of Supervisors in Speech-Language Pathology and Audiology), its nationwide research and education network, Supernet, and quarterly newsletter, *SUPERvision*, have linked supervisors nationwide in a common cause. Regional and state supervisors' interest groups have been formed and continue to be active, often in conjunction with meetings of state speech-language-hearing associations. Canadian supervisors, participating in supervision groups in the United States as well as in their own country, have brought innovation to the process. The recently established Centre for Studies in Clinical Education at the University of Alberta, has joined occupational therapy, physical therapy, and speech-language pathology and audiology in an interdisciplinary effort to promote graduate study and research in clinical education processes (Staff 1989).

Because of supervision information readily available from other sources, this chapter does not purport to offer a complete analysis of the topic. Instead, readers interested in comprehensive treatments of supervision in communication sciences and disorders (CSD) are referred to other texts: Oratio (1977); Rassi (1978); Crago and Pickering (1987); Anderson (1988); Casey, Smith, and Ulrich (1988); Farmer and Farmer (1989); and Leith, McNiece, and Fusilier (1989). This chapter, in keeping with the book's educational and teaching emphasis, highlights relevant features of the supervisory process, taking into consideration information from our own and other disciplines, and examining various instructional aspects of clinical supervision. Discussion is based on the premise that classroom, laboratory, and clinical instruction are parallel endeavors and that they must complement one another in order to effect an integrated curriculum.

DELINEATING CLINICAL COMPETENCIES

As stated in Chapter 3, the identification of competencies to be cultivated in students is a curriculum development task. Such competencies are usually general, however, awaiting specific delineation by the respective classroom, laboratory, and clinical instructors. Within the clinical realm, this task can be accomplished in three steps, each more specific than the preceding one: first, by a group of supervisors whose clinical responsibilities are similar; second, by each supervisor, for the purpose of specifying competencies unique to the supervisor's clinical work; and third, by each supervisor-student pair, as plans are made for a particular practicum assignment. These steps, in order of increasing specificity, are illustrated in the example shown in table I.

Identifying and Selecting Competencies

A competency statement not only serves as an indicator of knowledge or skill but, as the term denotes, a degree of competence is assumed. As clinical competencies are identified and selected, their contribution to competence in clinical work is taken into account. Some are more contributory than others, of course, and some, although essential for competence, may not be noteworthy because they are so basic that all supervisees are expected to have them. In any case, the identification of as many competencies as possible for each area of clinical activity is extremely helpful in supervisory planning. For a clinical teacher, a detailed compilation facilitates planning instructional strategies (An-

Table I. Delineating Clinical Competencies: Illustration of Increasing Specificity According to Decision-Making Source

Decision-Making Source	Competency Statement(s)
I. Departmental curriculum group	Provides appropriate audiologic informational counseling for adult clients and parents of child clients
Within Clinic:	
II. Audiology supervisors of students in diagnostic and hearing aid sessions	Explains audiometric results appropriately and clearly
	Explains acoustic immittance findings appropriately and clearly
III. Individual audiology supervisor	Relates pure-tone to speech audiometric results meaningfully
	Discusses individual hearing loss relative to average conversational loudness
	Discusses acoustic reflex findings only when necessary for client understanding of findings and recommendations
IV. Specific audiology supervisor-supervisee dyad	Uses lay terminology consistently in explaining degree and type of hearing loss
	Uses analogies in explaining communicative implications of hearing loss
	Ensures that explanations of findings having medical correlates are corroborated by physician

drews 1971). For student clinicians, the larger the number of indicators and the greater their specificity, the more information students will have to draw upon. This serves to de-mystify and, thereby, increase understanding of clinical and supervisory processes for students. Expectations become more realistic. Finally, the content of a thorough competency delineation provides both the clinical teacher and student with much subject matter for discussions and conferences, a basis for goal-setting and evaluation (Rassi 1987b), and, in essence, a context of the clinical-supervisory experience.

In the interest of an integrated curriculum, determination of clinical competencies should be made relative to classroom and laboratory competencies. That is to say, balance of clinical objectives with classroom and laboratory objectives can be achieved through selection of competencies that complement or supplement their counterparts. Although care should be taken to avoid redundancy in sets of competency statements, clinical teachers must understand the importance of reinforcing classroom- and laboratory-learning in the clinic.

Sequencing Competencies

Clinical learning, dependent to a certain extent on the orderly acquisition of knowledge and skill, can be facilitated by clinical instructors' determining the difficulty of specific competencies. The outcome of this determination, in turn, is used to calculate achievement levels expected of student clinicians at designated checkpoints (Carlson, Lubiejewski, and Polaski 1987). Time and experience intervals such as completed school terms or accumulated practicum clock hours, when linked to expectations, provide a means for both supervisor and supervisee to set clinical goals and monitor progress toward those goals. After accounting for difficulty and experience factors, clinical teachers can sequence individual competencies within each area according to the approximate order of their expected attainment. Here, consideration must be given to timing and sequence of classroom and laboratory work so that clinical expectations are not premature. Even so, certain clinical competencies are often attainable for students who have not yet completed all corresponding coursework. This may be accomplished through supplemental reading and modeling, demonstration, or one-to-one teaching by the clinical instructor. Although not a substitute for coursework, these instructional steps usually provide enough information for students to participate meaningfully in related clinical work until formal courses are completed.

Sequenced clinical competencies, similar in format and purpose to that of classroom learning objectives, provide direction for both teacher and learner. Notwithstanding the reality that clinical case problems do not always present themselves in a predictable, skill-building order, clinical teachers can look at the sequence as a guide for order of explanation or discussion (Popham and Baker 1963; Douglas, Hosokawa, and Lawler 1988), while student clinicians can use the sequence to identify knowledge or skill gaps to be filled before moving to a more advanced level. Sequencing thus reflects movement along a multi-dimensional continuum, answering the self-analytical question, "What do I need to know or be able to do before I can accomplish _____?" A possible sequencing of clinical competencies is illustrated in table II.

Table II. Illustration of Sequenced Clinical Competencies According to Assumed Level of Difficulty from Low to High

Competency-Area Example: Clinical Decision Making, Diagnostic

1. Makes diagnostic hypotheses on basis of history and other relevant background information
2. Selects category of diagnostic tests to administer
3. Selects specific tests to administer
4. Modifies test administration during testing on basis of client behavior and emerging test results
5. Adds tests to, and deletes tests from, battery on basis of results
6. Interprets individual test results, considering relevant history and other information, client behavior during testing, and other possible influencing factors
7. Interprets test profile, considering weight of individual test results based on relative diagnostic power of each and on contributory client factors
8. Determines clinical significance of test profile findings
9. Formulates speech, language, or hearing diagnostic impression(s)
10. Formulates intervention recommendations on basis of diagnostic impression(s)
11. Considers diagnostic and other findings that suggest the presence of problems unrelated to speech, language, or hearing disorders or problems related to these disorders but not appropriately managed by the clinician
12. Makes referral recommendations on basis of other-disorder impressions

ANDERSON'S COMPONENTS OF THE SUPERVISORY PROCESS

In her text on the supervisory process in speech-language pathology and audiology, Anderson (1988) identifies five major components of a collaborative supervisory style. The first of these, *understanding* the supervisory process, she believes, is important both to supervisors and supervisees in preparing them for their respective roles and providing a basis for their continuing discussion of the supervisory process with one another. The second component, *planning*, involves collaborative planning not only for the clinical process but also for the supervisory process. *Observing*, the third component in Anderson's conceptualization, consists of objective data collection and recording by both the supervisor and supervisee during a clinical or supervisory session. This leads to the next primary component, *analysis*, a stage in which collected data are analyzed by supervisor and supervisee to determine the nature of client and/or clinician change relative to the initial planning. *Integrating* is the final Anderson component, occurring typically in a supervisory conference when both parties view the previous components as a whole. (pp. 63–66)

APPROACHES TO SUPERVISION

Available approaches to clinical instruction or supervision are numerous, as described in the educational and training literature for business and industry; medicine, nursing and other health professions; counseling psychology and social work; and teaching. Virtually all supervisors, whatever their circumstances, are called upon to inform, explain, demonstrate, and tell; to question, challenge, interpret, and evaluate; and to encourage, support, confirm, and advise. Which of these behaviors become selected and implemented and how they are balanced or emphasized are the factors that differentiate supervisory approaches among persons and disciplines. Farmer (1989b) has categorized the supervisory process according to systems, theories, styles, forms, and types, indicating the extent of its complexity and the myriad ways in which it can be analyzed. A selected sample is discussed here.

Indirect versus Direct Styles

Supervisory behaviors have been categorized either as direct (e.g., giving information, evaluating) or as indirect (e.g., using supervisee's ideas, providing support) by supervision researchers in education (Blumberg 1974) and, more recently, in speech-language pathology (Brasseur and Anderson 1983). It has been suggested by these and other investigators that, depending on a supervisee's level of independence, combinations of direct and indirect approaches may be appropriate.

The Continuum

In general, for beginning student clinicians, an emphasis on direct supervision is often indicated; whereas, for more advanced supervisees such as student clinicians with practicum experience, or externs, or clinical fellows, supervision can and should become increasingly indirect, and, finally, for self-supervising peers, consultative. While intervening circumstantial and situational factors, including clinical service and time demands, may necessitate periodic adjustments (Rassi 1987b; Anderson 1988; Casey, Smith, and Ulrich 1988), the overall move from direct to indirect supervisory styles is appropriate as the supervisor moves along in parallel with the supervisee's progression from Anderson's evaluation-feedback stage to a transitional stage, and then to a self-supervision stage (1988, p. 62). This change in supervisory approach, matched to needs, is described variously as a continuum of supervision (Anderson 1988), as developmental stages of supervision

(Hart 1982), and as levels of supervision (Rassi 1978, 1987b). According to Anderson (1988), maintaining a collaborative supervisory style throughout the process is key to supervisee movement.

Style and Content Combinations

Rudisill, Painter, and Rodenhauser (1988), representing views from education in medicine, psychiatry, and psychology, have identified four major approaches to instruction in a clinical setting: (1) didactic—the supervisor shares knowledge with the supervisee; (2) consultative—the supervisor engages in a more collegial interaction with the supervisee and serves as a resource person; (3) organizational—the supervisor emphasizes supervisee conformance to rules and standards of clinical practice as required by the institution or profession; and (4) personal growth—the supervisor focuses on the development of the supervisee's personal growth and its effect on patient care (p. 11).

It can be seen in this particular classification that didactic is similar to the previously discussed direct style, whereas consultative implies an indirect style. Organizational and personal approaches focus on content or clinical competencies to be developed, as well as on the supervisor's approach; that is to say, one involves behavioral skill mastery, whereas the other is analagous to a psychotherapeutic approach. Any of these approaches, either in whole or in part, has application in the audiology and speech-language pathology supervisory process. Depending on situational and personal requirements, they may be employed alone or in style-content combinations, for example, didactic and organizational, or consultative and personal.

The Clinical Supervision Model

Another approach, this one used with on-the-job teachers, is called clinical, or in-class, supervision (Goldhammer 1969; Cogan 1973). Cogan's version of the model (1973, pp. 10–12), depicted as a "cycle of supervision," is made up of eight successive phases. In phase one, the teacher-supervisor relationship is established; phase two finds the supervisor and teacher planning together the lesson or activity, specifying their desired outcomes, anticipating any problems, and discussing the mode of evaluation and feedback to be used. In the third phase, the supervisor plans, first alone, then together with the teacher-supervisee, the strategy of observation, including objectives and processes, as well as arrangements necessary for the collection of observation data.

The supervisor observes the teacher's instruction in phase four, followed, in the fifth phase, by analysis of the teaching-learning process, first by each party separately, then together. During the sixth phase, the supervisor and supervisee plan a strategy of their upcoming conference; and, in the seventh phase, discuss further the teacher's instruction. The eighth and final phase consists of renewed planning wherein both parties end their discussion and analysis of previous work, and begin planning the next lesson or activity, which includes changes to be incorporated by the teacher. It should be noted that phases six, seven, and eight may occur within the same meeting and other phases may be combined or omitted as a working relationship between the supervisor and supervisee develops. Other models of clinical supervision in education (Goldhammer 1969; Mosher and Purpel 1972; Acheson and Gall 1980; Goldhammer, Anderson, and Krajewski 1980) are similar in concept but differ in the number of phases or stages (Shapiro 1985). As Oliva (1989) points out, however, all of them have three essential components: communication between supervisor and supervisee-teacher prior to observation; classroom (clinical) observation; and follow-up after the observation. Anderson's supervisory process components are analogous to those used in teacher education.

A Cognitive Behavioral Supervision System

Leith et al. (1989) have developed a system of supervision for speech-language pathologists and audiologists that is based on cognitive behavior modification theory and a corresponding clinical interaction model (Leith 1984). The latter, transformed into a supervisory clinical interaction model, wherein the supervisor and supervisee are seen, alternately, as stimulus and response provides the basis for clinical teaching in the supervisory conference. Another feature of the system is its incorporation of 43 clinical behaviors, or competencies, into six different categories. Supervisory tasks, goals, and teaching self-supervision are also addressed in this system.

Differential Supervision

S. Farmer (1989b, 1989c, 1989d) has presented the so-called trigonal model, a way of dissecting supervision in communication disorders into three components: constituents, that is, those involved in the supervisory process; concepts, that is, theories and models developed for understanding the process; and contexts, that is, work settings in which the process takes place. In his elaboration of interrelationships among components, Farmer describes differential supervision, a theoretical model that provides for approaches to supervision differentiated according to individual component variables.

The Integrative Task-Maturity Model

Also based on a premise of individualizing supervisory style according to a supervisee's needs, the Integrative Task-Maturity Model of Supervision (ITMMS), an eclectic approach developed for use in speech-language pathology by Mawdsley and Scudder (1989), incorporates an adapted leadership model having four supervisory styles. Each style, based on the amount of assistance and support a supervisor must give to a supervisee, is matched with the supervisee's task-relevant maturity, or skill and confidence, as determined through administration of the W-PACC (Shriberg et al. 1975) evaluation of supervisee performance. The ITMMS is then implemented, in a progressive sequence, within the framework of Cogan's (1973) cycle of clinical supervision. Specific supervisory techniques are suggested for each phase.

Application Decisions

As already suggested, these approaches, as well as others not discussed here, are sometimes used in audiology and speech-language pathology educational programs. Two sets of observations about this circumstance are noteworthy. First, because they represent different kinds of categorization (components, style, system, and model) and because they reflect overlapping philosophies and needs, it is clear that these particular supervisory approaches are not mutually exclusive. The same can probably be said of all supervisory approaches regardless of their origin. Second, individual and program variations are undoubtedly related to the fact that no single approach has been adopted as a standard for the field. Such a move, of course, must await results of efficacy research and, even then, may not be desirable. Meanwhile, systematic preparation of individuals for supervisory roles can help supervisors and programs become informed about the approaches they choose to use.

Notwithstanding the multiplicity of supervision approaches, a number of practitioners and researchers have found the clinical supervision model, and variations thereof, as practiced in teacher education, particularly applicable to supervision in speech-language pathology (Anderson 1988). It has meshed well with ongoing clinical planning, pre- and post-observation supervisory conferences, and data-gathering observations of clinical sessions central to speech-language pathology supervision. Supervisory practice in audiology, although parallel in its conceptualization, conforms more closely, for clinical reasons, to a different supervision approach. As revealed in findings from the ASHA study of clinical certification requirements (Lingwall 1988), audiologists spend 46% of their clinical work time performing client evaluations, nearly twice as much time as the 25% spent in providing client treatment. (The latter, typically consists of hearing aid evaluation, fitting, and dispensing, clinical activities that, when placed in a supervision framework, are more diagnostic than therapeutic in nature.) Conversely, the study found, speech-language pathologists spend 21% of their work time in evaluation and 52% in treatment. Among other significant comparative points (Rassi 1978; 1987b), it is important to state explicitly that much of an audiologist's time, whether spent in evaluation or treatment, involves the manipulation of equipment and instruments and, therefore, intermittent, rather than sustained, interpersonal communication with clients.

Because of these substantial differences in predominant clinical activities,[1] the majority of audiology supervision strategies are more appropriately patterned after those in areas such as medical, nursing, and health professions education (de Tornyay and Thompson 1987; Rassi 1987b; Douglas, Hosokawa, and Lawler 1988) where supervisor-supervisee interactions take place primarily during a clinical session rather than in separate, planned conferences; where observation is mixed with frequently spontaneous intervention and participation by the supervisor; and where, often, the supervisory approach is necessarily direct, near, and immediate. Time constraints and the newness of case after case often prevent a supervisor and supervisee from engaging in sequential collaborative planning and anticipatory or reflective problem solving, leaving fewer opportunities for the supervisor to operate in a collaborative continuum mode between the direct instruction and consultation styles. Nevertheless, whenever the reverse clinical situations occur, that is, when the speech-language session is diagnostic or the audiology session involves aural (re)habilitation therapy, the opposite kinds of supervisory models, in modified form, are likely to be more workable.

SELECTING CLINICAL TEACHING STRATEGIES

Equipped with instructional content and direction provided by competency statements; with access to applicable approaches to clinical instruction; and with the teaching-learning context of the clinical envi-

---

[1]Throughout this book, as stated in the preface, the terms, discipline and field, in singular form, are used in reference to audiology and speech-language pathology, combined. However, it should be noted that, during the time of manuscript preparation, the ASHA Legislative Council passed a resolution stating that audiology and speech-language pathology are to be viewed as two professions (ASHA 1990b). The implications, if any, of this declaration relative to defining the supervisory process and describing its similarities and differences in speech-language pathology and audiology are as yet unknown.

ronment, a clinical instructor and student clinician can proceed with joint clinical-supervisory planning. It is during this planning stage, and in later stages as well, that individual teaching strategies should be discussed. Many students, having experienced years of instruction in the classroom, and fewers years in the laboratory and clinic, are aware of their own responsiveness to various modes of teaching. They often know which modes are reinforcing and which are reassuring. As a result, these students may have definite preferences for learning styles (West and Kaufman 1981; Rudisill, Painter, and Rodenhouser 1988), many of which are adaptable to the clinical teaching-learning process. S. Farmer (1989c) reports the instruments that examine supervisees' cognitive styles, experiential learning, and related preferences can provide additional information about their learning styles. (By the same means, supervisors can gain an increased understanding of their own teaching preferences and supervisory styles.) One such instrument, the Supervisory Needs Rating Scale, developed by Larson (1982), can lead a supervisor and supervisee to a better understanding of the supervisee's teaching-learning needs. These insights, when shared by supervisor and supervisee, along with other pertinent background information, facilitate joint planning of instructional strategies (Jason and Westberg 1982; Wiles and Bondi 1989).

Before systematic planning can take place, clinical instructors must be aware of the wide range of applicable strategies. McCabe (1985), after reviewing the results of clinical teaching studies in nursing, medicine, and dentistry, concluded that professional educators in different fields need to pool their resources. Our own review of strategy options from a variety of settings and disciplines has led us to the same conclusion. Publications on the supervisory process in communication disorders, especially the comprehensive texts by Anderson (1988) and Farmer and Farmer (1989), show evidence of many different sources of information already being applied in our field. The following compendium is a representative sample of strategies, some of them content- or competency-specific, others more generic in nature. Furthermore, some strategies and certain content may be introduced in the classroom and/or in laboratory exercises, then reviewed and/or applied in the clinic, whereas others are more suitable for clinical teaching only. All are applicable or adaptable to some phase of clinical education in audiology and speech-language pathology.

The Teaching Clinic

Because supervision can occur in groups as well as in dyads, Dowling (1979) introduced to the field of communication disorders a form of peer group supervision referred to as the teaching clinic. In this model, supervisees (peers) meet voluntarily on a weekly basis with a supervisor (clinic leader) to view and analyze a videotaped therapy session involving one of the supervisees (demonstration clinician) in the group. Following a carefully planned set of rules monitored by one of the supervisees (group monitor), the supervisees discuss the observed session, under the supervisor's guidance, offering suggestions and support.

The Teaching of Charting

McPhee (1987) reports a system of teaching clinical nursing students how to write consistently correct SOAP notes, where: S = subjective data, that is, a patient's, and other knowing persons', reported complaints, symptoms, and responses, either quoted or paraphrased; O = objective data, consisting of measurable observations pertaining to a patient's problem; A = assessment, where a clinician speculates on the nature of a patient's problem, including its cause or status; and P = plan, the clinician's recommendations, referrals, and other planned actions. The SOAP method of charting, a representative example of problem-oriented clinical reporting, can be practiced by students, prior to their clinical involvement, according to McPhee, through a series of reading and writing exercises based on generic, published materials.

Frisch and Coscarelli (1986), in teaching charting skills, use a model of systematic instruction. Prerequisite skills are first identified, then placed into a hierarchy of perceived difficulty. On the basis of this hierarchy, a sequenced plan of instruction is organized. For actual instruction they follow the steps developed by Merrill (1983): presenting a skills concept or principle; elaborating on the explanation, that is, clarifying and drawing analogies; citing illustrative examples; providing additional help through explanation of rationale; giving students opportunities, in a variety of situations, to practice what has been taught; and giving learners feedback on their understanding and performance. The final phase involves evaluation of instruction, by administering a cognitive pre- and posttest and by asking students to evaluate the instruction qualitatively.

It can be seen that the McPhee method is more suitable for teaching a clinical writing task in the classroom, whereas the second set of instructional strategies is applicable to classroom, laboratory, and clinical teaching in any number of combinations. The decision as to who, how, and where clinical writing is to be taught becomes a curricular as well as methodological matter.

Cognitive Behavioral Techniques

In the counselor supervision literature, supervisory cognitive-behavioral techniques are presented (Kurpius and Morran 1988). Similar in principle to that underlying the system used by Leith, McNiece, and Fusilier (1989), these techniques focus on integration of knowing and doing. Believed to be applicable to a broad range of supervision situations, three such techniques are mental practice, covert modeling, and cognitive modeling. In the mental practice technique, based on imagery, supervisees are asked to recall a past interpersonal experience in which they imagine themselves as the counselor and the other person as the client, then to imagine themselves as facilitators in the interaction. This technique provides the supervisee with an unlimited number of experiences, practicable outside the clinical environment, and allows for self-evaluation. A variation of the mental practice technique, covert modeling, involves a supervisor who gives the supervisee specific instructions as to what client situation to imagine and which skills to employ in the imagined interaction. Reportedly effective for learning a new skill or improving a previously acquired skill, the technique can be adapted to a learner's needs.

In cognitive modeling, the third technique, a supervisor conducts a video- or audiotaped counseling session with a client, then reviews the tape with the supervisee while simultaneously telling the supervisee what thinking process was used during that session. A supervisor may share thought processes as explanations of reasoning leading to a certain initiative or response for recalling internal dialogue. This technique has proven an effective training strategy, allowing students to examine and compare their own thinking, inferring, and decision-making processes. Kurpius and Morran (1988) assert that, "Whereas behavioral modeling is an effective way to teach the mechanics of a given skill, cognitive modeling can help teach the proper sequencing, timing, and integration of skills as well as the conceptual process of thinking that experienced counselors use but is not observable directly" (p. 371).

Dual-Focus Supervision

Another effective technique in the clinical training of counselors is called dual-focused supervision (McBride and Martin 1986), where two supervisors assume equal responsibility for teaching, counseling, and consulting with supervisees. The two supervisors share their knowledge of clinical theory and methods with each other and with supervisees. Several students may participate in the related practicum. Each is required to read about the theory presented by the supervisors, as well as about related theories, and then to share what they have learned with one another and with the supervisors in individual and/ or group conferences, and, finally, to apply the theory in client practice. Applicability of the theory is then shared by supervisees with the supervisors. Among the advantages of this method are the multiple paths of information flowing from one participant to another. Professional knowledge grows as new theories and techniques develop from interaction of all the participants. Moreover, as with other group supervision techniques, supervisees and supervisors are exposed to several role models.

In a subsequent study of the use of co-equal supervisors in this paradigm, Martin and McBride (1987) found it to be effective in teaching beginning practicum students to use counseling theory "in a professional manner" (p. 155). These students were judged to have skills equal to, or higher than, comparable groups of counselors in training and of practicing counselors. In addition, students involved in this practicum assigned higher ratings to the experience than did their counterparts in traditional apprenticeship dyads.

Live Team Supervision

Another variation of the collaborative approach to counseling supervision is revealed in live team supervision (Sperling et al. 1986), a strategy in which a supervisor and a team of students observe via a one-way window a student counselor engaged in a real counseling session and, communicating with that student by microphone-to-earphone or in brief face-to-face conferences, provide support, suggestions, or other kinds of information. All team members and the student counselor are involved in therapy pre-planning, but the supervisor decides what kinds of observer roles student team members will play. Various views are represented in this team approach not only to the supervisory process but to the clinical process as well. Furthermore, the team of students, along with the supervisee, experiences and contributes to on-site problem-solving while being exposed to the thought processes of others. From an integrative curricular perspective, this innovative technique combines laboratory and clinical learning in a unique way. Many elements of the live supervision approach are similar to those used in audiology supervision.

Assignment Variations

A look at the different ways in which clinical assignments in nursing education are made to meet special needs of students provides a basis for devising inventive clinical teaching strategies. A dual assignment, for example, pairs two students, or a student with a staff member who is not the clinical instructor, to work as a team with one or more clients. These arrangements, according to de Tornyay and Thompson (1987), serve to reduce anxiety, develop mutually supportive relationships, and provide exposure to different role models. Through joint planning, shared responsibilities, and alternating roles as primary and secondary caretakers, student-student and student-staff pairs experience the give-and-take of professional teamwork. The clinical instructor in this system alternates individual and paired conferences with students.

The alternative assignment is used when special arrangements are required to meet a particular student's needs or when there are not enough patients available to meet all students' needs (de Tornyay and Thompson 1987). In such cases, an alternative assignment might find a beginning student working in a supportive role with a more experienced student. The helper, nonetheless, is required to participate in all aspects of patient care. In another illustration of an alternative assignment, this one suitable in a pediatric setting, one student may be assigned to conduct social activities within a group, whereas another may be involved in direct nursing care. In this instance, the first might pursue learning objectives related to child growth and development, while the second focuses on certain childhood illnesses.

Experimental Strategies

Novel arrangements borrowed from other disciplines can be used as blueprints to design nontraditional clinical teaching strategies. Those just described, for example, suggest such strategies as clinically based team projects; individualized tutoring; disorder- or procedure-focused clinical teaching linked to teaching modules; and layered supervision funneling from clinical instructor to staff clinician to advanced student clinician to beginning student clinician. These and other teaching-learning paradigms need to be explored, not only because the potential for experimental clinical teaching in this field has not yet been tapped, but also because significant demands are being created by an ever-changing health and education climate. These changes include, but are not limited to, shifting limitations imposed by student enrollment, patient populations, faculty, staff, supervisor-practitioners, work settings, and delivery systems; the prospect of part-time students and growing numbers of professionals seeking updated education; and the expanding knowledge bases and scopes of practice that cannot be accommodated without reform in our present system of clinical education.

This need for systemic change in clinical practica was recognized in a resolution proposed at the St. Paul Conference and supported by 101 of 111 voting participants (Rees and Snope 1983), and stated: " . . . resolved, that alternative models of [the] clinical practicum based on criteria other than a required number of clock hours distributed across specific disorders be investigated" (p. 116). Despite this strong support for exploring departures from existing practice, both the new CCC and new ESB standards, established since the 1983 conference, continue to contain stipulations that restrict imaginative experimentation with innovative clinical teaching strategies. There remains an emphasis on quantity rather than on quality, on conformity rather than on innovation.

INTEGRATING CLASSROOM, LABORATORY, AND CLINICAL TEACHING

As illustrated in the previous discussion of clinical teaching strategies, subject matter can be divided, for teaching/learning purposes, into classroom, laboratory, and clinical modes. These lines are not always clear-cut, however, and educators need to consider different ways of packaging information. For example, it can be emphasized in one mode and supplemented in others; it can be presented sequentially in the three modes with equal emphasis in each; or it can be packaged in a recurring series of trimodal presentations, such as classroom-laboratory-clinic sequences repeated for each appropriate subtopic. The mixing and timing of teaching modes relative to subject matter are critical factors in instruction.

The Clinical Seminar

In audiology and speech-language pathology programs, one of the most common places for merging classroom, laboratory, and clinical instruction has been the clinical seminar. It is often held weekly, is customarily conducted by a team of clinical supervisors and/or academic faculty, and involves a combination of lecture, discussion, demonstration, practice, and problem-solving. Often, there is an accompanying project in which students are required to write a paper on clinically observed cases or to prepare and present in class a case study on a particular individual with whom they may be working in a regular practicum assignment. Some of the weekly seminars may be devoted to students' reviews and presentations of ongoing cases. This combination of class, lab, and clinic represents, if executed properly, curriculum integration at its best and can be used as a model for other topical treatments within a particular program.

Invitational Education

In nursing education, an integrative program known as invitational education (Purkey and Novak 1984) has been successful not only in combining educational delivery modes but also in making students responsible for their own learning. Students are invited to perceive themselves as being responsible, able learners who are valuable and have limitless potential. Similar in philosophy to the collaborative approach to clinical supervision, invitational education is a teaching-learning process of "doing with" rather than "doing to" (Spikes 1987, p. 26). Used in a nursing course on synthesis, this approach invites students to identify their clinical strengths and needs and their individual clinical goals. On the basis of this background information, the course instructor pairs each student with a "clinical guide," that is, a nurse practitioner who is an expert in the student's area of perceived need. The clinical guide is provided with a syllabus and an overview of the clinical course being taken by the student.

Throughout the course and accompanying practicum, students are encouraged to engage in metacognition, that is, in thinking about their own thinking and about how this relates to their learning and participation in the nursing process. Reflecting on one's own thinking, particularly as it relates to personal experience, says Spikes (1987), is important to the realization of one's potential to think creatively, take risks, and solve problems. In addition to classroom and clinical components, each student completes a project based on a problem of a patient in the student's clinical practicum and the subject of which is agreed upon by the student, clinical guide, and course instructor. After identifying the patient problem, the student then concentrates on finding a creative solution, using all sorts of available resources, including literature, organizations, agencies, and professionals, as well as the clinical guide and course instructor. When refined and completed by the student through study, analysis, and discussion with classmates and others, the proposed solution is carried out with the target patient under the nursing student's care.

Case Presentation Within Supervision

In counselor education, Biggs (1988) discusses the merging of a case presentation into clinical supervision. The combination, he asserts, gives students an awareness of contextual relevance, while engaging, through the supervisory process, in mutual dialogue characterized by divergent thinking and the raising of questions. A supervisee is exposed to the supervisor's thinking process in their joint search for understanding the meaning of a particular case as it relates to similar cases in either or both parties' clinical experience. They "are involved in a similar cognitive activity that includes searching for a contextual understanding of the particular client problem and developing a treatment plan" (p. 24). Thus, a typical classroom activity has been introduced to the clinical setting with apparent success.

The Microtraining Approach

Another useful blending of methods and persons is seen in microtraining techniques, forms of peer supervision that involve more advanced students working with students having less clinical education and experience (for example, doctoral students assisting master's or undergraduate students; second-year master's students assisting first-year master's students; or master's students assisting undergraduate students). The helping or teaching activity is accomplished through laboratory practice in which participants are monitored by a staff supervisor. Both groups benefit from their respective participation in the process.

Although this method may be used for prepracticum laboratory teaching of almost any kind of clinical skill, it has been found to be particularly beneficial in preparing student clinicians for interactive clinical work, removing the pressure of first-time practice with a real client. Such a training method, called microteaching and involving graduate-student "supervisors" and undergraduate-student "teachers," has been used effectively in special education (Douglas and Pfeiffer 1971). In preparing speech-language pathology students, Auburn and Irwin (1979) successfully embedded microinterviewing into a carefully structured sequence of activities: study session, practice interviews, feedback, training, restudy period, reinterview, and feedback. There are probably any number of other applications, including microsupervising, which has some potential as one of several techniques for preparing students for the supervisory process in our field.

Role Playing and Bridging

Role playing has been used as a clinical teaching technique in classrooms, in laboratory situations such as those just described, and in clinics. Role playing is typically used as a means for teaching students to use, and giving them an opportunity to practice, desirable interpersonal skills as they engage in simulated interactive clinical activities such as interviewing and counseling patients. Patient roles can be played by supervisors, by the students' peers, or by volunteer patients. Medical education has employed actors or lay persons trained specifically for role playing (Flaherty 1985). Borrowing this method for the prepracticum preparation of speech-language pathology and audiology students, Godden and Fey (1990) have successfully used actors or drama majors from their university's theatre department.

Research in medical education indicates that the most effective methods for teaching interviewing skills are those that include observation of others' interviews; discussion groups; and actual patient interviews followed by immediate, specific feedback from a clinical instructor (Flaherty 1985). Programmed instruction (Enelow, McKinney, and Wexler 1970) has been particularly effective, providing simulated interview samples, supplementary instruction at strategic points, and immediate feedback in response to students' selections of program options.

Because interactive clinical activities such as instructing, interviewing, and counseling of patients are appropriately taught in all instructional settings, it is important that they be given careful consideration in a program's overall curricular plan. If they are not balanced and coordinated, then consistency, reinforcement, continuity, and thoroughness cannot be assured.

IMPLEMENTING CLINICAL TEACHING STRATEGIES

In our discussion of the need for supervisor-supervisee joint planning and selection of applicable clinical teaching strategies, several references have already been made to actual implementation. This section will probe additional aspects of implementation as they relate specifically to the process and procedures of clinical teaching.

Observation and the Recording of Data

Numerous authors, for example, Goldhammer (1969) and Cogan (1973) in teacher education, and Anderson (1988) in speech-language pathology, cite the difficulties that can arise when observing another individual engaged in interactive work. The purposes of observations vary, depending on their context and on the kind of information being sought by the observer and the observed. In the case of a supervisor who is observing a supervisee for teaching-learning purposes, the supervisor should record objectively the events and interactions taking place. Unless there is a specific reason, predetermined by the supervisor and supervisee during observation planning, to use judgmental statements in evaluating part(s) of a clinical session, it is recommended that an actual account of happenings be recorded as accurately as possible without interpretation. If recording has not been objective, the recapturing of valid information for subsequent review, analysis, and integration by the supervisor and supervisee is virtually impossible. Anderson suggests that supervisors heed these succinct instructions: "Perceptions—not inferences; description—not commentary" (Anderson, 1988, p. 124). To facilitate recording of data, a variety of instruments has been adapted for use in speech-language pathology supervision (e.g., McCrea 1980; Smith 1980). Audio- and videotaping procedures have also been utilized.

Notwithstanding a clinical instructor's attempts to record clinical activities accurately and objectively, human errors in judgment and perception, arising from personal beliefs, values, biases, and previous experiences, are likely to occur. Selectivity in recording behaviors, inventing happenings to fill in gaps not observed, and projecting one's own ideas into what is occurring create in an observer what Cogan (1973) calls "inferential set" (p. 36). Distorted perceptions result. It is, therefore, important that supervisors, as they prepare for clinical teaching roles, gain insight into what underlies their own inferences, then learn to modify or control their observational behaviors accordingly. See J. Farmer (1989), which has a chapter devoted entirely to "observation competence," and which suggests a number of strategies for supervisors to use as they seek to make changes.

It should be noted here that supervisors' observations of the many clinical audiology events that involve little or no interpersonal communication between clinician and client are not particularly conducive to recording. It is possible, of course, to record specific actions as they occur. However, if changes in the supervisee's actions are needed, immediate intervention by the supervisor is usually necessary to reinforce a behavior, to correct a miscalculation, or to prevent an error from recurring; that is, if valid test results and/or correct hearing aid settings are desired within the client's allotted appointment time. There may be no point in recording specific details (e.g., the steps of pure-tone threshold determination) for later discussion and analysis; but the supervisor and supervisee may need to note particular instructional points or clinical areas needing analysis in subsequent discussions. Data recording such as that recommended for supervisors in education and speech-language pathology is more appropriately reserved for those diagnostic audiology and hearing aid activities in which a supervisee instructs, interviews, or counsels a client. In any case, observation planning in audiology supervision is equal in importance to that in speech-language pathology supervision.

The Supervisory Conference

Much of the dialogue between supervisor(s) and student(s) takes place in the supervisory conference. Therefore, the bulk of research on the supervisory process in speech-language pathology has focused on content of, and interactions within, this conference. Findings have yielded information on supervisors' perceptions of each other and of the process; on their feelings and their interpersonal communication; on the kinds of dialogue; and on the contribution to changes effected in supervisors, supervisees, and clients.

Conferences are used for planning clinical and supervisory agendas, as well as the focus and methods of observations and data collection, and the content of future conferences. They are used to analyze collected data and to integrate clinical and supervisory information into a meaningful whole. They also provide a forum for the supervisor and supervisee to exchange evaluative feedback. They afford occasions for joint problem solving and decision making. The extent to which conferences are used for these purposes and the degree to which supervisees actively participate in them, in large measure determines the substance and direction of clinical teaching and learning.

Given that formal supervisory conferences with planned agendas are not the primary means for informational exchange between diagnostic and hearing aid audiology supervisors and their supervisees, the benefits ascribed to such conferences must often be derived in other ways. Depending on the clinical operation and the demands on an audiology supervisor's time, pre- and post-clinical session meetings can be held for planning and review or analysis. Although supervisory and clinical planning are somewhat limited when a caseload does not include regularly returning clients, ongoing contingency planning can be accomplished. This requires some ingenuity on the part of the supervisor who needs to be anticipatory and be available to discuss and analyze data with the student soon after a clinical session. In those instances where audiology or speech-language pathology supervisors cannot or do not hold even the briefest of meetings with students (except, perhaps, for midterm and end-of-term evaluation conferences), and where communication is limited to exchanges within clinical sessions, opportunities for systematic supervisory planning are minimal. Even so, supervising "on the run," if executed with attention to an orderly development of competencies, and frequent solicitations of student input, can become a workable compromise. In some clinical settings, this kind of supervisory modification, although far from ideal, may be the only option.

In other settings, group conferences, that is, one or more supervisor meeting with several supervisees who have supervisors and assignments in common, can save time and increase efficiency. Dealing with specific issues may be sacrificed in this format, but many clinical and supervisory matters common to all participants can be addressed in group conferences. Indeed, group problem solving fosters collaboration among students and exposes them to others' thinking (Werner-McCullough and L'Orange 1985). S. Farmer (1989b) has developed a comparative analysis of dyadic and group conferences that can be used to help decide the appropriateness of different conference forms for certain supervisory needs (pp. 65–66).

Process Teaching

Clinical education literature is replete with exhortations to teach students to think. As indicated in the chapters on classroom and laboratory teaching, this advice is not directed exclusively to those who teach in the clinic. Nor is it, for that matter, limited to those in professional education, or to those in higher education. Indeed, "teach them how to think," has become the catch phrase of those in this country who are calling for educational reform at every level in every setting. Perhaps our students do know how to think, but have not been challenged enough to use the thinking skills they already have. In any event, it is difficult to disagree with persons who say that our students, as future audiologists and speech-language pathologists, need to be able to think, to use sound judgment, and to base their professional decisions on defensible rationale and logical reasoning. In keeping with the specific context of this chapter, how do we cultivate student thinking in the supervised clinical practicum?

Some answers have already been presented. That is to say, problem solving, clinical reasoning, critical thinking, and effective decision-making skills in students are promoted by strategic, open-ended questions, challenging discussions, real and hypothetical case analyses, and shared thought processes. These are essentially the same techniques as those recommended for use in the classroom or laboratory (Regan-Smith 1987). The differences lie in: the number of persons involved in the thinking process; the instructional setting; and the reality of time frames that necessarily compress the decision-making process. Clearly, there is no lack of teaching material. But unless the clinical instructor stimulates and encourages student thinking, the full teaching potential of clinical material will not be realized. A model for such collaborative, creative problem solving in our field is described by Shapiro and Moses (1989), who related supervision principles to the facilitation of problem-solving skills, and recommended specific techniques for supervisors and supervisees in public school supervision.

Because teaching effective decision making is similar in the classroom, the laboratory, and the clinic, instructors can design lessons, learning objectives, and competency statements that complement and parallel one another. If implemented over time, progression from simple to complex decisions can be achieved in a student's program of study (Jenkins 1985). Further linking of the decision-making process to the research process, the clinical process, and the supervisory process—the linking of the latter three was proposed by Anderson (1988)—consolidates and clarifies for instructors and students the interrelatedness of these fundamental processes.

Assessing/Evaluating Knowledge and Performance

Assessment and evaluation procedures can be accomplished by noting a supervisee's progress toward the attainment of previously established competency-based goals (Rassi 1978; Rassi 1987b). A number of clinical instruments, competency- or behavior-based, have been developed for evaluating clinical performance of supervisees in speech-language pathology and audiology. Several have been described in articles or have been published, for example, the Wisconsin Procedure for Appraisal of Clinical Competence (W-PACC) (Shriberg et al. 1975); the UTD Competency Based Evaluation System (Lougeay-Mottinger et al. 1984); the UWO Clinical Grading System (Johnson and Shewan 1988), and the Cognitive Behavioral System supervision forms (Leith, McNiece, and Fusilier 1989). For the most part, reliability and validity data are available. Many educational programs have developed or adapted evaluations, either in the form of rating scales or checklists, to fit specific needs. Some instruments are designed to provide a means for assigning grades. Some are criterion-referenced; some normative-referenced; and some can be modified for either. A variety of forms has been devised to provide students with evaluative and nonevaluative feedback on performance in both diagnostic and therapy sessions. Additional tools have been developed in our field for other data-gathering or evaluative purposes such as: conference analysis, for example, the Individual Supervisory Conference Rating Scale (ISCRS) (Smith and Anderson 1982a, 1982b); self-supervision by supervisees, for example, Casey's Clinician/Supervisee Skills Self-Assessment Instrument (Casey, Smith, and Ulrich 1988); and self-supervision by supervisors, for example, Casey's Supervisory Skills Self-Assessment Instrument (Casey, Smith, and Ulrich 1988). Frank (1980) devised a skill-based evaluation procedure for tracking outcomes in an audiology practicum by computer. A competency-based oral, practical examination using an interactive format with audiology student clinicians also has been developed (Rassi 1987a).

A considerable portion of the literature in allied health professions education is devoted to analysis and evaluation of clinical performance and the clinical teaching or supervisory process. Much of this information has application to audiology and speech-language pathology. In nursing education, for example, McKnight et al. (1987) developed an objective, structured clinical examination in which the competency areas and evaluation criteria were based on coursework and clinical objectives. Students, rotating through a series of testing stations, each staffed by a clinical instructor, were asked to perform certain skills, answer questions, and solve problems in management, patient teaching, case history, data analysis, and physical examination. This is but one example of a summative evaluation, seen by a number of nursing educators as a reliable alternative to assessment of student clinical performance through observation during the practicum period when students are in a learning phase (Hillegas and Valentine 1986; Tower and Majewski 1987; Johnson, Lehman, and Sandoval 1988). Others seem to favor ongoing, formative evaluations (Brozenec et al. 1987; Novak 1988), or a combination (Beare 1985; Higgins and Ochsner 1989).

The type of standardized practical examination described above is not unlike that being developed and used in some states' examinations for hearing aid dispensers (Strand 1987). Performance testing is suitable for clinical professions, since it can be designed to accomplish both process and product evaluations, can be administered orally, and can evaluate a clinician's ability to identify appropriate materials and tools. It is especially appropriate for assessment of technical skills (Watts and Feldman 1985). If well designed and administered, a performance examination can be an objective, reliable, and valid measure. If designed in a series to assess clinical competency at increasingly difficult levels, a performance examination can be an indicator of students' progress throughout a clinical practicum and assess their readiness for succeeding levels and specific experiences such as externships. When combined with a written component, a performance test can provide information about an individual's knowledge and ability to perform as a clinician, and has been used in comprehensive examinations just prior to the conclusion of students' preparation programs.

Clinical contracts have been found to be useful in conjunction with the evaluation process. They provide specific information on how students' clinical performance will be monitored and evaluated, including the learning objectives, competencies to be developed, teaching strategies, evaluation criteria and process, expected learning outcomes, time frames, grading policy, and other pertinent details. A clinical contract emphasizes the collaborative effort and responsibility expected of both clinical instructor and student, giving the two parties an understanding of what to expect during the practicum experience. The document can be designed to be sufficiently flexible for individual needs (Beare 1985). In a study of contract use with speech-language pathology students, Larson, Hoag, and Schraeder-Neidenthal (1987) concluded that, for most student participants, " . . . the contractual component of the process yielded positive impressions about objectivity, explicitness and clarity of expectations, as well as feedback consistency" (p. 120).

Other forms of evaluation applicable in clinical education include the following: peer evaluation (Erickson 1987; Davis and Inamdar 1988); videotaping and audiotaping of clinical communication skills (Browning and Campbell 1987) and audiotaping of evaluation conferences (Watson and Vinnick 1986); direct, multiple observations of interpersonal skills (Wakefield 1985); written simulations; computer simulations; record review (Neufeld 1985); and the use of simulated patients in a performance-based assessment (Barrows, Williams, and Moy 1987). Douglas, Hosokawa, and Lawler (1988), in their evaluation of noncognitive attitudes and skills in medical students, have described the benefits of using a behavioral approach based on observation or performance indicators. In medical education programs for primary care physicians, the coupling of criterion-referenced measurements with competency-based education has been strongly endorsed (Knopke and Goodwin 1981). The selection of diverse evaluation methods, recommended by West, Umland, and Lucero (1985) seems especially important at postgraduate levels, where evaluation results are used to determine eligibility for clinical practice. Along with written examinations, performance and oral examinations can provide revealing and meaningful information about an individual's clinical competence.

Beyond the practicum evaluations of CSD students' clinical knowledge and performance lie, in probable succession, the already-mentioned comprehensive examination, the National Examinations in Speech-Language Pathology and Audiology (NESPA), the heretofore optional Clinical Fellowship Year Performance Rating Observation (PRO) Scale (ASHA 1990a), and professional licensure and certification examinations.

Although intended to be the ultimate gauges by which a student is judged, these various measures to assess clinical competence have been questioned by professionals and educators. Among means employed to remedy this problem, the evaluation and validation of ASHA requirements for certificates of clinical competence (Lingwall 1988) helped to launch important changes. Item content on subsequently revised national examinations, for example, has been designed to correspond more closely to validated clinical knowledge and skills. This same knowledge/skill base is also being used by a recently appointed ASHA panel to develop an appraisal system for use by clinical supervisors in evaluating the performance of clinical fellows (Amy Finch, personal communication 1991). Furthermore, the evaluation of clinical fellows will become mandatory and required on three occasions during the fellowship period (ASHA 1991). This combination of an improved written examination, i.e., the NESPA examination(s), and a widely used practical evaluation, i.e., the clinical-fellow performance appraisal series, appears to hold promise as a more comprehensive and meaningful effort to assess clinical competence at the professional level.

Research on assessment of clinical competence in all health professions is critical in today's litigious climate. In medical education, for example, Norman (1985) points out, "there exists no consensus about precisely what is clinical competence or clinical problem solving" (p. 332). Also, there are inherent problems of subjectivity, most apparent in rating scales with descriptive terms rated on a continuum of poor to superior performance (Streiner 1985). Similarly, as reported in Shaw and Dobson's review of competency scales in the training of psychotherapists (1988), there exist significant concerns about inter-rater reliability and predictive validity. In view of the many difficulties created by these kinds of measurement variables, it is not surprising that clinical grading is an often debated and unresolved issue. A related problem, this one identified in the evaluation of medical students' performance, is the reluctance of clinical instructors to write negative evaluations for students even though these instructors may acknowledge to colleagues that the same students' performance is less than acceptable (Stemmler 1986). This attitude may contribute to grade inflation and, ultimately, to passing and graduating marginal students. Or, in the converse situation, on the basis of insufficient or negatively biased information, a misguided decision to fail a marginal student may be reached. Anderson (1988) advises programs "to have an established procedure for dealing with such students" (p. 247). Many of the challenges encountered by educators in comparable professions in the evaluation of clinical competence are also encountered by audiology and speech-language pathology educators.

Communicating Information and Feelings

Communication of evaluation information to student clinicians is not an easy task. Neither is communication of non-evaluative information, teaching of clinical principles, explanation of abstract concepts and unclear behaviors, nor expression of feelings that involve real or perceived risk. In our field, the complexity of interpersonal communication, particularly that within the supervisor-supervisee relationship, is evidenced in S. Farmer's chapter devoted to communication competence in supervision (1989a) and in Pickering's many writings on interpersonal communication in clinical and supervisory relationships (e.g., Pickering 1977, 1984, 1987a, 1987b, 1987c, 1989–1990; Pickering and Van-

Rheenen 1984, 1984–1985). As already indicated, much of the super-vision research in this field has focused on analysis of supervisor-supervisee conference interactions (e.g., McCrea 1980; Smith 1980; Cimorell-Strong and Ensley 1982; Roberts and Smith 1982; Smith and Anderson 1982a, 1982b; Brasseur and Anderson 1983; Shattuck-Hansen, Kennedy, and Laiko 1986; McCready, Shapiro, and Kennedy 1987), sub-stantiating the singular importance of supervisory communication.

Because any summarizing effort would be superficial and, there-fore, potentially misleading, it is not the authors' intention to explore here the dimensions of supervisory communication. Rather, readers are advised to consult the above references. Let it be said, however, that interpersonal communication in clinical teaching is even more con-sequential than that between teacher and student in the classroom or laboratory because the one-to-one relationship must be sustained over time to effect an atmosphere conducive to teaching and learning. In addition, the interpersonal focus of the clinical elements within this instructional, role-modeling domain contributes another set of com-munication factors.

As emphasized by Douglas, Hosokawa, and Lawler (1988) in refer-ence to clinical teaching in medicine, there must be trust between learner and teacher before learning can be expected to take place. To establish trust, a clinical teacher must communicate through active lis-tening; confidence-building; verbal messages; and consistent nonver-bal messages. Additional supervisory strategies such as self-disclosure and emphasis on positive teaching-learning experiences also facilitate communication (Gelazis and Kempe 1986), as do mutual exchanges that are descriptive, specific, and based on observed behaviors (Crago 1987; Douglas, Hosokawa, and Lawler 1988). In short, clear, open com-munication, unconstrained by personal biases and professional or in-stitutional role assumptions, is critical to the clinical teaching-learning process.

CLINICAL TEACHING EFFECTIVENESS

The effectiveness of clinical teaching in general and its methods in par-ticular, continues to be questioned. As Scheetz (1989) notes, in refer-ence to clinical competence in nursing practice, students do not neces-sarily improve their performance by the mere passage of time in the clinical area. In a study of nursing students, for example, those who participated in a structured supervision program attained greater clini-cal competence than did those students who worked, for the same time, as nursing assistants in noninstructional clinical settings (Scheetz 1989). In counseling supervision, Leddick and Dye (1987) have observed that "supervision should be highly active, providing large amounts of observation, feedback, and instruction" (p. 150). In his review of efficacy studies in clinical psychology education, Garb (1989) found that on-the-job experience did not increase the validity of psychologists' clinical judgments, whereas clinical training did accomplish this, albeit to a minor degree.

Shapiro and Anderson (1989), using their analysis of student-written agreements to document change in speech-language pathology and audiology supervisees' behaviors following a supervisory conference, found that student clinicians did follow through on their commitments; that is, they realized their conference-based clinical goals. On the basis of trackable, measurable behavior-change, rather than on the basis of supervisors' or supervisees' perceptions, these investigators have demonstrated evidence of one kind of supervisory effectiveness. Efficacy studies are not only needed to determine if supervisory intervention effects a change in supervisees, but also to determine the relative effectiveness of specific clinical teaching methods.

SUMMARY AND CONCLUSION

The supervisory process in speech-language pathology and audiology has become a viable area of research and study. Combining information from this source with comparable data from other disciplines yields an extensive variety of applicable and/or researchable clinical teaching approaches. This is fortunate because the current status of educational products and professional practice in CSD demands experimentation and innovation in the clinical education setting.

REFERENCES

Acheson, K., and Gall, M. 1980. *Techniques in the Clinical Supervision of Teachers.* New York: Longman Inc.

American Speech-Language-Hearing Association. 1985. Committee on Supervision in Speech-Language Pathology and Audiology. Clinical supervision in speech-language pathology and audiology. A position statement. *Asha* 27(6): 57–60.

American Speech-Language-Hearing Association. 1990a. *Asha Membership and Certification Handbook* (rev.). Rockville, MD: Author.

American Speech-Language-Hearing Association. 1990b. Legislative Council Report (LC 7-89). *Asha* 32(3):18.

American Speech-Language-Hearing Association. 1991. Clinical Certification Board. Implementation procedures for the standards for the certificates of clinical competence. *Asha* 33(5):47–53.

Anderson, J. 1981. Training of supervisors in speech-language pathology and audiology. *Asha* 23:77–82.

Anderson, J. L. 1988. *The Supervisory Process in Speech-Language Pathology and Audiology.* Austin, TX: Pro-Ed.

Andrews, J. R. 1971. Operationally written therapy goals in supervised clinical practicum. *Asha* 13:385–87.

Auburn, S. K., and Irwin, R. B. 1979. *Microinterviewing in Speech Pathology.* Poster session presented at the annual convention of the American-Speech-Language-Hearing Association, Atlanta.

Barrows, H. S., Williams, R. G., and Moy, R. H. 1987. A comprehensive performance-based assessment of fourth-year students' clinical skills. *Journal of Medical Education* 62(10):805–809.

Beare, P. 1985. The clinical contract—An approach to competency-based clinical learning and evaluation. *Journal of Nursing Education* 24(2):75–77.

Biggs, D. A. 1988. Discussions on the case presentation. The case presentation approach in clinical supervision. *Counselor Education and Supervision* 27(3): 240–48.

Blumberg, A. 1974. *Supervisors and Teachers: A Private Cold War.* Berkeley, CA: McCutchan Publishing Corp.

Brasseur, J. A., and Anderson, J. L. 1983. Observed differences between direct, indirect, and direct/indirect videotaped supervisory conferences. *Journal of Speech and Hearing Research* 26:349–55.

Browning, E. M., and Campbell, M. E. 1987. Evaluating students' communication skills: Tape recording. *Nurse Educator* 12(1):28–29.

Brozenec, S., Marshall, J. R., Thomas, C., and Walsh, M. 1987. Evaluating borderline students. *Journal of Nursing Education* 26(1):42–44.

Carlson, D. S., Lubiejewski, M. A., and Polaski, A. L. 1987. Communicating leveled clinical expectations to nursing students. *Journal of Nursing Education* 26(5):194–96.

Casey, P. L., Smith, K. J., and Ulrich, S. R. 1988. *Self-Supervision: A Career Tool for Audiologists and Speech-Language Pathologists* (Clinical Series 10). Rockville, MD: National Student Speech Language Hearing Association.

Cimorell-Strong, J., and Ensley, K. G. 1982. Effects of student clinician feedback on the supervisory conference. *Asha* 24:23–29.

Cogan, M. L. 1973. *Clinical Supervision.* Boston: Houghton Mifflin Co.

Crago, M. B. 1987. Supervision and self-exploration. In *Supervision in Human Communication Disorders: Perspectives on a Process,* eds. M. B. Crago and M. Pickering. San Diego, CA: Singular Publishing Group.

Crago, M. B., and Pickering, M. (eds.). 1987. *Supervision in Human Communication Disorders: Perspectives on a Process.* San Diego, CA: Singular Publishing Group.

Davis, J. K., and Inamdar, S. 1988. Use of peer ratings in a pediatric residency. *Journal of Medical Education* 63(8):647–49.

de Tornyay, R., and Thompson, M. A. 1987. *Strategies for Teaching Nursing* (3rd ed). New York: John Wiley & Sons.

Douglas, J. E., and Pfeiffer, I. L. 1971. *Microteaching as a Practicum for Supervisor Education: The Effect on Supervisor Conference Behavior and Skills.* (ERIC Reproduction Service ED 046 248)

Douglas, K. C., Hosokawa, M. C., and Lawler, F. H. 1988. *A Practical Guide to Clinical Teaching in Medicine.* New York: Springer Publishing Company.

Dowling, S. 1979. The teaching clinic: A supervisory alternative. *Asha* 21:646–49.

Enelow, A. J., McKinney, L., and Wexler, M. 1970. Programmed instruction in interviewing. *Journal of the American Medical Association* 212(11):1843–1846.

Erickson, G. P. 1987. Peer evaluation as a teaching-learning strategy in baccalaureate education for community health nursing. *Journal of Nursing Education* 26(5):204–206.

Farmer, J. L. 1989. Observational competence. In *Supervision in Communication Disorders*, eds. S. S. Farmer and J. L. Farmer. Columbus, OH: Merrill Publishing Company.

Farmer, S. S. 1989a. Communication competence. In *Supervision in Communication Disorders*, eds. S. S. Farmer and J. L. Farmer. Columbus, OH: Merrill Publishing Company.

Farmer, S. S. 1989b. The trigonal model of communication supervision: Concepts. In *Supervision in Communication Disorders*, eds. S. S. Farmer and J. L. Farmer. Columbus, OH: Merrill Publishing Company.

Farmer, S. S. 1989c. The trigonal model of communication disorders supervision: Constituents. In *Supervision in Communication Disorders*, eds. S. S. Farmer and J. L. Farmer. Columbus, OH: Merrill Publishing Company.

Farmer, S. S. 1989d. The trigonal model of communication disorders supervision: Contexts. In *Supervision in Communication Disorders*, eds. S. S. Farmer and J. L. Farmer. Columbus, OH: Merrill Publishing Company.

Farmer, S. S., and Farmer, J. L. 1989. *Supervision in Communication Disorders*. Columbus, OH: Merrill Publishing Company.

Flaherty, J. A. 1985. Education and evaluation of interpersonal skills. In *The Interpersonal Dimension in Medical Education*, eds. A. G. Rezler and J. A. Flaherty. New York: Springer Publishing Company.

Frank, T. 1980. A skill-based clinical audiology practicum evaluation procedure. *Asha* 22:251–54.

Frisch, N. A., and Coscarelli, W. 1986. Systematic instructional strategies in clinical teaching: Outcomes in student charting. *Nurse Educator* 11(6):29–32.

Garb, H. N. 1989. Clinical judgment, clinical training, and professional experience. *Psychological Bulletin* 105(3):387–96.

Gelazis, R., and Kempe, A. 1986. Reducing stress in faculty and students. *Nurse Educator* 11(3):4.

Godden, A. L., and Fey, S. H. 1990. Simulation: A tool for teaching clinical and supervisory skills. Miniseminar presented at the annual convention of the American Speech-Language-Hearing Association, Seattle, November.

Goldhammer, R. 1969. *Clinical Supervision*. New York: Holt, Rinehart & Winston, Inc.

Goldhammer, R., Anderson, R., and Krajewski, R. 1980. *Clinical Supervision* (2nd ed.). New York: Holt, Rinehart & Winston, Inc.

Hart, G. M. 1982. *The Process of Clinical Supervision*. Baltimore: University Park Press.

Higgins, B., and Ochsner, S. 1989. Two approaches to clinical evaluation. *Nurse Educator* 14(2):8–11.

Hillegas, K. B., and Valentine, S. 1986. Development and evaluation of a summative clinical grading tool. *Journal of Nursing Education* 25(5):218–20.

Jason, H., and Westberg, J. 1982. *Teachers and Teaching in U. S. Medical Schools*. Norwalk, CT: Appleton-Century-Crofts.

Jenkins, H. M. 1985. Improving clinical decision making in nursing. *Journal of Nursing Education* 24(6):242–43.

Johnson, C. J., and Shewan, C. M. 1988. A new perspective in evaluating clinical effectiveness: The UWO Clinical Grading System. *Journal of Speech and Hearing Disorders* 53:328–40.

Johnson, G., Lehman, B. B., and Sandoval, J. B. 1988. Clinical exam: A summative evaluation tool. *Journal of Nursing Education* 27(8):373–74.

Knopke, H. J., and Goodwin, B. B. 1981. Assessing student competence. In *Approaches to Teaching Primary Health Care*, eds. H. J. Knopke and N. L. Diekelmann. St. Louis: C. V. Mosby Company.

Kurpius, D. J., and Morran, D. K. 1988. Aspects of counselor preparation. Cognitive-behavioral techniques and interventions for application in counselor supervision. *Counselor Education and Supervision* 27(4):368–76.

Larson, L. 1982. Perceived supervisory needs and expectations of experienced vs. inexperienced student clinicians. (Doctoral dissertation, Indiana University, 1981). *Dissertation Abstracts International* 42:4758B. (University Microfilms No. 82–11, 183.)

Larson, L. C., Hoag, L. A., and Schraeder-Neidenthal, J. 1987. Supervisor-supervisee satisfaction with a contract-based system for grading practicum. In *Clinical Supervision: A Coming of Age*, ed. S. S. Farmer. Proceedings of a conference held at Jekyll Island, GA. Las Cruces, NM: New Mexico State University.

Leddick, G. R., and Dye, H. A. 1987. Counselor supervision. Effective supervision as portrayed by trainee expectations and preferences. *Counselor Education and Supervision* 27(2):139–54.

Leith, W. R. 1984. *Handbook of Clinical Methods in Communication Disorders.* Austin, TX: Pro-Ed.

Leith, W. R., McNiece, E. M., and Fusilier, B. B. 1989. *Handbook of Supervision: A Cognitive Behavioral System.* Austin, TX: Pro-Ed.

Lingwall, J. B. 1988. Evaluation of the requirements for the certificates of clinical competence in speech-language pathology and audiology. *Asha* 30(9):75–78.

Lougeay-Mottinger, J., Harris, M. R., Perlstein-Kaplan, K. E., and Felicetti, T. 1984. UTD Competency Based Evaluation System. *Asha* 26(11):39–43.

Martin, G. E., and McBride, M. C. 1987. The results of the implementation of a professional supervision model on counselor trainee behavior. *Counselor Education and Supervision* 27(2):155–67.

Mawdsley, B. L., and Scudder, R. R. 1989. The integrative task-maturity model of supervision. *Language, Speech, and Hearing Services in Schools* 20(3):305–319.

McBride, M. C., and Martin, G. E. 1986. Dual-focus supervision: A nonapprenticeship approach. *Counselor Education and Supervision* 25(3):175–82.

McCabe, B. W. 1985. The improvement of instruction in the clinical area: A challenge waiting to be met. *Journal of Nursing Education* 24(6):255–57.

McCrea, E. 1980. Supervisee ability to self-explore and four facilitative dimensions of supervisor behavior in individual conferences in speech-language pathology. (Doctoral dissertation, Indiana University, 1980.) *Dissertation Abstracts International* 41:2134B. (University Microfilms No. 80-29, 239.)

McCready, V., Shapiro, D., and Kennedy, K. 1987. Identifying hidden dynamics in supervision: Four scenarios. In *Supervision in Human Communication Disorders: Perspectives on a Process*, eds. M. B. Crago and M. Pickering. San Diego, CA: Singular Publishing Group.

McKnight, J., Rideout, E., Brown, B., Ciliska, D., Patton, D., Rankin, J., and Woodward, C. 1987. The objective structured clinical examination: An alternative approach to assessing student clinical performance. *Journal of Nursing Education* 26(1):39–41.

McPhee, A. 1987. Teaching students how to chart. *Nurse Educator* 12(4):33–36.

Merrill, M. D. 1983. Component display theory. In *Instructional Design Theories and Models: An Overview of their Current Status*, ed. C. Reigeleuth. Hillsdale, NJ: Lawrence Erlbaum Associates.

Mosher, R., and Purpel, D. 1972. *Supervision: The Reluctant Profession.* Boston: Houghton Mifflin Co.

Neufeld, V. R. 1985. Implications for education. In *Assessing Clinical Competence*, eds. V. R. Neufeld and G. R. Norman. New York: Springer Publishing Company.

Norman, G. R. 1985. Implications for research. In *Assessing Clinical Competence*, eds. V. R. Neufeld and G. R. Norman. New York: Springer Publishing Company.

Novak, S. 1988. An effective clinical evaluation tool. *Journal of Nursing Education* 27(2):83–84.

Oliva, P. F. 1989. *Supervision for Today's Teachers* (3rd ed). New York: Longman Inc.

Oratio, A. 1977. *Supervision in Speech Pathology: A Handbook for Supervisors and Clinicians*. Baltimore: University Park Press.

Pickering, M. 1977. An examination of concepts operative in the supervisory relationship. *Asha* 19:607–610.

Pickering, M. 1984. Interpersonal communication in speech-language pathology supervisory conferences: A qualitative study. *Journal of Speech and Hearing Disorders* 49:189–95.

Pickering, M. 1987a. Expectation and intent in the supervisory process. *The Clinical Supervisor* 5(4):43–57.

Pickering, M. 1987b. Interpersonal communication and the supervisory process: A search for Ariadne's thread. In *Supervision in Human Communication Disorders: Perspectives on a Process*, eds. M. B. Crago and M. Pickering. San Diego, CA: Singular Publishing Group.

Pickering, M. 1987c. Supervision: A person-focused process. In *Supervision in Human Communication Disorders: Perspectives on a Process*, eds. M. B. Crago and M. Pickering. San Diego, CA: Singular Publishing Group.

Pickering, M. 1989–1990. The supervisory process: An experience of interpersonal relationships and professional growth. *National Student Speech Language Hearing Association Journal* 17:17–28.

Pickering, M., and VanRheenen, D. D. 1984. Interpersonal communication in clinical and supervisory relationships: Skills, research, theory. *SUPERvision* 8(2):2–7(Summary).

Pickering, M., and VanRheenen, D. D. 1984–1985. Supervisory conferences: A place for teaching interpersonal communication concepts, skills. *SUPERvision* 8(4):2–11(Summary).

Popham, J., and Baker, E. 1963. *Planning an Instructional Sequence*. Englewood Cliffs, NJ: Prentice-Hall.

Purkey, W. W., and Novak, J. 1984. *Inviting School Success: A Self-Concept Approach to the Teaching-Learning Process* (2nd ed.). Belmont, CA: Wadsworth Publishing Company.

Rassi, J. A. 1978. *Supervision in Audiology*. Baltimore: University Park Press.

Rassi, J. A. 1987a. Comprehensive examination of audiology graduate students: A competency-based practical component. In *Clinical Supervision: A Coming of Age*, ed. S. S. Farmer. Proceedings of a conference held at Jekyll Island, GA. Las Cruces, NM: New Mexico State University.

Rassi, J. A. 1987b. The uniqueness of audiology supervision. In *Supervision in Human Communication Disorders: Perspectives on a Process*, eds. M. B. Crago and M. Pickering. San Diego, CA: Singular Publishing Group.

Rees, N. S., and Snope, T. L. (eds.). 1983. *Proceedings of the 1983 National Conference on Undergraduate, Graduate, and Continuing Education* (Report No. 13). Rockville, MD: American Speech-Language-Hearing Association.

Regan-Smith, M. G. 1987. Teaching clinical reasoning in a clinical clerkship by use of case assessments. *Journal of Medical Education* 62(1):60–63.

Roberts, J. E., and Smith, K. J. 1982. Supervisor-supervisee role differences and consistency of behavior in supervisory conferences. *Journal of Speech and Hearing Research* 25:428–34.

Rudisill, J. R., Painter, A. F., and Rodenhouser, P. 1988. Clinical teaching modes: A usage guide. *The Clinical Supervisor* 6(1):3–19.

Scheetz, L. J. 1989. Baccalaureate nursing student preceptorship programs and the development of clinical competence. *Journal of Nursing Education* 28(1): 29–35.

Shapiro, D. 1985. An experimental and descriptive analysis of supervisees' commitments and follow-through behaviors as one measure of supervisory effectiveness in speech-langauge pathology and audiology. 1984. Doctoral dissertation, Indiana University. *Dissertation Abstracts International* 39:2889B. (University Microfilms No. 84-26, 682.)

Shapiro, D. A., and Anderson, J. L. 1989. One measure of supervisory effectiveness in speech-language pathology and audiology. *Journal of Speech and Hearing Disorders* 54:549–57.

Shapiro, D. A., and Moses, N. 1989. Creative problem solving in public school supervision. *Language, Speech, and Hearing Services in Schools* 20(3):320–32.

Shattuck-Hansen, D., Kennedy, K. B., and Laikko, P. A. 1986. Verbal interaction patterns in supervisory conferences: A preliminary investigation. *NSSLHA Journal* 13(1):20–29.

Shaw, B. F., and Dobson, K. S. 1988. Competency judgments in the training and evaluation of psychotherapists. *Journal of Consulting and Clinical Psychology* 56(5):666–72.

Shriberg, L., Filley, F., Hayes, D., Kwiatkowski, J., Schatz, J., Simmons, K., and Smith, M. 1975. The Wisconsin Procedure for Appraisal of Clinical Competence (W-PACC): Model and data. *Asha* 17:158–65.

Smith, K. 1980. Multidimensional Observational System for the Analysis of Interactions in Clinical Supervision (MOSAICS). In *Proceedings—Conference on Training in the Supervisory Process in Speech-Language Pathology and Audiology*, ed. J. Anderson. Bloomington, IN: Indiana University.

Smith, K. J., and Anderson, J. L. 1982a. Development and validation of an individual supervisory conference rating scale for use in speech-language pathology. *Journal of Speech and Hearing Research* 25:243–51.

Smith, K. J., and Anderson, J. L. 1982b. Relationship of perceived effectiveness to verbal interaction/content variables in supervisory conferences in speech-language pathology. *Journal of Speech and Hearing Research* 25:252–61.

Sperling, M. B., Handen, B. L., Miller, D., Schumm, P., Pirrotta, S., Simons, L. A., Lysiak, G., and Terry, L. 1986. The collaborative team as a training and therapeutic tool. *Counselor Education and Supervision* 25(3):183–90.

Spikes, J. M. 1987. Invitational education: A model for nursing. *Nurse Educator* 12(3):26–29.

Staff. 1989, March 9. Center for Studies in Clinical Education Established. *Folio*, p. 6.

Stemmler, E. J. 1986. Promoting improved evaluation of students during clinical education: A complex management task. *Journal of Medical Education* 61(9): 75–81.

Strand, T. 1987. A job analysis of Illinois hearing instruments dispensers. *Hearing Instruments* 38(5):120–21.

Streiner, D. L. 1985. Global rating scales. In *Assessing Clinical Competence*, eds. V. R. Neufeld and G. R. Norman. New York: Springer Publishing Company.

Tower, B. L., and Majewski, T. V. 1987. Behaviorally based clinical evaluation. *Journal of Nursing Education* 26(3):120–23.

Wakefield, J. 1985. Direct observation. In *Assessing Clinical Competence*, eds. V. R. Neufeld and G. R. Norman. New York: Springer Publishing Company.

Watson, M., and Vinnik, M. 1986. The tape recorder in clinical evaluation. *Nurse Educator* 11(1):30, 39.

Watts, J., and Feldman, W. B. 1985. Assessment of technical skills. In *Assessing Clinical Competence*, eds. V. R. Neufeld and G. R. Norman. New York: Springer Publishing Company.

Werner-McCullough, M., and L'Orange, C. 1985. Putting "oomph" into clinical conferences. *Nurse Educator* 10(6):33–35.

West, D. A., and Kaufman, A. 1981. Instructional strategies in the classroom and the clinic. In *Approaches to Teaching Primary Health Care*, eds. H. J. Knopke and N. L. Diekelmann. St. Louis: C. V. Mosby Company.

West, D. A., Umland, B. E., and Lucero, S. M. 1985. Evaluating student performance. In *Implementing Problem-Based Medical Education. Lessons from Successful Innovations*, ed. A. Kaufman. New York: Springer Publishing Company.

Wiles, J., and Bondi, J. 1989. *Curriculum Development. A Guide to Practice* (3rd ed.). Columbus, OH: Merrill Publishing.

Chapter 12

Using Media in Teaching

Glen L. Bull and Paula S. Cochran

Historically, a range of media has been used in the instructional process in communication disorders. This was the case for audiotapes in the 1970s, and for videotapes in the 1980s. As computing technologies play increasing roles in clinical applications, from augmentative communication to audiometric assessment, we may anticipate that they will be employed in a variety of instructional roles as well.

In the past, different types of instructional media have been classified by separate categories. In 1985 the Massachusetts Institute of Technology constructed the Weisner Building and founded the M.I.T. Media Laboratory based on the premise that all media are converging. The director, Nicholas Negroponte, used a diagram of converging circles of media to make the case for establishment of the media laboratory (Brand 1988) (see figure 1). By the end of the decade a complete evolution will have taken place. A 35 millimeter slide, an overhead transparency, or a set of lecture notes may be based on the same digitized image from a computer file.

Although projected computer images that create "electronic blackboards" will increasingly find their way into classrooms, print materials will continue to be instructional mainstays over the next decade and beyond. In former years, a chart or diagram might have been created with pen and ink. Later, press-on letters and symbol packages made it easier to correct mistakes by peeling off incorrectly positioned lines or lettering. Graphics software now makes it possible to do the equivalent electronically. The final product remains the same, but the decreased technical skills required make it possible to focus on content rather than production techniques. Decreased cost, in either personal time or remuneration of a professional illustrator, also makes day-to-day use of such instructional materials more practical. In an era of overlapping media, the same illustration can be projected on a screen in a computer slide show, presented during a lecture, and provided as a handout.

THE ACADEMIC WORKSTATION

Van Riper's first text began as a mimeographed collection of lecture notes. Very little changed in the development of lecture notes and related instructional materials until the advent of the word processor, when for the first time it was possible to revise instructional materials without retyping an entire set of notes. Now almost all instructional materials that appear in printed form are generated with a computer, but paper will continue to be the foremost instructional medium for the foreseeable future.

The first word processors were character-based. They could reproduce text, but graphics were not easily incorporated. Inclusion of illustrations required what an early ASHA presenter on technology laughingly referred to as a "poor man's word processor"—scissors and paste. Further advances in word processing and the academic workstation are dependent upon two related technologies: display technologies and the user interface.

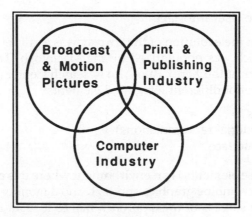

Figure 1. Circles of converging media.

Display Technologies

Widespread availability of word processors resulted from the advent of personal microcomputers in the second half of the 1970s. Early micro-computers that utilized the CP/M (Control Program/Microcomputers) operating system were often connected to separate display terminals that had no graphics capabilities. The Apple II computers had graphics capabilities, but low resolution of the display initially limited these systems to 40 columns of text per screen.

In the next generation of IBM-compatible microcomputers, the CP/M operating system was succeeded by the MS-DOS operating system. This generation of IBM-compatible computers has been characterized by graphics displays of increasing resolution: CGA (Color Graphics Adapter), EGA (Enhanced Graphics Adapter), and VGA (Video Graphics Array). The ultimate goal of a word processing display is to present an image as it will appear on a final printed version. All modern word processors espouse a "What You See Is What You Get" (WYSIWYG) philosophy. Increasing degrees of resolution on the screen make successive degrees of approximation to that goal possible. The two elements of a true approximation of the final printed output are:

- accurate representation of different typefaces and styles, such as **boldface**, *italics*, and varying sizes and fonts, and
- incorporation of graphics materials

The effort to make a screen image match the printed page exactly was pioneered on the Macintosh. However, the increasing resolution of IBM-compatible computers (CGA, EGA, VGA) soon made realistic displays possible on those systems as well.

Evolution of the User Interface

The next step in the evolution of the display was a graphics user interface (GUI), which was popularized by the Macintosh. This interface, inspired by work at the Xerox Palo Alto Research Center (PARC), consists of a number of different integrated elements:

- windows
- icons (pictorial representations)
- mouse interface

The sum of these elements is an environment where it is easy to create documents that combine graphics and text, and a monitor that can display them. The success of this approach makes it seem likely that all future microcomputer operating systems will utilize a graphics user interface. *Windows 3.0* and *OS/2 (Operating System 2)*, operating systems designated as successors to *MS-DOS* on IBM-compatible machines, incorporate this type of user interface, as do a number of other microcomputer operating systems under development.

Another highly desirable feature of an academic workstation is *multitasking*. This capability allows a user to run different programs in separate windows on the display. The capability of intermixing and displaying graphics and text on the same screen implies availability of a graphics program to complement the word processing program. In a few cases a graphics program and a word processing program may be combined in a single *integrated* program, but the capabilities of individual elements of an integrated program are often weaker than the same capabilities purchased separately.

Multitasking enables the user to run a word processing program in one window, a drawing program in a second, and a graphing program in a third. This allows a user to create a graphic in one window, and transport it to a word processing document in a second window. This capability was introduced with MultiFinder on Macintosh computers, and is a feature of the *Windows 3.0* and *OS/2* operating systems on IBM compatible computers.

Multitasking increases the importance of the size of the display monitor, an aspect of academic workstations often overlooked. The final output of the system is most often an 8½ by 11-inch sheet of paper. Many displays show only a portion of this page at any one time, an effect likened to an attempt to read the *New York Times* through a 4- by 6-inch window cut into a cardboard template that is moved around the newspaper as it is read. Ideally, a display should be the same size as the final document: an 8½ by 11-inch piece of paper.

Multitasking makes a full-page monitor even more desirable. The advantages of having several windows (each with a different program) are increased if it is possible to see more than one window at a time. The increased size of a full-page monitor makes this possible. Full-page monitors are now available for both Macintosh and IBM-compatible systems, and are highly desirable for production of instructional materials. The graphics user interface and graphics displays made incorporation of graphics and text practical in the production of lecture notes. In the next section some attention will be given to graphic illustrations.

GRAPHIC ILLUSTRATIONS

As microcomputer displays gained graphics capabilities, it became possible to integrate graphics and text in lecture notes. The following example (figure 2) illustrates the potential effect of incorporating graphics.

The addition of an illustration makes it easier to understand *visual and verbal* relationships. The illustration makes it clear that as more events per second occur, the time between events decreases. In the past, this type of graphic could be added to lecture materials with scissors and paste, or sketched freehand on a chalkboard, but the unwieldiness of the process made it difficult to update lecture notes. The two major categories of graphics programs are *illustration* programs and

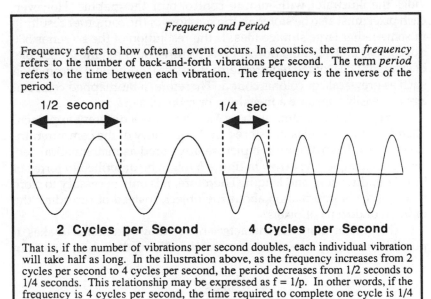

Figure 2. Lecture notes with graphics incorporated.

graphing programs. A graphing program is used for charts and graphs. An illustration program, as its name implies, can be used for creating illustrations, such as a drawing of the cochlea. Two major categories of illustration programs are *paint* programs and *draw* programs.

Paint and Draw Programs

A paint program stores its information in a bit-mapped format. A draw program, on the other hand, stores its representation in a vector-based format. Each type of illustration program has advantages and disadvantages. The names for the categories of graphics programs are drawn from two of the early programs that popularized this type of program on microcomputers, *MacPaint* and *MacDraw*. Each program has been followed by more sophisticated successors, but inspired the names that are used generically today.

MacPaint uses a bit-mapped approach, now often described as a *paint* mode. The individual picture elements (or *pixels*) of a bit-mapped display consist of a series of dots across the screen. If an illustration, such as the butterfly in figure 3, is enlarged, the individual pixels that make up the illustration can be seen as in figure 4.

Each pixel can be changed in a *bit-mapped* display. In a paint mode, it is possible to edit an illustration on a pixel-by-pixel basis. This provides the illustrator with minute control over the graphic. However, each pixel must also be stored in the memory of the computer resulting in some rather large storage files. If the resolution of the screen is 500 dots across and 400 dots down, each picture could require 20,000 bits of storage. The storage requirements increase if additional information such as grey-scale or color is coded. Therefore, a bit-mapped color image can easily consume a megabyte or more of storage.

Vector-based programs such as *MacDraw* use a different approach. Each individual pixel is not stored in the memory of the computer. Instead, lines that make up the picture are stored as mathematical vectors. For example, the arrow in figure 5 might be described in terms of its origin, direction, and length. Therefore, it is only necessary to store three pieces of information about the object, instead of recording the location of dozens of pixels.

This vector-mapped characteristic of draw programs makes it possible to change the sizes of objects without distorting them. In

Figure 3.   Butterfly.

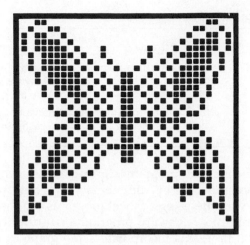

Figure 4. Picture elements (pixels) of a butterfly.

contrast, if the size of a bit-mapped image is altered, distortion often occurs. Because the illustrator works with entire objects instead of pixel-by-pixel as in a paint program, this program is sometimes described as an *object-oriented* approach (see table I).

Each approach has its advantages. More recent programs, such as *SuperPaint* and *Canvas*, provide both paint and draw modes. This provides the user with the best of both worlds. Even more sophisticated programs, such as Adobe *Illustrator* and Aldus *Freehand*, have been developed for professional illustrators, but they may require more time to master than the occasional user is willing to invest.

Graphing Programs

Paint and draw programs are general purpose programs allowing the user to determine the applications for which they will be used. It is possible to develop a chart or graph with a paint or draw program, but it would be more efficient to use a graphing program because it is designed to transform a table of numbers into a chart or graph. It can perform certain functions such as determining the overall scale for the graph, making it possible to quickly view the data from several perspectives.

There are three types of graphing programs: those provided with spreadsheets; graphing utilities incorporated with statistical programs;

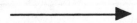

Figure 5. Vector-mapped arrow.

Table I.   Types of Illustration Programs

Mode	Advantage	Disadvantage
Paint (Bit-Mapped)	Individual picture elements (pixels) can be manipulated	Large amounts of memory may be required to store the image
Draw (Object Oriented)	Object can be transformed without distortion	Individual elements of each object cannot be altered.

and stand-alone graphics programs. Spreadsheets such as Lotus *1-2-3* or *Excel* are accompanied by rudimentary graphing programs. The charts created with these spreadsheet programs can then be imported into a general purpose drawing program for further enhancements. Many statistical programs incorporate some graphics capability, but most stand-alone programs have been designed solely for the purpose of generating charts and graphs. *Delta Graph* on the Macintosh and *Chart Master* on the IBM were designed for this purpose, as their names imply. The bar chart in figure 6, which shows the percentage of faculty

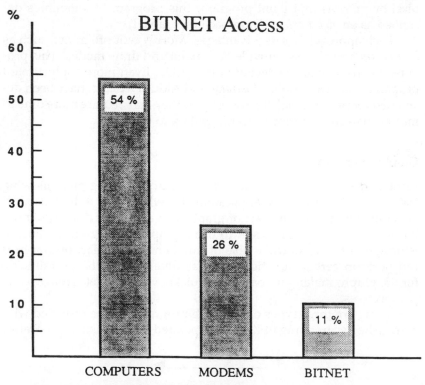

Figure 6.   Bar chart illustrating BITNET usage.

in 67 communication sciences and disorders (CSD) programs who have computers on their desks, was created with this type of program (Cochran and Bull 1991).

In addition to charting and graphing software, other types of specialized graphics programs are available for creating organizational charts, calendars, project management diagrams, and for almost every imaginable purpose. If a special function is required frequently, investing in an application for that purpose may be worthwhile. Otherwise, specialized programs are almost certain to sit on the shelf unused because the time required to learn them will not compensate for their infrequent use.

One feature of the Macintosh operating system is worth mentioning in the context of graphics. It is possible to transfer most graphics on the Macintosh from any program to any other program via the Macintosh electronic clipboard. By common convention, all programs even use the same commands to copy (⌘-C) and insert (⌘-V) graphics to and from the clipboard. As a result, it is unnecessary to learn different commands for copying and inserting graphics in different programs. This type of common user interface, which has the same structure across all programs and which enables programs to share information with one another, may also be a feature of *Windows* or *OS/2* when they eventually replace the *MS-DOS* operating system on IBM-compatible computers.

Sources of Graphic Images

The foregoing discussion implies that an entire illustration will be created by the user. This is not necessarily the case. Often portions of a graphic may be imported from other sources. There is no particular reason that every instructor in every CSD program in the United States should recreate a schematic diagram of a cochlea, for example. Libraries of electronic *clip art* in paint and draw formats have been created for this purpose. Rather than attempt to create an original drawing of the United States, one could purchase a disk of geography clip art. Soon departments of CSD may begin storing graphic libraries of clip art related to speech-language pathology and audiology, just as other instructional materials are made available to their faculty.

A video digitizer provides a means of converting a three-dimensional image to a digitized image stored in the computer. Any video source, such as a video camera or videocassette recorder (VCR), can be used as an input to the digitizer. If a videocassette recorder is used for this purpose, the machine must be able to generate a stable pause in which the image does not jitter as it is being digitized. A VCR with four heads is more likely to possess this capability.

A scanner provides another means of digitizing images. A scanner works much like a copy machine except that the original illustration or photograph is converted to a digital image in the computer. It is important to note that the same copyright laws that protect written materials also apply to graphics and illustrations. Some scanners can only be used to digitize text (to save the time required to retype the document), others can only digitize graphics, while others, with the proper software, can digitize text and graphics.

The resolution of the current generation of video digitizers and scanners places some limits on their utility, but these limits are shifting upward every year. Increased resolution produces increased storage demands, especially when color images are involved which may require several megabytes of storage space. Storage capacity is also steadily increasing, however. A CD-ROM (compact disk, read-only memory) can hold 650 megabytes. To provide a basis for comparison, the entire works of Shakespeare consume only seven to eight megabytes of storage. Once the digitized image is in the computer it may be manipulated in a variety of ways. *Autotrace* programs can trace outlines of a digitized image and convert a bit-mapped illustration to an object-oriented figure. The converted figure can then be resized or further altered. Other programs such as *Digital Darkroom* and *Image Studio* can enhance the images in much the same way that photographic processing techniques enhance images in a conventional darkroom.

DESKTOP PUBLISHING

The term *desktop publishing* refers to the capability that permits an instructor to produce handouts and lecture notes with graphics and text in a single document. There are a number of types of graphics materials relevant to communication disorders, e.g., speech waveforms, sound spectrograms, audiograms, and anatomical figures. With desktop publishing, it is possible to incorporate a speech waveform or an audiogram from last week's clinical session into today's lecture notes.

Initially, this degree of control over the appearance of materials involved a two-step process. The text was first generated by a word processor; then format and layout information were later added through a *desktop publishing* program. The era of desktop publishing, introduced in 1985 by the program *Pagemaker,* made it possible for anyone who previously required commercial typesetting services to produce newsletters and journals. Separate desktop publishing programs may still be advantageous for production of journals and newsletters, but word processing systems are now incorporating desktop publishing features sufficient for production of most lecture materials. Regardless of how the graphics and textual materials are integrated, the term *desktop publishing* implies that the final output will appear in printed form.

The first output devices for microcomputers such as Teletypes were character-based. Later, impact printers such as *Diablo* or *NEC Spinwriter* improved the level of output to letter quality, but still lacked graphics capability. Dot-matrix printers, which use a matrix of wires to form characters, have both text and graphics capabilities. Their limitation is that they tend to be noisy, and the print is not letter quality.

Laser printers provide the combination of high resolution, speed, flexibility, and quietness that is desirable for production of instructional materials. Until recently, laser printers fell into two classes: *PostScript* printers and non-*PostScript* printers. *PostScript* is a page description language developed by Adobe that translates computer output into a format understood by any *PostScript* printer. Most graphics software has this capability. The practical significance of *PostScript* is that production of documents incorporating graphics elements is considerably facilitated.

To see why this is so, it is necessary to reconsider the two ways in which a graphic design can be represented inside a computer: (1) as a bit-mapped image, or (2) a vector-based representation. The resolution of a laser printer is typically much greater than the resolution of a corresponding display. For example, the resolution of a Macintosh screen is typically 72 dots per inch, while the resolution of the Apple Laser-Writer is 300 dots per inch. If the screen output is simply printed, pixel by pixel, the appearance of the final document is relatively crude. However, *PostScript* makes it possible to take advantage of the increased resolution of the laser printer.

Manufacturers who incorporate *PostScript* into their laser printers must pay a licensing fee to Adobe. This makes the cost of laser printers that incorporate *PostScript*, such as the Apple LaserWriter, more expensive than other printers such as the Hewlett-Packard Laserjet. (It is possible to upgrade some types of non-*PostScript* printers to add *PostScript*.) For production of routine secretarial documents such as clinical reports, a non-*PostScript* printer may be quite adequate. However, *PostScript* was the final element necessary for the desktop publishing revolution, and production of any instructional document with graphic elements may be facilitated by access to a laser printer that supports *PostScript*. Recently, Apple and Microsoft initiated a collaborative effort to develop a product competing with *PostScript* which they named *TrueType*. The advent of *TrueType* has made the marketplace more confusing, but has also reduced the cost of *PostScript*, improved its quality, and made Adobe more responsive to consumer concerns.

DESKTOP PRESENTATIONS

Emphasis on desktop publishing stems from the fact that the dominant instructional medium used by an average faculty member is paper. Course outlines, syllabi, lecture notes, and examinations will continue to be provided in a paper format for the foreseeable future, although some journals are beginning to accept electronic submissions. Development of a document on an electronic system implies the potential for output in a number of other instructional media. A presentation developed and displayed with a desktop computer is sometimes described as a *desktop presentation* system.

Computer Projection Devices

A desktop presentation may be as simple as a word processing file displayed with a computer projection device that is distributed in the form of printed lecture notes. The computer image may also be projected on a screen at the front of the room. Printed notes and projected computer image complement one another nicely. Printed output ensures that the attention of a class is not diverted by the necessity of making notes of minute details. Projected output is flexible and can be altered on the spot. The image becomes an electronic blackboard. It becomes possible to revise a clinical report for instructional purposes as a class watches. It can be changed in response to "what if" questions from a class. Sentences can be altered, deleted, or moved. In addition to examples of clinical reports generated by an instructor, it can also be helpful to review word processed clinical reports created by class members. This provides a convenient way for everyone to see selected examples without an overhead projector and cost of making individual printed copies. It also becomes possible to implement class suggestions for revisions immediately to show the effects. All of this can be accomplished with a copy of the file while leaving the original intact in the event that not every suggested revision is adopted.

Until recently, computer projection devices were expensive, costing $5,000 to $10,000, limiting the number of classrooms equipped in this way. The advent of inexpensive liquid crystal display (LCD) devices, which can be used in combination with overhead projectors to display the computer image, has altered this situation completely. Now it is feasible to use this technology in any classroom that can be equipped with an overhead projector. Curiously, the use of this technology has outstripped the vocabulary available to describe it. The first device of this type, developed by Kodak, was called a "Kodak Datashow," and this term is sometimes used to describe other devices of this kind in the same way that the word "Kleenex" is sometimes inaccurately used as a descriptor for all facial tissues. The term "Data Projection Device" (DPD) is sometimes used, but seems cumbersome.

Two types of computer projection systems are available currently. One consists of three electronic beams projected through different colored lenses (red, green, and blue) onto a large screen at the front of a room. Sometimes the system may be placed on a cart that is moved from room to room, but often it is mounted from a fixed location in the ceiling to ensure a more accurate focus. This type of system has two advantages: (1) it can be used to display computer images in color; and (2) it can be used to project video images (videotapes, satellite downlinks).

The latter advantage is significant because clinical details that may be obscured on a smaller monitor are easily observed on a six-foot projection. As noted above, the primary disadvantage of this type of system is cost, typically $5,000 to $10,000, although instructional benefits may warrant the expense if the system is used by a high percentage of faculty. The second type of computer projection system consists of the same (LCD) screen placed on an overhead projector. The liquid crystals are similar to those found in an electronic wristwatch. When the light of the overhead projector shines through the crystals, the patterns of light and darkness are displayed on a screen at the front of the room (see figure 7).

Many LCD projection tablets are monochrome, and, therefore, cannot be used to display videotapes. However, they are inexpensive and can be acquired for less than $1,000. In addition, they are lightweight and can easily be transported for presentations at other locations. They can be used at any site where an overhead projector can be employed, although they require the type of overhead projector that utilizes a direct beam rather than the compact, collapsible projection system that utilizes an indirect beam.

For either projection system, bandwidth is an important consideration. Resolution and bandwidth are closely related. Bandwidth, in this context, refers to the speed with which an electronic beam of a monitor or projector can traverse the front of a cathode ray tube (CRT). Resolution refers to the total number of lines displayed on a CRT and the number of dots displayed on each line. As the number of lines per screen and the number of dots per line increase, the speed with which the beam must traverse the screen increases. Consequently, a computer projection device capable of displaying a CGA image may not be capable of displaying the higher resolution EGA image. The practical implication is that a projection system cannot be assumed to work with all types of computer displays. Some computer projection systems will operate with both Macintosh and advanced high resolution IBM displays, but are higher priced because of their higher bandwidth and greater flexibility.

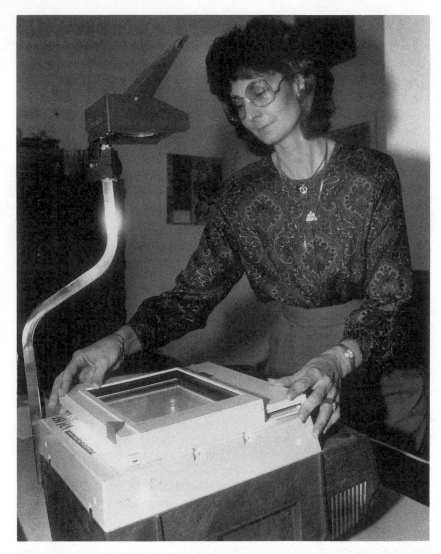

Figure 7.   LCD projection tablet placed on an overhead projector (Northeast Missouri State University).

Presentation Software

The capacity to display a word processing file by means of a computer projection device offers a number of useful instructional opportunities with little training required since faculty members are most likely to be conversant with their primary word processing program. A number of software programs, however, have been developed specifically to facilitate development of desktop presentations for use at professional conferences. If faculty members become familiar enough with these programs, they may begin to incorporate them in day-to-day classroom lectures as well. The concept underlying desktop presentation software is straightforward. The cost of conventional 35 mm slides prevents their use on a casual basis; the cost of an electronic computer slide is nil.

IBM *Storyboard* was one of the first programs of this genre for microcomputers. This program permits users to assemble text and graphics into a series of electronic slides that can be created within the program or imported from computer screens created with other programs. Another module permits a user to list the order in which slides will be presented. The presentation of electronic slides on the computer screen can be controlled manually by the presenter or automated for a self-running presentation. Dissolves and other special effects can be created during transition from one slide to the next, an option not available with conventional 35 mm slides.

Microsoft *Powerpoint* is a similar program for the Macintosh. This program has a particularly useful feature. Once a single background has been created, it can be masked into every slide in the series. Another program, Aldus *Persuasion*, combines this feature with another useful one. It can convert the outline of a set of lecture notes into a series of slides. The same outline can be used to list a sequence of topics to be discussed in a lecture and to create a series of slides for the presentation. Recently, *PowerPoint* and *Persuasion* have been adapted to run under the *Windows 3.0* operating system on IBM-compatible computers. Most programs of this genre offer the option of printing out copies of electronic slides, four to six to a page, for use as handouts. This makes it possible to supplement the electronic medium with printed notes for distribution after a lecture without the necessity of redoing materials in another format.

Desktop presentation programs will continue to evolve, adding more features and providing greater ease of use. They are ideally suited to classroom presentations depending on the instructor's style and the availability of a projection device. Because many of their functions can be replicated by word processing programs, albeit in a more cumbersome fashion, the necessity of learning another program may not warrant their uses in some instances. On the other hand, faculty members who use an appreciable number of slides either for classroom lectures or for formal professional presentations at conferences may find that the ease and flexibility warrant the time required to master a program of this type. Animated desktop presentations developed with writing tools such as *HyperCard* or *MacroMind Director* can also be used to present dynamic material less easily understood in static form.

SLIDES AND TRANSPARENCIES

Despite the advantages of animation, there are limitations to desktop presentations that may make transparencies or conventional 35 mm slides more appropriate for some presentations. If a computer projection device is not available, a desktop presentation is limited to three or four people who can comfortably gather around a computer monitor. This can be overcome by acquisition of an LCD- or CRT-based computer projection device for classroom lectures. Availability of such equipment at professional conferences, however, is still not routine although it is becoming more common. A second constraint is that the brightness of either type of computer projection device is limited, causing an audience to either drowse in the dark or strain to see the screen if the ambient room light is too bright. Transparencies and 35 mm slides also require that room lights be dimmed, but can be utilized in brighter light conditions than are currently practical for computer projection devices.

Under the proper conditions, a desktop presentation may have an impact that surpasses other types of presentations. Even so, a backup set of slides or transparencies is mandatory for a presentation of any importance. In contrast to the dozens of elements that can cause an inadequately supported desktop presentation to fail, a projection bulb that burns out is the most common source of failure for a presentation based on 35 mm slides or transparencies. Even that is fairly uncommon and can be addressed by ensuring that a spare bulb is on hand. Fortunately, electronic slides created for a desktop presentation are easily converted to conventional 35 mm slides or transparencies. It is not difficult to carry copies of slides in both electronic and conventional formats, ensuring that the presentation will be a success under any conditions.

Transparencies

Transparencies have several advantages over electronic or conventional 35 mm slides. It is possible to write on a transparency to highlight an element or to add a point suggested by a member of the audience, and the order of transparencies is more easily rearranged than either 35 mm or electronic slides. These characteristics can make a lecture based on transparencies more spontaneous than comparable lectures based on slides.

There are several ways to create a transparency with a computer. (See table II.) In most cases, the same figures created for a desktop presentation can be used to create a transparency as well. The simplest method is to substitute a transparency in place of a sheet of paper. This

Table II.   Methods of Producing Transparencies

Method	Characteristic
Laser printer	Monochrome output
Thermal transparency	Two-stage process
Color ink jet printer	Limited resolution
Color laser printer	Expensive
Plotter	Specialized software

produces black print on transparent film instead of the black print on a white sheet of paper that would have otherwise resulted. The advantage of this method is that it is fast and convenient. The printout can be proofread on regular paper. When the final draft is ready, laser transparencies are substituted for paper. This method is only slightly less convenient than electronic presentations, making it practical for day-to-day lectures. It is important to note that transparency film especially designed for thermal transfers must be used. If ordinary transparencies designed for marking pens are used, the heat of the printing process will melt the transparency, resulting in a mess on the platen of the laser printer.

At present, laser transparencies always produce black lettering on a transparent background. With a two-stage process, other colors, such as yellow printing on a blue background, can be achieved. The image in this case is first printed on a laser printer using ordinary paper. This printout, in turn, is sandwiched with a thermal transparency as it is sent through a thermal machine. This process, incidentally, can be used with any type of original, whether generated with a laser printer or not. If the original copy has been generated through some other means, a photocopy must be made to create an image that can be used with a thermal transparency.

The two methods described above are currently the most practical ones for day-to-day instructional applications. Their chief limitation is that the original colors of the screen are not reproduced in the transparency. Ink jet printers such as the Hewlett-Packard *Paint Jet* can be used to produce color transparencies. Unfortunately, the resolution of this particular technology is limited. Consequently, although the output may be acceptable for informal lectures, it may not meet standards for more formal presentations. There are a few high resolution thermal color printers that support *PostScript*, but they are fairly expensive and currently fall in the $5,000 to $10,000 range, a considerable decrease from the $30,000 to $50,000 price range of these devices only a couple of years ago.

A multipen plotter presents another means of producing a color transparency. This method produces a professional-looking transparency acceptable for any type of presentation. The chief drawback is that the production process may be slow and sometimes take five to ten minutes per transparency. In addition, not all software will support the plotter as an output device. Most word processing programs will not. In contrast, any program that can print to a laser printer can be used to generate monochrome transparencies.

To summarize, direct output to a laser transparency presents the simplest way to produce a transparency for everyday instructional use. It has the significant benefit of requiring no additional steps other than substitution of laser transparencies in place of paper. Other methods provide varying degrees of color that may be desirable for special presentations, but have the drawbacks of expense, limited resolution, or requirements for specialized software.

35 mm Slides

Thirty-five millimeter slides are likely to be the medium of choice under two conditions: (1) when accurate color renditions are required; and (2) when computer-generated images must be combined with other images. Thirty-five millimeter film has a range of color and a degree of resolution that exceeds other technologies, such as microcomputer displays and videotaped images. Consequently, when these qualities are important in a presentation, as in anatomy, slides may be the medium of choice. Slides also present a practical means of faithfully rendering the colors of computer displays.

In some cases, it may be desirable to interweave computer-generated graphics with other images. For example, a slide presenting the degree of a patient's facial paralysis might be followed by a computer-generated graph displaying the level of recovery after treatment. In that instance, the most practical approach would be to transfer the computer image to a 35 mm slide; to digitize the slide would mean the loss of some degree of resolution. Creating a slide of the computer graph would make it possible to conduct the entire presentation in a single medium.

There are several ways in which a computer display can be transferred to a 35 mm slide. (See table III.) One of the simplest is to print the image using a laser printer, and then transfer it to film using a copy

Table III. Methods of Transferring Computer Displays to Slides

Method	Output
Printout and copy stand	Professional but monochrome output
Direct screen shot	Color, but reflects screen curvature
Electronic transfer	Requires slide transfer device
Slide bureau	Professional but high cost per slide

stand and camera. This results in monochrome slides, and, if done properly, meets all professional standards. Many desktop presentation programs provide options that allow the user to select the intended output device and automatically adjust the corresponding aspect ratio. If it is known in advance that the final output will be a slide, this should be considered when the graphic is created, since the aspect ratio of a 35 mm slide is different from a transparency or a computer display. A slide has a 3:4 aspect ratio while a printed page or transparency has a ratio of 8.5:11 inches.

Another method consists of placing a camera in front of the computer display and taking a picture. Some experimentation with focal length and shutter speed may be necessary, but usable images can be obtained in this way. Inexpensive hoods, which fit over some computer displays to block out extraneous light and glare, are available. The chief drawback of this method is that the resolution of the slide can be no better than the resolution of the screen.

There are also devices that convert computer displays to slides electronically, through connection to the serial port. The chief advantage is that the superior resolution of film can be utilized, reducing the jagged look of diagonal lines that otherwise may be present. The cost of these types of devices naturally increases as higher resolution computer displays are employed. A device that supports output from the relatively low resolution of a CGA display may cost as little as $2,000, while more sophisticated units may cost as much as $10,000. Although it may be difficult to justify acquisition of one of these units by an individual department, acquisition by a school, college, or computing center may be feasible.

If only a few slides are needed each year, an electronic slide conversion service bureau provides another alternative. Telecommunications software is used to transmit the computer image to the service bureau via modem. In the case of some desktop presentation programs such as Aldus *Persuasion*, the necessary telecommunications software is included with the program. The images are converted to 35 mm slides by the service bureau and mailed to the user by overnight delivery if desired. The cost of this service is typically $10 to $20 per slide, but the result is a professional quality slide that can rival graphics produced by professional illustrators and, therefore, is justified for major presentations.

AUDIO AND VIDEO

Many aspects of communication disorders have their foundations in audio technologies. Audiology, as it is practiced today, would not be possible without the ability to deliver a calibrated stimulus of known frequency and intensity. The development of the tape recorder played a significant role in speech audiometry and has a number of therapeutic applications in speech-language pathology. Video technologies have had a greater impact on academic instruction than upon professional practice, but are widely used in most CSD programs. Significant changes are occurring in both audio and video technologies, but the most significant change is a shift from analog to digital processing and storage. This has resulted in increased fidelity and dynamic range, and improved editing capabilities. Another change is the availability of random access capabilities.

Audio

Early audio recordings were made with wire recorders that stored the audio information on a strand of wire. Later, audiotape quickly became the medium of choice. Both audiotape and videotape consist of an iron oxide film embedded in a strand of plastic. The same technology is used to construct floppy disks for computers except that a circular disk is used in place of a continuous strand of plastic. A magnetic record head produces a magnetic field embedded in the film of iron filings.

In an analog recording, there is a one-to-one correspondence between the original sound and the magnetic recording. As the intensity of sound increases, the length of the magnetic line extends further across the tape. Thus, intensity of the loudest sound that can be recorded is limited by the width of the tape. As the frequency of the sound increases, the number of magnetic lines on the tape also increases and the magnetic lines on the tape are eventually crowded so close together that a distinct resolution of separate lines is no longer possible, and the frequency limits of the tape are reached.

When a sound is digitized, amplitude of the waveform at each point can be stored as a number representing the height of the waveform at that point. In binary form, these numbers can be stored as a series of ones and zeroes. In a digital recording, a series of magnetic dashes can be used to represent these ones and zeroes on the audiotape. There is no longer a one-for-one correspondence between the original sound and the magnetic lines that represent it. Instead, the sound has been encoded as a series of binary numbers stored on the tape.

The dynamic range of a digital recording can be much greater than that of an analog recording. Moveover, an exact duplicate of a digital recording can be made with no degradation in quality. In contrast, with each successive generation dubbed from an analog audiotape, a further deterioration in quality occurs. As might be imagined, these characteristics could be important in distinguishing a correctly articulated /s/ or determining a vocal characteristic. In the 1950s and 60s, audiotape recorders were a major investment for a clinic, but now they are so inexpensive that every clinician has one. A similar trend will occur with digital audiotape recorders as mass production eventually drives the cost down.

One of the constraints on use of an audiotape in a lecture is the necessity for identifying the location of a desired example on the tape. Analog tape counters only provide an approximate index and differ from machine to machine. When information is encoded digitally, it becomes possible to construct a counter that can track movement of the tape in minutes and seconds. This may prove a considerable aid in location of clinical examples. Even when the exact location of a sample on an audiotape is known, it is still necessary to go through the remainder of the tape to get to that point, regardless of whether a digital or analog tape is employed. The rate at which access will occur depends on the speed of the transport mechanism and the distance separating the two points. This type of access is termed *serial access.*

Compact disc players with microcomputer interfaces were designed to play the CD-ROM disks described in the earlier section on graphics, but can also control and play compact music discs in some instances. The implications for audiology are apparent. Any point on a compact music disc (CD) can be randomly accessed, and it is possible to go directly to a specified location without going through the remainder of the recording. Rather than rewinding a tape to replay a stimulus, an audiologist can simply tap a key on a computer console. A range of different instructional applications is also feasible. For example, the exact element of a desired dysarthric voice sample could be presented in a lecture by selecting a check box on the computer screen. It is also possible to link electronic slides from a desktop presentation to specific audio samples on a compact music disc. The chief limitation of a compact music disc is that, in contrast to audiotape, no recording capability is available. Compact discs must be pressed at a factory much as phonograph records are. Therefore, it is necessary to re-master existing commercial audiotapes in communication disorders and re-release them in the CD format before instructional applications will be possible. This is already being done in some instances.

A *sound digitizer* is a different type of random access digital recording currently available to individual instructors. It digitizes sound and stores it in the memory of the computer. Sound digitizers such as *Mac-Recorder* can be obtained for as little as $200. As an added benefit, *Mac-Recorder* is provided with accompanying software that can display a sound waveform, the spectrum of a sound, or a limited version of a sound spectrogram. Digital editing capabilities for electronically cutting and splicing a sound are also provided. The primary limitation of a sound digitizer is the amount of disk space required to store a sound. For applications in communication disorders, the highest quality sound is often desired. As might be expected, increased sound resolution is associated with increased storage requirements. Under those circumstances, digitized speech may consume 20 kilobytes of storage per second. In other words, less than a minute of speech per megabyte could be stored. Methods for storing speech in compressed formats and increased storage capabilities will reduce this constraint in time. An advantage of storing digitized speech directly in the computer is that both an electronic slide or graphic and an associated speech sample can be stored on the same disk. This dimension of a desktop presentation cannot be duplicated on paper.

Video

Many aspects of video recording technology parallel those of audio technologies. The chief difference is that the bandwidth required to record a video signal is much greater than that necessary for an audio signal so the video capabilities have lagged behind audio capabilities. Television followed radio. Affordable videotape recorders became available more than a decade after their audio counterparts. Even today a videotape recorder is significantly larger and more expensive than an audiotape recorder. The gap in size and cost is steadily decreasing, however. Digital videotapes share all of the advantages of digital audiotapes, but are currently several times the price of analog videotape recorders. This difference should diminish in time. The chief limitation of digital videotape is the same as that of digital audiotapes—sequential access to information.

Modifications of the CD-ROM format called "CD-I" (compact disc-interactive) and "DVI" (digital video-interactive) have been developed that permit computer data and video information to be stored on the same compact disc. Video sequences can be randomly accessed and replayed on the computer screen. Thus far, however, it has not been possible to create a video image that fills the entire screen, and the resolution of the picture has been limited as well. These factors have discouraged commercial acceptance of this technology.

The greater bandwidth required by the video signal has also meant that, thus far, the ability to digitize and store a continuous video signal on a microcomputer in the same way that it is possible to digitize an audio signal has been limited. Although no random access digital storage medium has yet been a commercial success in the video format, a random access analog format is available. The *videodisc* was pre-empted by the videotape recorder for home entertainment use primarily because it lacked the recording capability of the VCR. However, the higher resolution and random access capabilities of the videodisc make it ideal for instructional use.

Videodiscs are available in two formats. The constant linear velocity (CLV) format provides a longer playing time but lacks random access capabilities. The constant angular velocity (CAV) format provides random access capabilities that are particularly useful in models of videodisc players with a computer interface, such as the Pioneer 2200 or the Sony 1200 videodisc players. In the CAV format more than 50,000 still frames, one-half hour of still video, or any combination thereof, can be stored on one side of a videodisc. In contrast to a typical slide tray for conventional 35 mm slides, the practical capacity of a videodisc for instructional use is essentially unlimited. (If each slide were viewed for 10 seconds, it would take a month to review 50,000 slides, watching eight hours a day.) Further, once the appropriate database is constructed, any one of the slides can be displayed by typing its name on a computer console. This allows the instructor to construct an electronic slide tray in advance in much the same fashion as slides are sequenced for a conventional slide presentation, or to access randomly any of the slides in response to class feedback and questions.

An ideal recording medium for video or audio would consist of a digital format with random access capability and no practical limitation on storage capacity. As table IV indicates, no recording medium yet meets all three requirements. Steady and continued advances in recording technologies will eventually remove these limitations, however.

MULTIMEDIA APPLICATIONS

Multimedia applications combine elements of several different media in one presentation. A slide-tape presentation, in which 35 mm slides are accompanied by a sound track from an audiotape, is an example of one type of multimedia presentation. Microcomputers have created

Table IV. Different Types of Video and Audio Recording Media

Medium	Method	Access	Recording	Characteristic
Audio	Audiotape	Serial	Read/write	Digital or analog
	Compact disc	Random	Read only	Sound or data
	Computer	Random	Read/write	Limited storage
Video	Videotape	Serial	Read/write	Digital or analog
	Videodisc	Random	Read only	Analog
	CD-I	Random	Read only	Partial screen
	Computer	Random	Read/write	Limited storage

new possibilities for integrating several types of media in a random access format known as *hypermedia*. *HyperCard* was the program that popularized the concept of hypermedia applications on microcomputers, in part because a copy of *HyperCard* is provided with every Macintosh. Comparable programs are available for other computers, such as *Link-Way*, sold by IBM, and *Toolbook*.

Hypermedia applications often incorporate audio and video resources as well as computer graphics and text. For example, one *Hyper-Card* program for medical students presents the pages of an anatomical text on the screen of the computer. If a student selects an unfamiliar term, such as *corpus callosum*, a videodisc player controlled by the computer presents a picture of that anatomical structure. In this hypermedia application, the student can go directly to the image of the corpus callosum. (See Chapter 13 for more examples of hypermedia applications in communication disorders.)

The enormous capacity of videodiscs offers great potential for sharing information across CSD programs. If faculty from 100 training programs each contributed 1,000 of the most frequently used slides from their programs, a visual database of 100,000 slides would be created for the profession. Because a slide costs approximately a dollar to duplicate, it would be impractical to make a set of slides for each educational program. The cost, at $100,000 per educational program, would be millions of dollars. In addition, most educational programs would lack the space to store a slide library of this size or personnel to maintain the library. However, the visual database of 100,000 slides would fit onto two sides of a videodisc, with room to spare. Once a master copy of a videodisc has been pressed, at a cost of about $2,000, additional copies are twenty dollars each. This would make it feasible for each educational program to acquire several copies.

This hypothetical example is described to suggest the potential of the medium. In practice it costs about a dollar per slide to transfer a 35 mm slide to videotape (the intermediate step for creating a videodisc), although savings can be realized by placing this step in the hands of graduate students if local slide conversion facilities are available at a university. The primary costs of such a project would be the managerial ones of organizing receipt, conversion, and return of slides from educational programs across the country.

Although the example of a common visual database for programs in communication disorders is a hypothetical one, multimedia applications combining computer-generated text with video slides have been developed for specific courses. Zahrl Schoeny, a faculty member at the University of Virginia, has transferred a series of cross-sectional slides of the temporal bone to videodisc in this manner, and uses a hypermedia program created with *HyperCard* in his instruction (see figure 8).

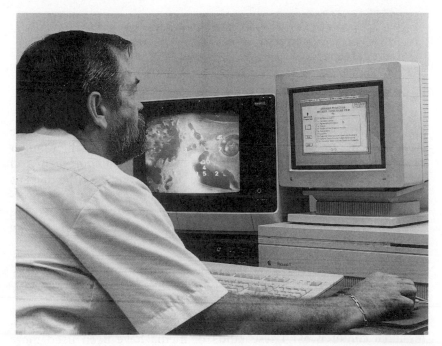

Figure 8. Using hypermedia to learn temporal bone anatomy (University of Virginia Communication Disorders Program).

In addition to the benefits that a hypermedia application of this kind has for direct classroom instruction, it also enables students to view the slides outside class using a videodisc player and computer.

We will conclude by returning to the relationship between frequency and period used to illustrate several types of media. The ideal way of displaying this relationship is to illustrate it interactively. We formerly demonstrated this relationship by connecting an oscillator to an oscilloscope and a speaker. A camera placed in front of the oscilloscope screen transmitted the picture to a video monitor that displayed the signal for the class (figure 9).

The drawback of this "multimedia" display was that it was necessary to move several pieces of equipment (oscillator, oscilloscope, amplifier, speaker, camera, monitor) to the classroom. If n cables were needed to connect all the components, only n-1 cables were usually available. Also, the sine wave tended to etch its image on the monitor permanently if the camera was left in place for any length of time. Today, a program such as *MacRecorder* can be used to generate the sine wave and display it on the computer screen while simultaneously playing back the corresponding sound. An LCD computer projection tablet

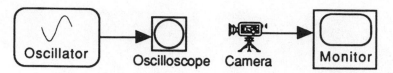

Figure 9. The previous generation of multimedia displays.

placed on an overhead projector displays the image on a screen at the front of the room. The frequency is specified by typing in the number of Hz required. This method requires fewer pieces of equipment and interconnections, while affording more precise control of the display. As an added advantage, any given screen can be captured and incorporated into the lecture notes. Thus, the class has the benefit of seeing the display interactively, while also possessing a printed copy to take home for further review.

SUMMARY

Historically, a variety of media has been used for presentations at professional conferences. These kinds of media have been used more sparingly for classroom instruction because of the time and expense associated with their production. A series of technologic innovations is now placing in the hands of instructors capabilities that were formerly available only to professional illustrators and media specialists. Terms such as *desktop publishing* and *desktop presentations* are finding their way into the vocabulary of instructional technology. Presentation format can never be an adequate substitute for appropriate content, but graphic displays and illustrations can often illuminate points that might otherwise be obscure.

REFERENCES

Brand, S. 1987. *The Media Lab: Inventing the Future at MIT.* New York: Penguin Books.
Cochran, P. S., and Bull, G. L. 1991. The use of BITNET in communication disorders programs. *Asha* 33 (1):55-58.

Chapter 13

Computer-Assisted Learning and Instruction

Paula S. Cochran and Glen L. Bull

INTRODUCTION

The first part of this chapter focuses on teaching *with* computers. It is not necessary to be a computer expert in order to use computers effectively for classroom or clinical instruction. Effective instructional use of computers is much like using chalkboards, slides, or overhead projectors and does not require vast hardware and software resources. Several methods for using computers to teach core content in communication sciences and disorders (CSD) can be implemented by instructors who have no more computer experience than word processing. It is necessary, however, for instructors to have their own computers in their offices so that complete familiarity with instructional applications is facilitated. As is detailed in Chapter 12, one computer attached to an appropriate projection device can be used with even a very large class. The power of a computer to provide flexible, instantaneous examples may dramatically enhance an introduction, discussion, and review of concepts or clinical procedures.

The last part of this chapter addresses the challenge of teaching students *about* computers and how to use them effectively as administrative, clinical, research, or personal tools. This information is intended for instructors with a special interest in computer applications, and for those who participate in departmental planning and curriculum revisions incorporating new technology. Several approaches and suggested goals for facilitating clinical computing competency are presented.

Computer Usage in Communication Disorders

Since 1983, the American Speech-Language-Hearing Association (ASHA) has surveyed a sample of its membership annually to gather data about employment trends. These Omnibus surveys reflect the rapid changes in the availability and uses of computers among ASHA members over the past few years. In 1983, about 30% of survey respondents reported that they used computers at least occasionally. By 1989 that percentage had doubled, and nearly 70% of respondents reported that they used a computer at work (ASHA 1989).

Although the Omnibus survey results for the past five years indicate changes in the level of computer use among all major employment groups, the group working in university settings is of particular interest. In the most recent survey, nearly 90% of respondents working in universities reported using a computer at least occasionally. According to a 1987 survey of program directors (Lorendo 1988), many departments were still planning for the integration of computers. Of the 164 communication disorders program directors responding, 52 indicated that computer courses were taught within their departments. Ninety others either recommended or required coursework offered outside their departments. Respondents indicated a significant discrepancy, however, between the *ideal* level and type of computer usage in their programs and the *actual* current use in academic, clinical, and administrative activities (Lorendo 1988).

Program directors indicated that about 56% of their faculty seldom or never used a computer for in-class teaching. Forty percent seldom or never prepared instructional materials with a computer, 48% seldom or never used a computer for clinical service delivery, and about 39% seldom or never used a computer for clinical information management such as report writing. In summary, in 1987 more than 70% of ASHA survey respondents working in university settings claimed to use computers at least occasionally (ASHA 1989); but, program directors that year perceived 40% to 60% of their faculty as seldom or never using computers for instructional or clinical activities (Lorendo 1988).

Barriers to computer use by faculty may be as simple, but as critical, as computer access. In a 1988 survey by Cochran and Bull (1991), the program directors of 40 Educational Standards Board (ESB) accredited educational programs indicated that only 283 out of 522 faculty (55%) had access to computers (or mainframe terminals) in their own offices. This level of access is likely to change as it becomes apparent that adequate resources are prerequisite for integration of technology and state-of-the-art instructional methods. Such resources include not only hardware and software, but also technical support (Bull et al. 1985; Bull and Cooper 1989). Having succeeded in facilitating faculty use of computers for teaching within a school of education, Bull and Cooper (1989) pointed out that "several experiments within the school have demonstrated that the computer must be placed on the desk before it is integrated into the instructor's routine, and it is important that students observe this routine use" (p. 7). Although the use of computers within CSD departments has increased dramatically over a short time, changes are likely to continue at a fairly rapid rate.

USING COMPUTERS TO TEACH

Sharing the Wealth of Instructional Materials

As instructors use newer technologies to generate teaching materials, sharing materials with other instructors will become easier. New instructional media for teaching are described in Chapter 12, including the use of computers to generate lecture notes, illustrations, overhead transparencies, and slides. The use of a computer to manipulate the large amounts of material available on CD-ROM and videodiscs are also discussed. As producing and distributing professional-quality materials becomes easier, more specialized teaching materials will become available, and faculties will likely increase their use of computers in the preparation and use of computer-based materials during instruction.

In the past, the exchange of personally developed course materials was limited not only by cost but also by the difficulty of customization. Now, computer files on disk allow easy editing of text and even customization of diagrams. Computer networks linking most colleges and universities facilitate the exchange of such files among instructors across the country in a matter of hours. In fact, students at two or more geographically distant universities could complete the same experiment, transmit their data over the network, then compare their results. This ability to exchange large amounts of detailed information almost instantly has the potential to change how and what instructors teach.

Focusing on Content Rather Than Computers

When computers first appeared in public schools, some teachers protested that they did not have time to teach yet another "subject," that computers would take time from the already meager amount devoted to core content areas like math and spelling. If and when teachers did think about computer-assisted-instruction (CAI), they usually assumed that the computer would function as the teacher, in a one-computer-per-student model. The phrase "electronic workbook" was born. Depending upon their expectations, teachers were either disappointed or gratified by the early lack-luster software designed to function in their places. As personal computers have become routinely available, their power and potential have increased substantially, and so has our understanding of how to use them effectively in instruction. The image of the computer as a repetitive, all-knowing, impersonal teaching machine persists only in the minds of those who do not actually use computers for teaching or therapy.

Now it is possible to take a broader perspective. Computers can play many roles in instruction to enhance content teaching, such as serving as audio/visual aids to provide more realistic examples or demonstrations during class sessions. This way of using computers for teaching requires that the instructor be familiar with software applications, but the focus remains on the content of the lesson rather than on how the computer works. Students need no computer training to benefit from this kind of activity. The importance of their skills increases, however, when computers are used for individual or small group activities. Table I presents a summary of the instructional computing alternatives most frequently used in CSD courses, types of software required, and an indication of computer expertise required of students or the instructor, or both.

Using a Computer to Facilitate Large-Group Instruction

The possible computer activities described in table I are not intended to be exhaustive, but merely representative of a variety of ways in which computers enhance instruction in CSD courses. Nearly every course in audiology or speech-language pathology includes some content that can be effectively presented using a computer and a projection device (see Chapter 12 for technical information). In some cases, it may be a matter of convenience and economy to project revised lecture notes instead of producing new overhead transparencies or extensive handouts for large classes. In other cases, the use of a computer for classroom demonstrations and simulations adds dramatic impact by increasing active participation of students and flexibility of the instructor.

Consider a typical introduction to clinical report writing. Possibly, the instructor makes use of handouts showing positive and negative examples of important points and uses an overhead projector with transparencies to focus the class on the text in question. Now consider how the instructor can engage students more actively in this lesson with the help of a computer. Rather than transparencies, the instructor uses the computer to present word-processed reports to illustrate major points. (See Chapter 12 for a discussion of devices that project the computer screen for large audiences to read.) The cursor highlights the text under discussion and focuses the attention of the group. Instead of having students imagine corrections, or writing all possibilities on a chalkboard, the instructor solicits and immediately makes changes suggested by the class, showing how revisions improve the actual report. Multiple solutions to the same question or problem are likely to arise and can be compared.

A similar approach can be used in classes covering how to write behavioral objectives, how to analyze a language sample, or how to write an individualized education plan (IEP). (Tip for instructors: you may want to recruit a class member to type students' suggestions as

Table I.   Examples of Computer-Based Instructional Activities

Instructional Computing Alternatives in Communication Disorders

Class Type	Computer Activity	Software Category	Computer Expertise
Large group— lecture	Lecture outline/ notes presented overhead Demonstration or illustration	Utility such as word process- ing or outliner Specialized soft- ware depend- ing on topic, such as speech analy- sis program or videodisc slide show	Instructor must have minimal expertise. Instructor must have famil- iarity with specialized program, and must plan or prepare demo.
Large group— review or discussion	Interactive prob- lem solving and *what-if* examples	Simulation, data analysis, or specialized clinical soft- ware	Instructor must be able to move quickly through soft- ware options, respond to student input for examples.
Small group— seminar	Interactive dem- onstrations	Simulations, clinical soft- ware, some tutorials	As above. Could involve stu- dents more directly in computer con- trol (such as making screen choices) in some cases.
Small group— labs	Experiments or special projects	Microcomputer- based lab soft- ware, clinical applications, or data collec- tion/analysis software	Instructor must be well versed in correct soft- ware opera- tion as well as likely student errors. Students must have at least minimal com- puter famil- iarity (such as disk care, printer opera- tion) and ex- plicit lab instructions.

continued

Table I. *continued*

Instructional Computing Alternatives in Communication Disorders

Class Type	Computer Activity	Software Category	Computer Expertise
Individual instruction	Computer as a tool Computer as instructor	As above Tutorials, simulations, or drill-and-practice	Each student must have basic computer familiarity and must be given explicit instructions Beyond basic computer familiarity, the student should have access to documentation or online help. Instructor needs minimal computer experience.

you facilitate the discussion.) With appropriate software, computers provide alternative ways to explain the decibel as a unit of measurement, or to demonstrate easy onset as a principle of fluency therapy. A single computer with a projection device can be used to focus a review session in a large class or to stimulate an in-depth discussion. Later, students might be asked to explore a concept or procedure further in a small-group computer-based exercise or in an individual laboratory assignment.

Using Computers to Facilitate Small-Group Instruction

In general, both instructors and students require additional computer skills to make small-group instruction successful (see table I). Such instruction often involves interactive demonstrations that help students grasp new information by providing novel problems or contrasting examples. Small-group instruction provides the opportunity for individuals to try their own ideas but also learn from group trial and error. Instructors may find simulation software especially useful for small-group instruction.

The main objective of a computer-based simulation is to provide an opportunity for users to experience the consequences of their actions under conditions that "simulate" a real situation. A clear benefit of a simulation is that no lasting negative effects result from mistakes. Flight simulators are a classic example. In communication disorders, commercial software that simulates audiometric testing is available. Given the frequently encountered difficulty of describing a preferred procedure for applying masking in a testing situation, instructors may choose to use a computer-based simulation to demonstrate the effects of correct and incorrect use of the procedure. Using a simulation, a group of students can pool their skills to obtain correct pure-tone thresholds for a sample case, or failing that, observe the consequences of overmasking.

The notion of a simulation is not new to preparation in speech-language pathology and audiology. For many years, audiometer simulators have been available for practicing audiometric testing procedures. New technology has greatly expanded the range of clinical situations that can be simulated with some degree of realism. Meyers, Strang, and Cartmell (1987) demonstrated the use of a computer-based simulation to instruct speech-language pathology students. When student clinicians provided appropriate verbal responses to young stutterers in the simulation, less disfluent synthesized speech was generated by the computer, and vice versa.

The use of videodiscs to provide more realistic sights and sounds for computer-based simulations is likely to continue to increase. (See Chapter 12 for an explanation of laser videodisc technology.) Examples of the instructional use of interactive videodisc technology abound in medical, industrial, and military settings, with new applications appearing at a fast rate. Medical students have used videodiscs to study the assessment of neuromotor dysfunction in infants (Reeves 1988), and archeology students study the mysteries of ancient China via videodisc (Chen 1989). It is important to note that the presence of a videodisc does not imply that the instruction was designed as a simulation; videodiscs are also frequently used to enhance a more traditional, tutorial approach to instruction. Rule, Salzberg, and Schulze (1990) reported the successful use of videodisc materials to introduce special education teachers-in-training to basic teaching and behavior management techniques. They stressed that learning about such techniques should never be confused with actual, supervised practice in a classroom.

A well-designed simulation, however, can provide practice in performing many of the skills required in a real clinical situation. One such acquired skill is accurate observation of client behavior. Horner et al. (1987) demonstrated a videodisc-based simulation for introducing student audiologists to infant hearing screening using Visual Reinforcement Audiometry (VRA). VRA relies on the audiologist's skill in observing infant behaviors and knowing how to develop and evaluate a conditioned infant response (head-turning). Usually, such skills must be developed in live practicum situations, where the student's errors may result in inaccurate or inconclusive findings with an infant client. Using simulation, however, students can prepare themselves to handle real situations more effectively.

Computer-based simulations are useful for large-group, small-group, and individual instruction. Small-group activities can be developed around other kinds of computer tools as well, such as the speech and voice analysis systems now available for major brands of microcomputers. Teams of speech and hearing-science students can be assigned to record their speech using a sound digitizer, and then examine the resulting speech waveform to identify periodic and a-periodic segments. With group assignments, instructors must be thoroughly familiar with whatever special software or hardware is needed, and should be aware of likely student errors. It is often useful to have a student control the computer during small-group activities, even if the instructor is present. Typical misconceptions and questions are more likely to be addressed, which will increase student confidence about continuing the activity independently. It is important to note that at least one student in each group should have basic computer skills, so that the group can focus on content rather than mechanics.

Using a Computer to Facilitate Individual Instruction

Most computer applications designed for use by individual learners are either computer-assisted-instruction (CAI) or tools. CAI generally consists of programmed instruction in which the computer functions as the instructor and in which specific, pre-defined instructional objectives are addressed (e.g., "The student will identify and label the major parts of the middle ear"). In contrast, computer tools function under the direction of the learner, and often have wide varieties of possible outcomes. Specific instructional goals may be addressed by activities in which students use computer tools, but such objectives are defined and modified by the instructor rather than pre-set by a software designer. For this and other reasons, CAI applications often fall short of instructor and student expectations. As many as 200 man hours are required to design, produce, evaluate, and revise just one hour of high-quality CAI. Such an investment in time and expertise is rare, and, therefore so is excellent CAI software.

When training demands and access to resources are high, such as in many military and industrial training programs, the investment in high-quality CAI may be deemed cost-effective. Computer-based instruction independent of an instructor has the advantage of consistency (every participant receives exactly the same information) and temporal flexibility (it is not necessary to have all learners available at the same time for instruction). Although requirements for careful instructional design will not change, at least the cost of including realistic speech and video examples in CAI will likely decrease in the foreseeable future (Bull, Cochran, and Snell 1988; Bull 1989). Programmed instruction is increasingly taking advantage of mixing media (computer/video/audio) and mixing approaches such as simulations with elements of drill and practice.

At the present time, university-level instructors in CSD are more likely to find existing CAI software that is appropriate for supplementing rather than replacing classroom sessions on a specific topic. The four most common types of CAI software are described in table II.

Readily available CAI of the tutorial/drill-and-practice type includes programmed instruction in anatomy, understanding audiograms, and English grammar. A newer approach to individual instruction is based on hypermedia (also see Chapter 12). Hypermedia applications often integrate graphics, sound, and text, and may include other peripheral devices such as a videodisc player or CD-ROM player/disk drive. Besides the integration of media, hypermedia applications are often distinguished by a non-linear organization of information. That is, users are permitted access to most parts of the program at any time so that individual interests and needs can be addressed without proceeding through a sequence of information in lock step. Examples of hypermedia software include *HyperCard* for the Macintosh, *Linkway*

Table II.   Common Types of CAI Software for Communication Disorders

CAI Software	Characteristics
Tutorial	Presents *new* information; provides opportunity to practice; tests learning; may provide review for errors; maintains student performance records. Sequence of material predetermined by programmer.
Drill and practice	Provides opportunity to practice a previously introduced skill; tests learning; maintains performance records; may allow instructor to modify practice items.
Simulation	Presents the factors, events, or materials typical of a real situation, problem, or experiment. Learner makes choices and observes the consequences of various actions. Extent of learner control and flexibility of outcomes vary. Examples: flight simulators, chemistry experiments, emergency medical procedures, audiometric testing.
Hypermedia	New category of instructional software well-suited for individual use. Takes advantage of nonlinear organization of data and easy integration of graphics and sound. Allows learner to explore content in self-directed manner.

and *Toolbook* for the IBM, and *HyperStudio* and *TutorTech* for Apple II computers. Such software provides the foundation for development of content-specific applications.

As access to hypermedia resources increases, it is likely that examples for instruction in communication sciences and disorders will proliferate. Prototypes pertaining to voice disorders, anatomy, and phonetics already exist. Miller et al. (1987) demonstrated a system designed to improve audiology instruction at the university level. Their system used a Macintosh computer to control a videodisc player for presenting instruction on sign language and audiometric testing. Instructors interested in identifying CAI appropriate for use with their students are encouraged to consult other institutions as well as sources that regularly announce and review instructional software (see Resources).

Computer tools and utilities are frequently used for instruction on an individual basis. In contrast to most CAI, such software does not have a testing component and does not track user performance. Rather than *simulating* tasks, computer-based *tools* help users *to accomplish* tasks such as analyzing a language sample or measuring fundamental frequency. The effective use of computer-based tools, therefore, often requires not only familiarity with the computer, but also previously acquired information in a relevant subject area. Although computer-based tools and utilities do not evaluate students in a traditional way, student achievement can be assessed through products. The instructor who designs an assignment requiring the use of a computer-based tool should have a clear notion of what the product of the assignment should be and of how the student should present it for evaluation. Products can include a lab report, a graph of results, or a printout of data from a computer program. As multi-media and hypermedia tools become widely available, students may produce multi-media "reports" or presentations to demonstrate their grasp of new material or share new discoveries with other learners.

Many computer-based tools have been developed that can be effectively integrated into coursework in communication disorders. Some are generic tools such as statistical packages, sound digitizers, or database software. For example, databases and spreadsheets may be used to teach content such as IEP generation, management of hearing screening data, elementary statistics, or billing procedures. (See Seaton 1990, for many *AppleWorks*® applications specific to communication disorders.) Another example of a generic tool includes microcomputer-based-labs (MBL) in which a probe or other device is attached to the computer in order to collect data. MBL software permits the experimenter to collect and store data collected by the computer via a light, heat, motion, or touch sensor, for example. Some MBL systems are expensive and highly technical; some are designed for use by students as young as third graders.

An example of the latter, available for about $50, is *The Science Toolkit* by Broderbund. This software has been used with students to provide a non-technical, memorable introduction to the concepts of frequency, period, and amplitude. A light sensor (included with the software) is connected to the gameport of an Apple II computer. The software acts as a strip chart that records perceived changes in light. A student with a bright flashlight walks back and forth near the light sensor, creating the pattern of waveforms on the strip chart as it records the increases and decreases in light. As the student walks faster, more cycles appear (frequency increases). As the student walks farther, the amplitude of the waveform increases. The students are challenged to decrease the period. By trial and error, students learn that the period of a waveform decreases when frequency increases. Active experience with these concepts promotes their later transfer to more sophisticated instrumentation and experiments. *The Personal Science Lab* from IBM includes a sonic transducer which, in a similar fashion, records the distance travelled by a student. Using such tools, instructors can bring abstract concepts to life during small-group sessions or in large classes when a computer projection device is available. Some computer-based tools designed especially with clinical and research applications in mind, also offer effective means for teaching basic information in CSD courses. Specialized tools of this type include computer-based voice analysis systems, speech and language sample analysis software, and data-bases for hearing aids or assistive listening devices. Table III presents possible content-related assignments requiring individual computer uses by students in a variety of courses.

The successful use of computer-based tools by students requires them to have higher levels of computer familiarity and more instruction in the use of specific computer software than does the use of more structured, less flexible CAI. It may be necessary to experiment with computer tools in a particular course in order to determine if the benefits are worth the time invested by students and instructors.

The Importance of Prerequisite Skills

When instructors plan assignments and course activities requiring students to use computers either individually or in small groups, they should ensure that students have prerequisite computer skills. Instructors should be cautious about relying on the abilities of students who are self-taught or who claim that they learned *about* computers in high school. It is quite possible that they learned about computers, but did very little with computers. Such students may readily recite the defini-

Table III. Using Computer Tools to Enhance Individual Instruction

Instructional Objective	Computer Tool	Assignment	Results or Product
Discover rise/fall intonation typical of declarative sentences in English	*Visi-Pitch* (Kay Elemetrics, Apple or IBM compatible)	Record and print screens showing pitch and intensity changes for each phrase in the Pledge of Allegiance.	Turn in all screen printouts and a one page explanation of the results.
Given a language sample transcript, learn to calculate *Mean-Length-Utterance* and *Type-Token Ratio* (different words/total words)	*SALT* (Systematic Analysis of Language Transcripts, University of Wisconsin, Apple or IBM compatible)	Using the transcription file provided, obtain *MLU* and *Type-Token Ratio* (TTR), then compare to results obtained manually.	Provide worksheets showing how MLU and TTR were obtained manually, and print screen of *SALT* results.
Understand the probable outcomes of a hearing conservation program	Any database software	Review screening results for 100 mock clients and recommend next phase of program.	Mock memo recommending next phase of program, using data from database to support a plan of action.

tion of RAM, but are often misinformed about the care of diskettes, for example, or basic printer functions. Lack of information, not just carelessness, accounts for much student frustration and wasted time and money for maintenance in university computing facilities. When students are adequately prepared to complete computer-based assignments, the risk of creating or reinforcing negative attitudes about computers can be avoided and students can focus on the content of the assignment.

Instructors have several options for providing prerequisite computing experiences, other than using content instruction time. Many academic computing (AC) centers in colleges and universities regularly offer free introductory workshops for faculty, students, and staff. The AC staff might, if asked, offer a special introduction for students in the communication disorders field. Alternatively, computer-wise faculty could offer periodic introductory workshops for student majors. Graduate-student assistants or work-study students can provide assistance for novices. Other suggestions for integrating computer-related instruction into a communication sciences and disorders curriculum are offered later in this chapter.

TEACHING STUDENTS TO USE COMPUTERS

Toward Clinical Computing Competency

So far this chapter has focused on the ways in which computers can effectively enhance content instruction in CSD. Faculty members in many speech-language pathology and audiology programs would like to take this process further; they would like to focus more on computer applications and on teaching each student to use computers effectively as personal and clinical tools. For some programs, the first challenge will be to acquire sufficient equipment, technical support, or faculty expertise. Success at this stage usually requires the energy and commitment of one or more faculty members in a leadership position within a department. Program directors and other faculty members will find practical, getting-started suggestions in "Technology Infusion: A Resource Guide" (Bull et al. 1985).

The availability and sophistication of computer applications for diagnosis, treatment, and research in communication disorders have changed rapidly during the past few years, and will continue to do so (Goldman and Dahle 1985; Schwartz 1986; Bull 1989). Long-term curriculum goals, therefore, should be flexible enough to incorporate new technology, yet specific enough to facilitate clinical computing competency. Toward this end, the ASHA Committee on Educational Technology has developed guidelines for educating speech-language pathologists about computer applications (Cochran et al. in preparation). Guidelines suggested by the Committee include broad goals that can be accomplished through the achievement of specific objectives. Because the use of computer technology depends on available resources in the form of hardware, software, and technical expertise, specific objectives should be determined locally.

Broad curriculum goals for speech-language pathologists should include competency with administrative, diagnostic, and rehabilitative applications of computers. Although clinical computing enthusiasts until recently have had only anecdotal evidence to suggest the efficacy of computer applications in therapy, data-based studies now suggest that certain computer applications are as effective or more effective than traditional approaches. During a therapy session a computer might function in the role of instructor, materials generator, biofeedback device, data keeper, alternative/augmentative communication device, or as a context for therapy. The latter use of a computer stresses the verbal interaction between client and clinician as they use the computer together to accomplish a shared goal (Bull, Cochran, and Snell 1988). Clinical applications are likely to continue to proliferate. Again, it is important that emphasis be placed on helping clinicians gain clinical computing competency rather than merely "computer literacy" (Cochran 1989).

Clinical Computing Advances in Audiology

Many of the broad clinical computing goals suggested by the ASHA Committee on Educational Technology, such as awareness of resources or use of administrative tools, are just as appropriate for audiologists as for speech-language pathologists. The wide range of other computer applications especially useful for speech-language pathologists is reflected in frequently appearing software and hardware reviews in *Asha* magazine and the *Journal for Computer Users in Speech and Hearing*. Computer-related technology has also resulted in new tools for nearly every aspect of audiometric testing and aural rehabilitation (Sims et al. 1985; Kent 1986; Mahshie 1987). A few examples serve to illustrate the potential impact of computers on clinical practice in audiology and, therefore, on the training of student clinicians.

Stach (1989) described the development and testing of a microcomputer-based speech audiometer designed to "replace the technologies of magnetic-tape and live-voice signal presentation that are in common use today" (p. 3). The software system makes use of the stereo output capability of a Macintosh computer to deliver a variety of digitized speech-audiometric stimuli (PB words, spondee words, and sentences). According to Stach, "the system is designed to control monotic and dichotic stimulus presentation, to control interstimulus interval, to randomize stimulus presentation, to allow easy [instantaneous] repetition of speech targets, and to provide data storage and analysis" (Stach 1989, p. 3).

New technology has affected the fitting of hearing aids by providing a means of identifying the optimal response curve of an aid for a specific client, a response curve that takes into consideration factors such as pure-tone thresholds and the actual resonance of the client's ear canal. This curve is plotted on a computer screen. The output of the aid can then be plotted on the same screen and adjusted to match the target curve. The ability of an audiologist to make more informed adjustments of hearing aid settings has particular impact on services provided to young children who cannot convey preferences and to elderly clients who cannot easily manipulate hearing aid controls (J. Paul Hunt, personal communication). Computer-based clinical tools for audiologists also include applications for aural rehabilitation. For example, Hurvitz and Goldojarb (1987) studied the use of a CAI program to teach nursing home residents about the ear, audiograms, management of hearing problems, speech reading, hearing aids, and communication skills.

In communication disorders, researchers interested in aural rehabilitation have led the way in the use of computer-controlled interactive videodisc technology (Sims et al. 1985; Kopra et al. 1987; Mahshie 1987; Tye-Murray et al. 1988; Hull 1989; also see Chapter 12 for an introductory explanation of this technology). Programs for teaching speechreading, fingerspelling, sign language, and visual tracking, have been developed and tested with normal-hearing and hearing-impaired children and adults. (See Mahshie 1987, for an especially good overview.)

Recently developed computer-based applications suggest the need for curriculum revisions that integrate new technology into speech-language pathology and audiology programs. Instructors in communication sciences and disorders may choose from several strategies for achieving such integration.

Creating a Clinical Computing Culture

It is recommended that faculty consider strategies for creating a computing culture within their department, in which students and faculty support each other throughout the process of acquiring new technical and clinical skills (Cochran 1989).

Provide Models of Appropriate Clinical Uses of Computers. Student clinicians need specific examples of how to integrate a computer application into audiology or speech-language pathology services. Positive examples should address specific, individualized clinical objectives by using resources available within the department. Videotapes could emphasize appropriate client-clinician interaction and effective pre/post computer activities.

Provide a Supportive Environment for Computer Users. A supportive environment includes easy access to equipment and software for pre-therapy practice or clinical planning and the availability of faculty and student assistance. Faculty and students should be encouraged to ask for help and, in return, to be generous with their own expertise.

Provide Recognition of Computer Use as a Clinical Skill. Both administrative computing skills (such as word processing) and clinical computing skills (such as using a computer-based hearing aid configuration protocol) should be recognized as clinical skills. They should be included in a comprehensive clinical competency checklist maintained for all student clinicians.

Provide Supervision and Consultation as Clinical Applications Are Attempted. Clinical supervision is an essential part of helping student clinicians gain competency. Supervisors should encourage students to consider factors that cause computer applications to succeed or fail during a session. Use of computer-based procedures for diagnosis or therapy is only one available alternative. Supervisors should emphasize the need for matching computer applications to predetermined objectives for the client.

Provide Active Participation in a Professional Culture, via Electronic Communication. An ideal clinical environment with direct supervision may not be available to student clinicians after graduation. One way in which students can receive and provide professional support is by becoming active participants in electronic communication (e-mail system, bulletin board, and/or conference). Most universities provide faculty, supervisors, and student clinicians with access to a major electronic network through which individuals can stay in touch with other interested professionals in an informal, convenient way.

Curriculum Options

Administrative and clinical applications of computers can be integrated into a communication disorders curriculum in the following ways:

- General computing course offered *outside* the department
- Specialized computing course or series of courses offered in-house
- Computer-related units offered within existing courses
- Periodic workshops or guest speakers focusing on computers

Some combination of these options will be the best approach for most programs. As the expertise of faculty and incoming students changes, plans may require revision. Some of the advantages and disadvantages of each option are indicated below.

Coursework Offered Outside the Department. Recommending or requiring *carefully selected* computer-related coursework offered by other academic departments may be a good way to provide a broad-based introduction for students in communication disorders. The kind of course to look for emphasizes hands-on experience with what is often called "productivity software," such as word-processors, data-bases, spreadsheets, and electronic mail. Such courses generally have names like "Introduction to Personal Computing," "Survey of Computing," or, when offered by an education department, "Introduction to Instructional Computing." Beware of sending computer novices to courses taught in math or computer science, with names like "Introduction to Programming" or "Introduction to (name of computer language)." These courses may be ideal for students expressing interest in computer programming, but are generally not appropriate as an introduction for using a computer as an administrative or clinical tool. In addition to introductions to the use of computers, more advanced courses offered outside the communication disorders department are sometimes appropriate for advanced graduate or doctoral students pursuing related areas. For example, students interested in health administration might benefit from computer-related coursework offered by business faculty. Similarly, technology courses offered by regular or special education faculty are likely to be valuable to communication disorders graduates.

Units within an Existing Course or Courses. A unit of instruction focusing on computer skills may be fairly easy to incorporate into an existing communication disorders course on clinical procedures or management. Developing introductory units is especially important in situations where orientation to computers and word processing instruction are not offered in convenient forms elsewhere on campus. A unit in a course for freshmen or sophomores may ensure that all communication disorders majors have the minimum skills in order to use computers in more advanced coursework. For example, introduction to word processing can readily be incorporated into an introduction to report writing. Approaches to computer-based intervention can also be appropriate for courses on aphasia, voice disorders, fluency, or aural rehabilitation. Whenever possible, hands-on activities and detailed examples of appropriate clinical use should be included.Instructional materials in communication disorders are available (Seaton 1990), as well as self-instructional computer literacy modules developed through ASHA's Project IMPACT (see Resources).

Advanced or Specialized Coursework in Clinical Computing. When faculty expertise and computing resources are available, a specialized course in clinical computing may be an appropriate way to address curriculum goals. Such a course helps students become aware of technology available within the department, and gives advanced students opportunities to explore the uses of new clinical tools enabling them to acquire levels of expertise and confidence that will continue to grow as they encounter new technology. These students can serve as resources for other students, clinical supervisors, and instructors within the department. It is excellent preparation for assuming a leadership role in technology after graduation.

Guest Speakers, Workshops, and Electronic Communication. Faculty may be surprised to find local clinicians who have already developed levels of expertise in administrative and clinical uses of computers. Many get started by attending workshops at regional and national conferences; some have friends or spouses who have stimulated their interest; and others have come from undergraduate and graduate programs where clinical computing competency was highlighted. Student and faculty contact with such clinicians can be initiated through field trips or guest presentations at universities. Local or regional workshops can supplement the computing expertise to which students have access, and local workshops on very specific topics—such as how to make single switches and/or adapt battery-operated toys for handicapped children—can double as educational opportunities and service projects.

One of the most widely available yet under-utilized resources among communication disorders faculty is electronic communication (Cochran and Bull 1991). A series of networks (the Internet) links all major colleges, universities, and research centers in the United States and around the world. Generally, access to the network for an individual faculty member or student is as simple as getting an account (electronic mail address) on a university main-frame computer, and logging on to the local electronic mail system. From there, the system sends messages, documents, or data through appropriate networks to the destination (electronic mail address) specified by the sender. Most users of word processing software find that they already know most of what they need to use electronic mail successfully. At most colleges and universities, the network can be accessed from a terminal on campus or via phone lines from any personal computer equipped with a modem. The exact procedures for doing this usually can be provided by the university academic computing staff.

Clearly, the ability to transmit informal messages, documents, or data to colleagues across the country will affect the scholarly activities of faculty members who participate. Maintaining long-distance partnerships, for example, is greatly facilitated. As it was drafted, this chapter was electronically transmitted between the author in Missouri and the author in Virginia several times. Frequent, informal communication between people with similar research interests is also facilitated by the network. Users may join on-line discussion groups in which on-going written "conversations" are regularly sent to all interested participants for their comments. Some large academic computer facilities also permit distant network users to access their data libraries.

The instructional potential of electronic communication has barely been tapped. As previously suggested, classes at two universities can perform the same experiment, exchange their data, and compare their findings in a matter of hours. A seminar class might "converse" in writing with a well-known expert. For example, an audiology seminar in

Montana used the CONFER electronic conferencing system at the University of Michigan to interview Charles Berlin at the Kresge Labs in New Orleans (Michael Wynne, personal communication 1988). During the fall semester of 1989, students in a clinical computing class in Missouri were paired with electronic mail pen-pals in a software design class in Virginia. Students in both courses reported that the experience not only demonstrated the convenience and potential of electronic communication, but also gave them new perspectives on computer applications (Cochran and Bull, personal communication). Electronic communication can greatly enhance the resources available to faculty, staff, and students in a communication disorders program.

SUMMARY

Teaching *with* a chalkboard is quite different from teaching *about* a chalkboard. Instructors should also recognize the distinction between teaching with the assistance of computers versus teaching about computers. Instructors with minimal computer expertise may, nevertheless, find that computer-based instruction greatly enhances classroom presentations in communication disorders. Instructors are especially encouraged to explore computer tools that they or their students direct, rather than rely on traditional CAI. When instructors teach *with* a computer, it is important to focus on the content, not the computer. This is facilitated by careful preparation and consideration of the skills that students may need prior to completing an assignment requiring computer use.

Some university programs in communication sciences and disorders will choose to revise their curricula in ways that will help student clinicians acquire clinical computing competency. This will require instruction *about* computers and opportunities to integrate computer applications with clinical practice. Several strategies besides offering specialized computer courses are recommended for facilitating clinical computing competency in speech-language pathology and audiology.

REFERENCES

American Speech-Language-Hearing Association 1989. *Omnibus Survey Trends 1984–1989.* Rockville, MD: Author.
Bull, G. L. 1989. Computer applications in speech and hearing: Perspectives for the 1990s. *Journal for Computer Users in Speech and Hearing* 5(2):105–109.
Bull, G. L., and Cooper, J. M. 1989. New technologies in teacher education. *The American Association of Colleges for Teacher Education Briefs* 10(2):7–8.

Bull, G. L., Cochran, P. S., and Snell, M. E. 1988. Beyond CAI: Computers, language, and persons with mental retardation. *Topics in Language Disorder* 8(4):55–76.

Bull, G., Cochran, P., Lang, J. K., Pierce, B. R., Seaton, W., Smaldino, J. J., Mahaffey, R. B., and Chial, M. 1985. Technology infusion: A resource guide. *Journal for Computer Users in Speech and Hearing* 1(2):96–116.

Chen, C. 1989. The first emperor of China's ancient world uncovered: From Xian to your electronic screen. *Academic Computing* 10–14, 54–57.

Cochran, P. S. 1989. Clinical computing in the 1990's: There's more to it than which key to press. *Journal for Computer Users in Speech and Hearing* 5(2): 110–13.

Cochran, P. S., and Bull, G. L. 1991. The use of BITNET in communication disorders programs. *Asha* 33(1):55–57, 66.

Cochran, P. S., Dustrude, S., Krupke, D., Mills, R., and Schwartz, A. In preparation. Suggested goals for educating speech-language pathologists about clinical applications of computers. A report by the Committee on Educational Technology. Rockville, MD: American Speech-Language-Hearing Association.

Goldman, R., and Dahle, A. J. 1985. Current and emerging applications of microcomputer technology in communication disorders. *Topics in Language Disorders* 6(1):11–25.

Horner, J. S., Halpin, C., Tarrant, M. R., and Pho, Q. 1987. Interactive videodisc simulation of infant VRA test. Scientific exhibit presented at the annual convention of the American Speech-Language-Hearing Association, New Orleans, November.

Hull, R. H. 1989. Training in visual tracking and synthesis through interactive laser technology. Paper presented at the annual convention of the American Speech-Language-Hearing Association, St. Louis, November.

Hurvitz, J. A., and Goldojarb, M. F. 1987. Comparison of two aural rehabilitation methods in a nursing home. Paper presented at the annual convention of the American Speech-Language-Hearing Association, New Orleans, November.

Kent, R. D. 1986. Technology: New tools for the clinic and laboratory. In *Speech-Language-Hearing Pathology and Audiology: Issues in Management*, ed. R. M. McLauchlin. Orlando, FL: Grune & Stratton, Inc.

Kopra, L. L., Kopra, M. A., Abrahamson, J. E., and Dunlop, R. J. 1987. Lipreading drill and practice software for an auditory-visual laser videodisc system (ALVIS). *Journal for Computer Users in Speech and Hearing* 3(1):58–68.

Lorendo, L. C. 1988. Computer implementation in communication sciences and disorders. Paper presented at the annual convention of the American Speech-Language-Hearing Association, Boston, November.

Mahshie, J. J. 1987. A primer on interactive video. *Journal for Computer Users in Speech and Hearing* 3(1):39–57.

Meyers, S. C., Strang, H. R., and Cartmell, D. J. 1987. A simulation for training stuttering intervention. Scientific exhibit presented at the annual convention of the American Speech-Language-Hearing Association, New Orleans, November.

Miller, G. D., Slike, S. B., Bailey, H. J., and Hobbis, D. H. 1987. Interactive videodisc technology: Audiometric testing and sign language instruction. Scientific exhibit presented at the annual convention of the American Speech-Language-Hearing Association, New Orleans, November.

Reeves, T. C. 1988. Evaluation review: Assessment of neuromotor dysfunction in infants. *The Videodisc Monitor* 6(4):26–27.

Rule, S., Salzberg, C. L., and Schulze, K. 1990. The role of videodiscs in special education methods courses. *Journal of Special Education Technology* 10(2):80–85.

Schwartz, A. H. 1986. Microcomputer applications: What changes hath this tool wrought? *Texas Journal of Audiology and Speech Pathology* 12(1):4–9.

Seaton, W. H. 1990. *Managing Information in Communication Sciences and Disorders with Appleworks Software*. Hudson, OH: Seaton & Sibs.

Sims, D., Kopra, L., Dunlop, R., and Kopra, M. 1985. A survey of microcomputer applications in aural rehabilitation. *Journal of the Academy of Rehabilitative Audiology* 18:9–26.

Stach, B. A. 1989. The building bridges project: A microcomputer-based speech audiometer. Paper presented at the annual convention of the American Speech-Language-Hearing Association, St. Louis, November.

Tye-Murray, N., Tyler, R. S., Bong, B., and Nares, T. 1988. Computerized laser videodisc programs for training speechreading and assertive communication behaviors. *Journal of the Academy of Rehabilitative Audiology* 21:143–52.

SUPPLEMENTARY READINGS

Bull, G. L., Harris, J., Lloyd, J., and Short, J. 1989. The electronic academical village. *Journal of Teacher Education* July–August: 27–31.

Bull, G. L., and Rushakoff, G. E. 1987. Computers and speech and language disordered individuals. In *Computers and Exceptional Individuals*, ed. J. D. Lindsey. Columbus, OH: Merrill Publishing Company.

Dean, R., and Pickering, J. 1989. Accessibility to BITNET for communication disorders institutions. Paper presented at the annual convention of the American Speech-Language-Hearing Association, St. Louis, November.

Harris, J. 1989. Teacher-LINK: An electronic culture. In *Proceedings of the National Educational Computing Conference*, ed. W. Ryan. Boston: International Council on Computers for Education.

Mills, R. H. 1986. Computerized management of aphasia. In *Language Intervention Strategies in Adult Aphasia*, ed. R. Chapey. Baltimore: Williams & Wilkins.

Russell, S. J., Corwin, R., Mokros, J. R., and Kapisovsky, P. M. 1989. *Beyond Drill and Practice: Expanding the Computer; Mainstream*. Reston, VA: Council for Exceptional Children.

Schrader, M. 1990. *Computer Applications for Language Learning*. Tucson, AZ: Communication Skill Builders.

Shriberg, L. D., Kwiatkowski, J., and Snyder, T. 1989. Tabletop versus micro-computer-assisted speech management: Stabilization phase. *Journal of Speech and Hearing Disorders* 54:233–48.

Updegrove, D. A., Muffo, J. A., and Dunn, J. A. 1990. Electronic mail and networks: New tools for university administrators. *Cause/Effect* 13:41–48.

RESOURCES

Teaching *with* Computers in Higher Education

For research findings, innovative strategies, and nationwide trends, consult:

- Collegiate Microcomputer (a quarterly journal devoted to microcomputers in higher education curriculum)
- *EDUCOM Review* (a quarterly publication of EDUCOM, a nonprofit consortium of 590 colleges and universities and 120 corporate associates)

For software and hardware reviews, product announcements, and professor-developed software, consult:

- *Asha*
  American Speech-Language-Hearing Association
  10801 Rockville Pike
  Rockville, MD 20852
- The Boston Computer Society (world's largest personal computer users' organization)
  One Center Plaza
  Boston, MA 02108
- Wisc-Ware (a consortium of educational institutions that distributes research and instructional software for IBM/MS-DOS microcomputers)
  Academic Computing Center
  University of Wisconsin-Madison
  1210 West Dayton St.
  Madison, WI 53706
- Intellimation (Apple Academic Software/Courseware Exchange)
  1-800-346-8355
- Infostack (HyperCard-based directory of all Macintosh products available for higher education)
  c/o Syllabus
  P.O. Box 2716
  Sunnyvale, CA 94087

Teaching *about* Computer Applications in Communication Disorders

For self-instructional modules (Apple or IBM):

- ASHA Project IMPACT
  ASHA Publication Sales
  10801 Rockville Pike
  Rockville, MD 20852

For clinical software information, reviews, product announcements, and research results, consult:

- *Closing the Gap* (national newspaper about technology for special populations)
  P.O. Box 68
  Henderson, MN 56044
- *Child Language Teaching and Therapy*
  Edward Arnold, Publisher
  Cambridge University Press
  32 East 57 Street
  New York, NY 10022
- *Journal for Computers Users in Speech and Hearing*
  CUSH Business Office
  Attn: William Seaton, Ph.D.
  P.O. Box 2160
  Hudson, OH 44236
- *Journal of Special Education Technology*
  A publication of the Council for Exceptional Children, Technology and Media Division
  Peabody College of Vanderbilt University
  Box 328
  Nashville, TN 37203

For technical information about specific devices or software for persons with special needs consult:

- Brandenburg, S. A., and Vanderheiden, G. C . (eds). *Communication, Control, and Computer Access for Disabled and Elderly Individuals: Resource Books 1, 2, and 3.*
  Little, Brown and Company
  34 Beacon Street
  Boston, MA 02108
- IBM National Support Center for Persons with Disabilities
  P.O. Box 2150 (A06S1)
  Atlanta, GA 30055
- National Special Education Alliance
  Apple Computer, Inc.
  20525 Mariani Ave., MS 36-M
  Cupertino, CA 95014

SECTION IV

EDUCATIONAL CONTEXT AND CONTINUUM

Chapter 14

Counseling and Advising Preprofessionals

Robert L. Schum and John E. Bernthal

Educators often interpret the term *student counseling* to mean academic advising and consulting with students. However, it is important to distinguish *counseling* from *advising* because each signifies a different aspect of student-faculty interaction.

COUNSELING

The need for counseling is particularly apparent in professional education programs that focus on a student's personal interactions with clients, supervisors, and colleagues. In this context, students and faculty are more sensitive to personal behavior of students. Speech and hearing education programs emphasize attention to interpersonal relationships and habilitation of clients. In this educational context, a student might be more willing to identify personal problems and seek help from faculty members.

At the same time, most educators deal with students' personal problems. Sometimes these interactions are initiated by the student in search of assistance. At other times, this help begins with the faculty member who believes that it is important, for the educational progress and/or the welfare of the student, to discuss concerns about the student's adjustment. In either case, the faculty member has a professional responsibility to provide counseling to the student regarding personal problems.

A legitimate question exists as to the proper nature and extent of the faculty member's assistance in a student's personal problems. It is often difficult to determine if a student's personal problem is related to academic difficulty. Beyond the challenge of looking for a clear boundary that probably does not exist, one needs to recognize that the most important resources in an academic/professional discipline are the people involved.

Common Problems

Certain problems are common to students partly because of the academic situation, and, partly and probably more importantly, because of their developmental stage as young adults. One common cluster of problems centers on students' adjustments to college including living away from home, adapting to an intensive social environment, and defining their adult identities in the context of many people who are the same age. Students also may have trouble understanding what is expected of them scholastically and socially. In adapting to the roles demanded in higher education, students may find that measures of academic success—grades, degree, theses, dissertations—cause particular stress. At times, a student may have trouble meeting academic standards or deadlines. At other times, although a student's progress is adequate, he/she might have difficulty accepting certain grades and constantly strive to do better.

Some students have problems establishing appropriate relationships with faculty members. A student, although an adult, may perceive adult/adolescent relationships with faculty members, as inordinately dependent on, or resistant to, guidance from a professor. The faculty member may be the focus point of the student's efforts to learn how to relate to an authority figure when both are adults.

Some students experience financial difficulties that affect their academic progress; others face problems related to their families. Students have parents who are ill or die, and other family members who need attention. Sometimes students, in their emerging roles as adults, feel responsibility for family members, including spouses and young children, and therefore become involved in managing family problems. The time, emotional drain, and financial demands of caring for family members may cause personal problems or stress. Students also have to deal with interpersonal relationships outside the family. Traditional students are, typically, young adults who are establishing relationships with others in their lives. The demands of such relationships often create problems as they try to establish their adult identities. Students may experience problems with roommates and find that these problems interfere with other aspects of their lives.

Particular problems occur for nontraditional students, such as older students returning to school, minority students, and foreign students. Older students may have concerns about re-establishing their student identity, and competing with younger classmates, who sometimes seem brighter and better prepared. Minority students may feel lonely and isolated within a department or a college community. A cultural/racial difference can create a situation in which the minority student, or members of the majority, accentuate the differences of the student. In seeing differences, rather than similarities, the student may feel even more separate and distinct, creating the special stresses one experiences with loneliness or isolation. Foreign students may have similar experiences, which are then exacerbated by being isolated from a culture they understand. They are often unable to visit families during holidays or breaks, and may not even regularly communicate with their support network.

In addition to the general types of problems listed above, some particular problems merit specific mention because of their frequency and relationship to young adults. Speech and hearing programs, with a large proportion of female students, probably have a significant number of students who experience eating disorders, such as anorexia and bulimia. For example, Kubistant (1982) estimated that 5% to 25% of young women experience eating disorders. A significant proportion of college students have difficulties with alcohol and drug abuse, as well as with suicidal behavior. Whitaker (1989) reported that the leading form of death among college-aged persons is automobile accidents, many of which are caused by alcohol abuse. The second leading cause of death among this age group is suicide. Bernard and Bernard (1982) reported that depression and isolation are common feelings reported by students. Among students who expressed these feelings by suicidal behaviors, the most frequently reported reasons were social difficulties, followed by family problems. These two reasons were given as causes of suicidal behavior 75% of the time. Academic problems were reported less frequently as causes of suicidal behavior.

Faculty members might reason that suicidal behavior is usually not related to academics and that drug and alcohol abuse, as well as eating disorders, are private matters for students. They may not believe that these issues are within the purview of the faculty-student relationship. Faculty members must remember, however, that often they are the authority figures and role models who have the most contact with the student. They are the persons who can most likely spot warning signs and discuss the students' need for help.

Causes

Besides identifying common student problems, one can also consider different mechanisms that cause certain problems. A primary cause is related to age or life development status. Grayson (1989) points out that there are certain developmental tasks associated with college students. These tasks include separating from parents, forming one's adult identity, experiencing intimacy with peers (including coping with romantic breakups), dealing with authority, coping with uncertainty and ambiguity, and finding security and self-esteem. Grayson suggests that these developmental challenges arrange themselves in a sequence, thus characterizing each year of college by the particular developmental challenges. Brown (1989) reminds readers that spiritual development is part of personal development, although people often avoid mentioning this topic. During the period of undergraduate or graduate studies, students often grapple with the development of personal identity and the meaning of their lives.

Another cause relates to the type of students who are attracted to graduate programs. Such students may have a tendency to carry out compulsive behaviors. A student in the speech and hearing field, for example, needs to organize his/her life, prepare for exams and papers, and meet deadlines for class work and clinical reports. A compulsive person is more likely to be successful. However, when people experience personal problems, the problems often exacerbate pre-existing methods for coping with stress. Under stress, such students are likely to become more compulsive in an effort to restore or maintain order in their lives. When compulsive tendencies are exacerbated, a student may experience problems with making simple decisions, feelings of inferiority, or fear of exposing flaws. Fear of exposure can be manifested by difficulty in writing a thesis or dissertation. Because of concern with producing a flawed document, and thereby exposing inferiority, a student may be obsessed over the paper or may procrastinate in completing it, in an effort to stave off a presumed disaster.

A third cause that might account for some reports of student stress is a variant of the "medical student syndrome." In a clinical education program, which emphasizes the examination of problems and pathological processes, a student might personally identify with the problems, which need not be confined to specific communication disorders. Rather, a broader concept of having difficulty adjusting to challenges might cause the student to question introspectively his/her own ability to cope with a life challenge. A student might find that a clinical problem discussed in class triggers reactions to personal events in the student's life. For example, one writer's experience is that after class lectures on physical and sexual abuse, students will stop by to talk about their own histories in the context of seeking help to come to terms with suppressed memories. With sexual abuse this should not be surprising, given the preponderance of females in speech and hearing programs. Summit (1985) reported that 20% to 30% of girls are sexually victimized by 13 years of age. Given that base rate, when the topic of sexual abuse is brought up in clinical training, perhaps one quarter to one third of the class can identify personally with the problem.

Interactions between faculty and students can create situations in which personal problems are revealed. For example, a teacher can create an atmosphere of trust and rapport in which a student feels safe revealing concerns or seeking counsel. Sometimes this openness is communicated directly to the student. At other times, the student may infer it from the teaching model demonstrated in dealing with clients. In other instances, the faculty/student interaction may be a negative one. For example, excessive academic demands, or the student's *perception* of excessive demands, can create a stressful situation. Often students in clinical training are not used to receiving detailed, specific critiques of their personal attributes, such as the ways in which they interact with other people. In their early academic training, they were used to more impersonal feedback given in academic courses. As they become involved in professional training, however, they find attention focused on their personal style. This novel circumstance may cause them discomfort, and students may require assistance in learning how to deal with this issue of the supervisory process.

Another cause that does not receive much acknowledgment in the literature regards sexual, romantic, and other personal complications between faculty members and students. Pope, Levenson, and Schover (1979) investigated sexual relationships between students and faculty/supervisors in psychology training programs. In their survey, 13% of the educators reported sexual contact with students, and 25% of female graduate students reported sexual contact. The authors commented that studies such as theirs were few. During the subsequent decade, this still seems to be the case. One can assume that this problem exists in speech and hearing departments. Where it does, it not only creates personal problems for the individual students involved, but can also create a climate of unrest among other students aware of such activities.

Recognition of these various causes can help faculty members understand why certain problems might occur among students in their department. Rather than focus on particular symptoms, one can recognize that behind the symptoms is an ongoing process creating the problems. By identifying the source of problems, one can better determine methods of intervention and problem resolution.

Intervention

Faculty members, as individuals and as a group, can address counseling issues with students at many levels. These include direct assistance from a faculty member, referral to specialized services, procedures implemented throughout a department, and procedures implemented campus-wide. Assistance can be chosen depending on the nature and severity of the student's problem. Some faculty members may be better able than others to provide individual services to a student. Or a campus counseling center may be more prepared to help students with particular types of issues.

One thing to keep in mind is the distinction between *process* and *content* in dealing with student problems (Schum 1986). Focus on the particular content of the student's problem can cause one to lose sight of the underlying process. A student may have a problem that in itself may not be the important underlying issue. It, nonetheless, enables the student to initiate a conversation with a faculty member concerning treatment. For example, a student who is concerned about a course grade may actually be struggling with the issue of leaving school.

Another aspect of process is that the precipitating problem reflects the broader issue of how the student deals with other people or events across a variety of situations. Or a student who is angry about a midterm evaluation in a clinical practicum might actually have difficulty accepting imperfection or flaws, particularly if they are obvious to others. This difficulty can be heightened when a student becomes involved in clinical education. In previous classroom courses, the emphasis was on mastering academic material. However, the educational process shifts in practicum training. The focus is often on the student him/herself, and how well he/she can manage situations and apply certain knowledge in a timely and appropriate manner. A student might find this personal focus more challenging and harder to accept and to master, requiring practice under the tutelage of a supervisor. The personalized evaluation might trigger a response whereby the student feels threatened by this scrutiny.

An *empathic understanding* of the student's situation can enhance the faculty member's counseling relationship. Using a developmental model of student problems, one realizes that what are important issues for a faculty member may be different from what is important for a student. For example, a faculty member may have long ago resolved issues of establishing intimacy or working out a relationship with parents. But these are two important issues for college-aged students. A faculty member may be financially secure and not be so immediately sensitive to a student's more precarious financial situation. An empathic perspective gives the faculty member the opportunity to focus on the most relevant dimensions of the student's dilemma.

One problem in counseling students is the *dual relationship*, which can occur in academic settings. For example, a student might seek counsel from a faculty member and, in that context, the two might establish a confidential and special relationship that focuses on personal counseling. The faculty member, however, may have another relationship with the student—course instructor, research supervisor, academic adviser, department administrator—and this second relationship may conflict with the first because the academic relationship may require the faculty member to provide a critical appraisal of the student's academic performance. In such cases, the faculty member's two roles may come into conflict with each other.

If a student seeks counsel from a faculty member, and the faculty member determines that such help requires more than a single conversation, the faculty member should carefully evaluate the potential problems of a dual relationship and help the student seek counseling from another person. An important counseling issue in itself is helping a student learn to trust other people.

Other potential problems for faculty members who counsel students are *transference* and *countertransference* issues. These involve the client's or clinician's transference of feelings and needs he/she has for other people to the other person in the counseling relationship (Schum 1986). Transference can be manifested in both positive and negative fashions. For example, a student may fall in love with the faculty member, decide that the faculty member can become a best friend, or consider that person as an idealized role model. Or the student might project onto the faculty member bitter feelings of being rejected by other people or anger towards an authority figure. Common countertransference difficulties of faculty members might include the needs for love, affiliation, or validation that student relationships might fulfill. It is common for people to confuse caring with love. In a counseling relationship, either the student or the faculty member may confound a caring attitude with a perception of more intense love. In other situations, it may be that faculty-student sexual entanglements reflect a sincere, but poorly chosen manner of fulfilling one's personal needs for intimacy.

A variation on academic countertransference is illustrated by George Bernard Shaw's *Pygmalion*, in which Professor Higgins tries to re-create Eliza in his own image and likeness. As a result, he becomes attached not to the real Eliza, but to his reflected image. Sometimes academics get involved in this type of countertransference; acting as mentors to students eventually causes them to become enamored of the qualities or ideas they, themselves, have fostered. Eventually the tension builds in this transformed relationship; either the student matures into a professional who rejects the role of slavishly following in the intellectual footsteps of the professor, or sometimes the professor narcissistically falls in love with his/her reflected image. In either case, the tension becomes too great for the relationship, and one or both parties find the need to back away and reduce the intensity.

In addition to individual faculty assistance, a department can address some of the students' counseling needs by creating a helpful, positive climate for its students. This carries a clear message to the students that the department expects that the students will be successful in their work and that the faculty offer opportunities to assist them in this endeavor.

A department can also help students by creating an atmosphere that enhances rapport among students and faculty. With better rapport, people feel comfortable bringing up concerns when they first occur, rather than waiting until they become more serious. An atmosphere in which people have friendly and respectful dialogue with one another provides a model of openness and trust for students. As part of creating trust, students find it important that departmental actions are communicated to them in a timely and thorough manner. When departmental actions are not fully explained, students may fill in the missing information with their own interpretations of the situation. By keeping them informed and giving them participation in decision processes (e.g., sitting on departmental committees), the department helps to reduce the students' feelings of helplessness that often exacerbate stress-related problems.

Opportunities to use persons outside the department to provide services include staff development activities and student educational forums. For example, a university may have a student counseling service that could provide staff training programs. Such activities might include methods for fostering a better climate of trust for students, methods for dealing with common academic problems, or methods for spotting subtle student problems and making appropriate referrals. Personnel from the counseling center may also offer forums to students on common student issues such as test anxiety or substance abuse.

Most universities and colleges recognize the need for centralized services to students, which usually includes student counseling. Delworth and Hanson (1989) and Grayson and Cauley (1989) delineate the scope of problems and the breadth of services available to college students. Such services include alcohol and drug abuse counseling, dealing with personal relationships, abuse and assault victim assistance, help with social skills development, and assistance with academic issues such as test anxiety and study skills. The philosophy of a campuswide counseling service is that the university/college is a small community of its own, with the counseling center providing a range of services to meet the needs of its citizens. It is prudent for faculty members to be aware of available services, so that when the need arises, a faculty member has a referral resource.

Besides a formal counseling service, many campuses have ancillary services that provide support for students. Campus ministries and religious centers offer assistance to students. Minority and foreign students sometimes find assistance in special support groups established at minority/cultural and international centers. In addition to campus-based programs, there are community mental health centers, private mental health specialists, self-help groups that specialize in treatment of particular problems such as alcohol and drug abuse, crisis lines for assistance to students who present acute problems, and community religious centers.

Referral

Sometimes a big hurdle in counseling students is the issue of how to refer a student to somebody else. A faculty member might use *projection* to explain that it is an awkward moment for the *student*—when he/she is confronted with a problem that is serious and needs special assistance. But it may be that the faculty member is also feeling awkward. Because we have been conditioned not to call attention to people's personal problems, it is difficult for us to look someone in the eye and say that he/she needs help. Yet the faculty person has a professional responsibility, as an academic and, in some cases, as a clinician, to be honest with the student. In a supportive manner, the faculty member must tell the student that a problem is apparent and that the student needs help. If the faculty member keeps in mind the student's needs, and communicates that attitude, he/she does not have to worry about being too blunt with the student. The faculty member can talk about what has been observed and how it affects the student's welfare. Often, when students are engaged in such conversations with a faculty member, their resistance is a result of their anxiety about their problems and their fear of things becoming worse if they try to change. A method for combating such anxiety is to provide structure and support to the anxious person (Schum 1986). The faculty member does so by describing the problem as it appears to others and by providing help with a referral to a specialist.

Benefits

A number of benefits can accrue to a department that addresses the student counseling issues discussed in this chapter. Attention to the student as a whole person creates a healthier work environment for both students and faculty members. There is understanding that people, as part of life, face obstacles and challenges that may prove difficult for them. An atmosphere is created in which people are willing to seek methods for helping other people find choices and alternatives in dealing with problems. This attitude is a good way to handle the most vital and important resource in an academic setting—people. Furthermore, a department with this focus provides an excellent model for students who are being taught how to provide clinical services for others.

ADVISING

As long as there have been colleges, there has been a need for students to receive guidance and assistance as they plan their programs of study, become adjusted to the college environment and its unique academic, social, and psychological demands, and face the rigors of growing up. In earlier days, such guidance was frequently the responsibility of college presidents and deans. With growth in the size and complexity of postsecondary institutions, much of the guidance has been assumed by 'academic advisors'—usually a faculty member assigned the role of academic advisor. Many people perceive that much of the personal attention shown students in the past has been lost and with it a change in the students' educational experience (Winston et al. 1984, p. ix).

Quality academic advising should be a high priority of departmental heads and upper-level administrators. However, in surveys of students and college administrators, there is general dissatisfacton with both the quality and effectiveness of academic advising on most campuses. Riesman (1981) stated, "faculty advising of students, including freshmen . . . is at most large institutions, including my own, at least an embarrassment, at worst a disgrace" (p. 258).

Ender, Winston, and Miller (1984) reported a renewed interest in academic advising during the 1980s. They cite several reasons for this interest, including (1) changes in the size and complexity of the institution, (2) a renewed sense of consumerism fueled by the competition for students, (3) student bodies with increasing numbers of first-generation college students, minorities, and returning adults, and (4) interest in student satisfaction and retention. Ender, Winston, and Miller (1984) recommended a model called "developmental academic advising" to meet the advising needs of today's students. Such an advising model calls for the adviser to be responsive to students and their changing needs as they progress through the institution. In other words, academic advising should be individualized and focus on the total well-being of each student. This view of academic advising expands that held by many faculty who see their advising roles as assisting students to matriculate in a timely manner and develop plans of study that meet the institutional and departmental graduation requirements.

What is Academic Advising?

The literature offers many definitions of the advising process. Developmental academic advising is defined

> . . . as a systematic process based on a close student-adviser relationship intended to aid students in achieving educational, career, and personal goals through the utilization of the full range of institutional and community resources. . . . Developmental advising relationships focus on identifying and accomplishing life goals, acquiring skills and attitudes that promote intellectual and personal growth, and sharing concerns for each other and for the academic community . . . (Ender, Winston, and Miller 1984, p. 19).

Ender, Winston, and Miller (1982) presented seven principles that are essential for developmental advising:

1. Must be a continuous process of personal contacts that have direction and purpose between the adviser and student.
2. Must concern itself with quality-of-life issues—advisers should be aware of and communicate to students resources and services

available to enhance the quality of the students' educational experiences.

3. Establishes student's goals encompassing academic, career, and personal development areas.
4. Establishes a caring human relationship—adviser must take primary responsibility for initial development.
5. Adviser models behaviors that lead to self-responsibility and self-directiveness.
6. Seeks to integrate the services and expertise of both the academic and student affairs professionals.
7. Adviser utilizes as many campus and community resources as possible.

These principles are not followed by many individuals who serve as academic advisers. Ender, Winston, and Miller (1984) point out that academic advising is not primarily an administrative function and that well-organized records are not ends in themselves; nor is it a matter of providing students with a computer printout of an educational plan and, from that point, merely affixing a signature to students' class schedules. Academic advising depends as much on the educational and academic needs of students as on the good intentions of the adviser. Academic advising should focus on a student's search for academic and personal competence and not be confused with personal counseling. When personal counseling or remedial intervention is required, students should be referred to campus offices with personnel who have specialized knowledge and skills to address such concerns.

Advising should begin during the freshman year and should be continued during a student's entire academic career. Freshman year is the time when students are most receptive to and most likely to take advantage of the educational opportunities of the institution. (In many undergraduate programs in communication sciences and disorders (CSD), a departmental adviser may not even see a student during this important year in the student's education.) Contact with a departmental adviser should help students mesh general education requirements with academic and career goals. The academic unit in CSD must keep in close touch with academic advisers who serve beginning students planning to major in CSD, or else provide advising assistance to such students so that appropriate information and recommendations for general education courses can be provided.

Organizational Structure

Centralized and decentralized structures exist for undergraduate advising. Centralized advising can be found campus-wide, in individual departments, or even in academic programs. The advising staff varies, ranging from professional advisers and trained paraprofessionals to faculty members who are assigned advising as an extra duty. On many campuses, an academic advising center is responsible for advising most students until general education or core curriculum requirements are met. Eighty percent of academic advising is provided by the faculty (Crockett and Levitz 1984). With faculty advising, there is a natural tendency for interactions to be subject-matter oriented. In addition to that limitation, many faculty advisers often are inaccessible, lack necessary skills, and have difficulty keeping up to date on institutional policies, procedures, and rules.

Larson and Brown (1983) reported that faculty and students agreed that advisers should be involved in facilitating student interaction with the bureaucracy, acting as referral agents for financial aid and part-time employment, and providing information about campus activities. Students indicated that they wanted advisers to assist in class selection (but not make decisions for them), to assist in career selection, and to be knowledgeable about all aspects of the institution, not just about academic matters. Winston and Sandor (1984), on the other hand, stated that although students want interest and support from advisers about academic and out-of-class activities, they do not want their freedom curtailed. In other words, "students wished to be partners in the advising process, not recipients of advice" (Ender, Winston, and Miller 1984, p. 28).

Two national surveys, both conducted by the American College Testing Program, examined undergraduate academic advising practices in colleges and universities (Carstensen and Silberhorn 1979; Crockett and Levitz 1984). Administrative recognition of the importance of advising was perceived by survey respondents to be the most important advising need at their respective institutions so that faculty could justify the time spent in this endeavor. Over half indicated there was no formal recognition or reward system for advising at their institutions. Other highlights of these two national surveys revealed that faculty continued to be the major providers of academic advising (80%), with most respondents reporting advising loads of 19 or fewer students. The vast majority of institutions did not have a systematic appraisal system; group advising was an under-utilized strategy even though it has been shown to be effective; 60% of the institutions had advising handbooks; about half of the institutions centrally set advising policies and procedures; the most common method for assigning students to advisers was by academic major; advising centers were more common in public than private colleges; and about 20% of the institutions had a director or coordinator of academic advising.

The Advising Process

Helping Students Make Decisions.   Students need assistance in making academic choices as well as in learning skills for decision making. Effective decision-making techniques not only influence academic success but are important skills for life, helping students develop interpersonal relationships, independence, and build vocational identity.

Some of life's critical decisions occur when a student chooses an academic direction and/or career path. Stages during the decision-making process have been described by Harren (1979, p. 121). The first stage is an *awareness* phase where students do self-appraisals in their new environment. The next is a *planning* stage where the students search for information and weigh past experiences and new data. Students may need help in gathering relevant information and examining the data that they find. Students with rational decision-making styles will approach this planning phase in a logical, orderly way; whereas students with intuitive styles may make the decision on the basis of emotional feelings. If students have enough information, they may choose a specific alternative and move to the *commitment* stage. Students frequently do not commit themselves publicly to decisions until they have discussed it in general terms with others and have gotten reactions. It is during this period that students begin to integrate the commitment with their self-concepts. In the final stage, students begin to *implement* their plans with specific actions.

Critical Academic Decisions

One of the most immediate decisions for students is the selection of a major; choosing the specific courses for a major is another important task. Many students equate the choice of a major with a career decision. Some students select a major on the basis of its identification with an occupation, whereas others, such as many arts and sciences students, choose a major that is fairly independent of the career goal. It is probably safe to assume that majors in CSD are typically vocationally oriented. It is important for advisers to encourage students to develop a strong liberal arts orientation in order to broaden their perspectives beyond a narrow occupational focus. A strong liberal arts component is consistent with the position taken by the Council of Graduate Programs in Communication Sciences and Disorders as well as the ASHA Ad Hoc Committee on Undergraduate Education (see Chapter 4).

Developing an Educational Plan

An adviser can play a key role in helping students develop and implement their educational plans. While most advisers view themselves primarily as information-givers, they also need to see themselves as sounding boards for ideas; they should provide a climate so that students feel free to share their ideas, and provide support so that students know someone has an interest in their future. Students, on the other hand, must make decisions for their plans of study and take responsibility for modifying them when needed.

Most students' initial decisions about their courses of study change at least once during their college years. At the institution of one of the authors of this chapter, the average student changes his/her major two or three times between the freshman and senior years.

The educational plan for students in CSD may differ a great deal depending on the institution. A comparison of the degree requirements for undergraduates from the co-authors' two respective institutions reveals that, at one, calculus is a required course, whereas at the other, the only math requirement beyond that necessary for general education is a statistics course. In one institution, an undergraduate clinical practicum is required; in the other, no undergraduate practicum is required. It is probable that the curriculum for majors in CSD is fairly prescriptive in nature, partially because of the preprofessional nature of the programs and the coursework requirements for the Certificates of Clinical Competence (CCC). (See Appendix A.) In addition to meeting preprofessional education requirements for study at the master's degree level, students who want to obtain certification for working in schools must meet certain college-of-education requirements. Students in many CSD programs have few electives, tend to focus on vocational skills, and sometimes lack strong liberal arts backgrounds.

Students who are rejected by master's programs or who decide not to apply to graduate school, even though that was an initial goal, merit special assistance. If they are upper-class students, they need to understand how their CSD program can be applied to other fields and how they can investigate occupational alternatives. Some of these students may also pursue graduate programs in other fields. The adviser can help identify realistic alternatives and appropriate resources, and provide support for these students as they explore alternative programs. Many universities have counseling and advising centers that assist students with changes in majors and career goals.

Students with Special Advising Needs

The increasing diversity of student populations, in terms of age, ethnic background, status, and academic preparation, reflects the changing demographics of higher education. No single advising approach will meet the needs of such diverse student populations. If academic advisers are to serve as true advisers rather than as mere "schedule makers," they are going to need knowledge and skills to promote effective development for an ever-broadening diversity of students.

Academic Underpreparation. The student who is academically underprepared is not new or unknown to higher education. In fact, prior to the beginning of this century, Wellesley College had a program designed to assist students with reading and study skills. Today, it is even more important that underprepared students be encouraged to seek assessment of their academic skills and to participate in appropriate remediation. There are more available resources, and more students who need them. Beginning with the 1960s, a high proportion of postsecondary students began to show deficits in basic skills needed for postsecondary study. At the same time, some colleges and universities began accepting students with lower standardized test scores and grades than had been done previously.

Academically underprepared students have been reported to have low motivation, are easily distracted, and may have poor work habits (Mitchell and Piatowska 1974). These characteristics may lead to low levels of confidence in academic abilities. Academically underprepared students experience more difficulty in educational planning and may have unrealistic images of school (Saunders and Ervin 1984). Some such students attribute academic success to luck rather than to ability or hard work (DeBoer 1983).

The subpopulations within this academically underprepared group are students with basic skills deficiencies, non-native English speakers, older and returning students, economically disadvantaged, and learning-disabled students. Academic advisers for such students may need to be proactive and even willing to make the initial contact with a student if he/she does not seek the adviser's help.

Other Topics

Part-Time Students/Students with Major Family and/or Job Responsibilities. Part-time students who are enrolled at institutions where most students reside on campus are likely to experience social isolation. Many part-time students with major family and/or job responsibilities frequently spend considerable time in activities that directly compete with their academic work. It is not uncommon, then, for such students to give their academic responsibilities lower priorities than their nonacademic responsibilities. In addition, adult learners who have not been in school for a long time may have low self-confidence about their ability to perform academic coursework. One common need for all students with multiple responsibilities is efficient and effective study skills and time management. These students may need assistance in the development of study plans, schedules, and estimates of time required for various assignments (Saunders and Ervin 1984). We have found academic advising especially challenging with students who attempt to combine full-time academic loads and time-consuming outside (nonacademic) obligations. Such a combination is frequently a ticket for student discouragement and academic failure. The creation of a plan that balances academic responsibilities with a student's other obligations is critical for academic success. Advisers must appreciate the demands of nonacademic responsibilities placed on these students and attempt to assist them in balancing the many claims on their time and resources.

Cultural Diversity. The number of students who are members of a minority group continues to be under-represented in American postsecondary education in general as well as in CSD programs. Although minorities account for approximately 20% of the total population, only 15% of the total college student enrollment in 1986 were minority group members (Bureau of the Census 1989). In CSD programs, the number of students who are minority group members is even less than that for the general college population. In the 1988–89 academic year, Cooper, Bernthal, and Creaghead (1989) reported that 8.4% of the undergraduates, 6.4% of the master's students, and 13% of the doctoral students in CSD programs were from minority groups. These data represent a decline in the percentage of minority students in CSD when compared to data reported just two years previously. Recruitment and retention of students who are members of minority groups must continue to be high priorities for academic programs in CSD as well as in the professions of speech-language pathology and audiology.

Research on attrition of minority students indicates that inadequate preparation and poor academic performance account for only about half of the attrition (Pantages and Creedon 1978). Feelings of alienation, frustration, and helplessness contribute significantly to attrition rates of minority students on predominantly white campuses.

The danger of generalizing about racial minorities obscures the uniqueness among their different cultures. However, there are some generalizations that can be made concerning racial minorities: (a) they tend to view the world differently from white students (Atkinson, Morton, and Sue 1979); (b) they may have a sense of oppression and racial discrimination (Suen 1983); (c) they may feel estranged and alienated; (d) they may experience language differences; and (e) they may hold values not shared by other students (Atkinson, Morton, and Sue 1979). Minority students when confronted with an academic concern are likely to seek help from minority professionals rather than from white faculty. Unfortunately, minority students in CSD have a small number of minority faculty available to them, as only 5.2% of the full-time faculty in CSD are members of minority groups (Creaghead, Bernthal, and Gilbert 1991). Advisers should make certain that minority students are aware of opportunities and support available from university-wide student services, as these students tend to under-utilize resources of student affairs and believe that such services are directed toward white students. Perhaps the best advice that can be given to advisers who work with students from differing cultural backgrounds is to seek information about these students' native culture.

Master's Students. The role of the academic adviser for a master's student in CSD is similar to that for advising undergraduates although the students' needs are quite different. Graduates are often treated as adolescents and have many of the same university restrictions as undergraduates. Most have middle-class backgrounds but lack the incomes required for middle-class life styles. Although they share common academic backgrounds, intellectual interests, and similar pressures with their fellow students, they are required to compete with them. This competition can be destructive and increase stress among students.

The first role of the adviser to master's students is to be a reliable source of information. Requirements for the Certificate of Clinical Competence (CCC), state licensure, state education certification, as well as those of the department and institution, must be met. All of these components have myriad rules and deadlines, in addition to coursework and practicum requirements. Although most programs have student handbooks that list these requirements, it is not uncommon for the student to miss critical deadlines for filing a program of study, registering for a comprehensive exam, or even applying for graduation. Entering master's students often have a need for structure, a low need for autonomy, and a high need for achievement. However, graduate study requires acceptance of responsibility for self, and some students have much difficulty assuming that responsibility for themselves and their program.

In a small master's degree program, there may be few options or electives that a student can take to meet CCC and institutional degree requirements. However, large programs may provide a smorgasbord of course offerings consistent with students' requirements, interests, and goals. A major decision for most master's-level students is whether or not to complete a thesis. Several programs have etablished areas of emphasis or tracks such as adult disorders or school-aged children's disorders. Advisers need to assist students in making appropriate decisions based on students' abilities, interests, and goals.

Doctoral Students. Doctoral study, quite different from study at either the undergraduate or master's level, does not focus on classroom experiences or completion of courses. For doctoral students, graduate study is a time of intensive mentoring in the skills and attitudes required for a career of scientific inquiry. Doctoral programs are typically characterized by few course requirements, a minimum of structure, and much research. Typically doctoral students have an adviser who is a mentor. Success in completing the program frequently is tied to how well the adviser is able to guide the student through the program. The doctoral adviser may also evaluate written and oral examinations, and direct a majority of the student's research. Winston and Polkosnik (1984) list five roles and functions essential to successful doctoral advising: (1) reliable information sources; (2) departmental socializer; (3) advocate; (4) role model; and (5) occupational socializer.

CONCLUSION

Counseling and advising are integral components of preprofessional education. Depending on the formal organization and assignment of duties within an educational program or, perhaps, simply on the basis of a student's choice of a helper, such responsibilities may, at different times, be assumed by administrators, researchers, classroom instructors, clinical supervisors, or any combination thereof. Given the importance of sensitive counseling and intelligent advising in the preparation of students for life and career, program personnel need to understand and coordinate their individual roles.

REFERENCES

Atkinson, D., Morton, G., and Sue, D. 1979. *Counseling American Minorities: A Cross-Cultural Perspective*. Dubuque, IA: Brown.

Bernard, J. L., and Bernard, M. L. 1982. Factors related to suicidal behavior among college students and the impact of institutional response. *Journal of College Student Personnel* 23(5):409–413. San Francisco: Jossey-Bass.

Brown, R. D. 1989. Fostering intellectual and personal growth: The student development role. In *Student Services: A Handbook for the Profession* (2nd ed.), eds. U. Delworth and G. R. Hanson. San Francisco: Jossey-Bass.

Bureau of the Census. 1989. *Statistical Abstract of the United States 109th Ed.* Washington, DC: U.S. Government Printing Office.

Carstensen, D. J., and Silberhorn, C. A. 1979. A national survey of academic advising final report. Iowa City, IA: American College Testing Programs.

Creaghead, N., Bernthal, J., and Gilbert, H. 1991. *The Council of Graduate Programs in Communication Sciences and Disorders 1990–91 National Survey*. Minneapolis, MN: Council of Graduate Programs in Communication Sciences and Disorders.

Crockett, D. W., and Levitz, R. S. 1984. Current advising practices in colleges and universities. In *Developmental Academic Advising*, eds. R. B. Winston, Jr., T. K. Miller, S. C. Ender, T. J. Grites, and Assoc. San Francisco: Jossey-Bass.

DeBoer, G. E. 1983. The importance of freshman students' perceptions of the factors responsible for first-term academic performance. *Journal of College Student Personnel* 24:344–49.

Delworth, U., and Hanson, G. R. (eds.). 1989. *Student Services: A Handbook for the Profession* (2nd ed.). San Francisco: Jossey-Bass.

Ender, S. C., Winston, R. B., Jr., and Miller, T. K. 1982. Academic advising as student development. In *New Directions for Student Services: Developmental Approaches to Academic Advising* (no. 17), eds. R. B. Winston, Jr., S. C. Ender, and T. K. Miller. San Francisco: Jossey-Bass.

Ender, S. C., Winston, R. B., Jr., and Miller, T. K. 1984. Academic advising reconsidered. In *Developmental Academic Advising*, eds. R. B. Winston, Jr., T. K. Miller, S. C. Ender, T. J. Grites, and Assoc. San Francisco: Jossey-Bass.

Grayson, P. A. 1989. The college psychotherapy client: An overview. In *College Psychotherapy*, eds. P. A. Grayson and K. Cauley. New York: Guilford Press.

Grayson, P. A., and Cauley, K. (eds.) 1989. *College Psychotherapy*. New York: Guilford Press.

Harren, V. A. 1979. A model of career decision making for college students. *Journal of Vocational Behavior* 14:119–33.

Kubistant, T. 1982. Bulimarexia. *Journal of College Student Personnel* 23(4):333–39.

Larson, M. D., and Brown, B. 1983. Student and faculty expectations of academic advising. *National Academic Advising Association Journal* 3:31–37.

Mitchell, K. R., and Piatowska, O. E. 1974. Effects of group treatment for college underachievers and bright failing underachievers. *Journal of Counseling Psychology* 21:494–501.

Pantages, T. L., and Creedon, C. E. 1978. Studies of college attrition: 1950–1975. *Review of Educational Records* 48:49–101.

Pope, K. S., Levenson, H., and Schover, L. R. 1979. Sexual intimacy in psychology training. *American Psychologist* 34(8):682–89.

Riesman, D. 1981. *On Higher Education: The Academic Enterprise in an Era of Rising Student Consumerism*. San Francisco: Jossey-Bass.

Saunders, S. A., and Ervin, L. 1984. Meeting the special advising needs of students. In *Developmental Academic Advising*, eds. R. B. Winston, Jr., T. K. Miller, S. C. Ender, T. J. Grites, and Assoc. San Francisco: Jossey-Bass.

Schum, R. L. 1986. *Counseling in Speech and Hearing Practice*. Clinical Series No. 9. Rockville, MD: National Student Speech Language Hearing Association.

Suen, H. K. 1983. Alienation and attrition of Black college students on a predominantly white campus. *Journal of College Student Personnel* 24:117–21.

Summit, R. 1985. Causes, consequences, treatment, and prevention of sexual assault against children. In *Assault Against Children*, ed. J. H. Meier. Austin, TX: Pro-Ed.

Whitaker, L. C. 1989. Suicide and other crises. In *College Psychotherapy*, eds. P. A. Grayson and K. Cauley. New York: Guilford Press.

Winston, R. B., Jr., and Polkosnik, M. C. 1984. Advising graduate and professional school students. In *Developmental Academic Advising*, eds. R. B. Winston, Jr., T. K. Miller, S. C. Ender, T. J. Grites, and Assoc. San Francisco: Jossey-Bass.

Winston, R. B., Jr., and Sandor, J. A. 1984. Developmental academic advising: What do students want? *National Academic Advising Journal* 4:5–13.

Winston, R. B., Jr., Miller, T. K., Ender, S. C., Grites, T. J., and Assoc. (eds.) 1984. *Developmental Academic Advising*. San Francisco: Jossey Bass.

Chapter 15

Continuing Education

Gloria D. Kellum and Ellen C. Fagan

RATIONALE FOR CONTINUING EDUCATION

"Degree obsolescence is today's way of life. The half-life of knowledge in any given profession may now be as little as two to three years"

(Frandson 1980, p. 61). Twenty years ago, it was estimated that within 10 to 12 years of receiving their professional education, human services professionals became approximately half as competent to meet the demands of their profession as they were upon graduation (Dubin 1972). With the explosion of new knowledge and technological advances occurring in the fields of speech-language pathology and audiology, degree half-life of two to three years may well be a reality. With the rapid changes taking place in our professions today, our degrees will not "keep us in the same place" very long. It is imperative to recognize that today's degree merely marks the beginning of the education continuum.

Graduate education alone cannot be expected to produce, immediately upon graduation, practitioners ready to function independently as professionals. This has been recognized by the American Speech-Language-Hearing Association (ASHA) Clinical Certification Board's requirement of the Clinical Fellowship Year prior to certification. It was also emphasized in ASHA's role delineation study in which practicing professionals identified at least six major skill areas that were acquired on the job (Wilcoxen 1989). In this age of rapid growth in new knowledge and technology, it is unrealistic to think that completion of graduate education equips professionals with skills, knowledge, and experience to function competently throughout the course of their careers (Moll 1983). ASHA's Certificate of Clinical Competence (CCC) represents attainment of entry-level requirements for professionals coming into the fields of speech-language pathology and audiology. Once professionals obtain the CCC, continuing education and professional development are expected, and the ASHA Code of Ethics requires that "individuals shall continue their professional development throughout their careers" (ASHA 1990, p. 91).

Continuing one's professional education beyond the graduate training level is no longer a luxury but a necessity. The public's call for competent professionals demands it; our professional association's standards and ethical codes require it; and the individual professional's pride in his or her work should dictate it (Queeney 1984).

HISTORY OF CONTINUING EDUCATION

Continuing education had its roots in Greek society (Gratten 1955). Much of what would come to America as adult education began in the 1700s in Great Britain. After the American Revolution, the religious aims of education gave way to citizenship training, trade skill development, and information about science (Stubblefield and Keane 1989). Following the Civil War, universities, social-political organizations, and public libraries became the major avenues for continuing education for adults. The primary aim of adult education in the early 1900s changed from making up educational deficits prior to World War I to social reform in the 1930s to economic reconstruction and basic literacy in the 1940s and 1950s (Apps 1985). By the 1960s, predominant continuing education activities centered on continued professional education with the primary focus on the improvement of competence and performance of health care professionals (Apps 1985).

Although ASHA does not currently require continuing education to maintain certification, there is a long history of voluntary participation by the members in continuing educational activities. Organized educational activities in the form of short courses for an ASHA meeting were first suggested in 1929 (Paden 1975), but did not become a reality until the 1939 annual convention.

The need for an organized effort by the association to meet the continued educational needs of members was recognized in 1966 when the ASHA Executive Board created the Continuing Education Committee. In 1974, that committee's proposed plan for mandatory continuing education was rejected by the Legislative Council in favor of a plan for voluntary continuing education that was finally approved in 1979. The two-phase plan established the Continuing Education Board, the implementation of a Sponsor (provider) review and approval system, a national Continuing Education Registry, a Continuing Education Information Clearinghouse, ASHA-Sponsored Continuing Education activities, the Award for Continuing Education, and the independent study and distant learning components of the program.

The number of participants in ASHA-Approved Continuing Education (CE) activities has steadily increased. In 1986, the CE Registry held records on 28,568 participants in CE events, while in 1990 the number of registered participants increased to 44,919 (Shewan and Fagan 1990, p. 83). Shewan and Fagan (1990) also reported an increase in the number of ASHA-Approved Sponsors, up from 276 in 1986 to 340 in 1990. The number of events offered by these Sponsors has gone from 915 activities in 1986 to 1,452 offerings in 1989.

THE ROLE OF CONTINUING PROFESSIONAL EDUCATION

What is continuing professional education and how does it differ from graduate education? Continuing professional education is an extension of higher education that meets the needs of a changing profession. Its intent is to remediate deficiencies, foster growth, and facilitate change for professional practitioners (Scanlon 1985). To be effective, continuing professional education should relate directly to professional competence by improving skills through knowledge reinforcement, mastery of recent developments, and the review of new trends in order to provide high quality service to clients (Bess 1983). Continuing professional education should be practice oriented, and provide professionals with knowledge and skills that they can immediately integrate into established service delivery models.

Bridging the Education Continuum

Although continuing professional education differs from graduate education, a bridge between the two is critical if the continuum is to be maintained. It is the responsibility of universities to prepare students with the understanding that entry-level education is only the first step in what will be a lifelong learning process (Smutz and Queeney 1990). Unfortunately, it is unlikely that students making the transition from graduate education to professional practice will immediately transform themselves into independent self-directed learners (Smutz and Queeney 1990). Recent research (Brookfield 1984) indicates that most professionals do not easily identify their learning needs, select educational programs to meet those needs, and chart an integrated educational course for themselves. Professionals require guidance and assistance in structuring their continuing professional education so that it will benefit their practice (Smutz and Queeney 1990). Professional societies should provide leadership and develop mechanisms for assisting professionals in continuing education.

Education: A Lifelong Endeavor

In order for a profession to grow and survive, its members must maintain their state-of-the-art skills and competencies. Continuing professional education is the vehicle that facilitates maintenance of those skills. *Lifelong learning* refers to the purposeful activities professionals undertake to increase their knowledge, develop and update their skills, and modify their attitudes throughout their lifetimes (Advisory Panel on Research Needs in Lifelong Learning During Adulthood 1978, p. 7). Learning may occur in formal settings, such as college and university campuses, or in less formal settings, such as home or work. The instructor may be a professional educator or some other knowledgeable person—a master clinician, a supervisor, a mentor, or a colleague. The instructional materials may be traditional textbooks or may include the newer technologies, such as videoconferencing and computers, or a combination of all of these. Learning experiences may occur in a classroom or in the field, as internships or as site visits.

As professionals expand their knowledge through continued

education, a resulting expansion in the profession's scope of practice occurs. Typically "emerging practices" are first introduced and addressed through continuing education and incorporated into practice long before they are added to the preprofessional educational curricula. An example of this phenomenon in speech-language pathology is seen in diagnosis and treatment of dysphagia. Continuing education providers have offered workshops and seminars on dysphagia since 1982; however, university educational programs have only recently begun to add courses to their curricula to specifically address the diagnosis and treatment of dysphagia (Fagan 1990a).

Motivation for Continuing Education

Professionals in the field of communication sciences and disorders (CSD) have ethical and legal reasons to pursue continuing education. ASHA members are ethically bound to participate in continuing education activities on an ongoing basis. In 20 states, speech-language pathologists and audiologists are required by law to document their continuing education for annual renewal of licensure (Lynch 1990).

TYPES OF CONTINUING EDUCATION ACTIVITIES IN THE PROFESSIONS

Historically, speech-language pathologists and audiologists have been offered an array of continuing education opportunities and formats. Continuing education activities offered by ASHA-Approved Sponsors have traditionally fallen into two distinct categories: sponsor-initiated activities and participant-initiated activities. Sponsor-initiated activities are developed by an Approved Sponsor and presented for group instruction or for individual study. The most frequent activities offered by Approved Sponsors include:

Conventions
Short Courses
Miniseminars
Technical sessions
Poster sessions
Round table discussions
Journal groups
Study groups
Videoconferences and
   satellite television
Correspondence courses
   and programmed study

Traditional
   academic courses
Journal/newsletter study
Conferences
Forums
Symposiums
Workshops
Seminars
Teleconferences
Inservice courses
Grand rounds

Participant-initiated activities (independent studies) are designed to meet the needs of practicing professionals who choose alternatives to group instructional activities. An independent study is planned by the learner and approved and monitored by an Independent Study Sponsor. In 1990, such sponsors numbered 167 (Fagan 1990a). Examples of activities for independent study (participant-initiated) are:

Home study through journals and newsletters	Professional visitations
	Computer assisted instruction
Literature reviews	Texts and workbooks
Course design and instruction	Audio- and/or videotape instruction
Research and publication	
Clinical case study/record review	

In a recent survey, when speech-language pathologists and audiologists were given a wide array of continuing education options from which to choose, professionals overwhelmingly chose workshops and conferences as the preferred form (66.5%). Videotaped presentations (8.7%) ranked second in popularity. Home study (6%) and site visits (5.7%) ranked third and fourth (Fagan 1989b).

PROVIDERS OF CONTINUING EDUCATION IN THE PROFESSIONS

The major providers of continuing professional education in speech-language pathology and audiology are: (a) colleges and universities; (b) state and national professional associations and public agencies; (c) hospitals and clinics; and (d) independent providers such as publishers and equipment manufacturers. Of 340 ASHA-Approved Sponsors of continuing education in 1990, 95 were colleges and universities, 73 were state and national professional associations or public agencies, 120 were hospitals or clinics, and 42 were independent providers (Fagan 1990b). Shelton and Craig (1983) found that half of the continuing education in health care is provided by employers. Speech-language pathology and audiology follow similar trends. Fifty-one percent (51%) of the CE activities offered in 1989 by ASHA Continuing Education Sponsors were provided by hospitals and clinics. Professional associations and public agencies sponsored 21% of the offerings; universities, 19%; and independent providers, 8% (Fagan 1989a).

Independent providers represent a wide range of institutions and constitute the most rapidly growing category for continuing professional education. Manufacturers and suppliers offer conferences to increase consumer interest and understanding of their products and clinical procedures. Publishers are also moving into continuing education as another way to serve well-defined audiences to whom they currently furnish printed materials. Other independent providers include the so-called "privates," institutions organized on a free-standing basis that treat continuing professional education as a business (Suleiman 1983), and publishers of journals and newsletters. Three Approved Sponsors, often referred to as providers of distance learning materials or journal study materials, are: Sarah Blackstone (1990), editor of *Augmentative Communication News;* Katherine Butler (1990), *Topics in Language Disorders;* and Jerry L. Northern (1990), editor-in-chief of *Seminars in Hearing.* Northern is also Approved Sponsor for *Seminars in Speech and Language,* of which Richard F. Curlee (1990) is editor-in-chief (Fagan 1990a).

ASHA-Approved Sponsors of Continuing Education offer a wide variety of continuing education. Several sponsors have ventured into audioteleconferencing and have reported this format to be an effective method of reaching a national audience in a cost-effective manner. Independent study has also increased in popularity among providers and consumers of CE.

THE CONTINUING EDUCATION UNIT (CEU)

Definition

The Continuing Education Unit (CEU) is the internationally recognized standard unit of measure for a continuing education activity. The CEU is defined as ten contact hours under responsible leadership, capable direction, and qualified instruction, excluding meals and breaks. The contact hour is defined as a clock hour, or a typical 50-minute classroom instructional session. A CEU is recorded to one decimal point. For example, a program meeting for 14½ hours would be recorded as 1.4 CEUs. Half-hour increments are dropped when computing the total number of CEUs for an activity (Award for Continuing Education 1990).

Educational activities that are offered for non-degree credit are often designated as CEU activities. For several decades, colleges, universities, businesses, and providers of continuing education have used CEUs to designate a learner's participation in a course for which university academic credit hours were not granted (The Continuing Education Unit 1970). Only those organizations or individuals designated as ASHA-Approved Sponsors of Continuing Education are granted authority to award ASHA CEUs to participants and approval is contingent upon many factors (Continuing Education Board 1988), some of which follow:

applicant's experience and expertise in the area of adult continuing
    education

applicant's administrative abilities and experience

budgetary resources available to the potential sponsor to plan and implement quality continuing education activities

continuing education goals and objectives of the organization

criteria or process by which the applicant will assess learner needs, qualifications of the instructional staff, and instructional outcomes

applicant's commitment to providing quality continuing education to speech-language pathologists and audiologists.

Once the Continuing Education Board grants Sponsor approval to an applicant, the Sponsor must adhere to stringent guidelines and requirements. Every three years, Sponsors undergo a formal review by the Board to determine the continuation of Sponsor approval (Continuing Education Board 1988).

The benefits of being an ASHA-Approved Sponsor of CE are the national recognition and credibility extended to the provider, access to a market of more than 62,000 speech-language pathologists and audiologists, marketing through ASHA's nationally accessible CE Activity Database Search (ADS), free publicity in the *Asha* journal with a circulation exceeding 75,000, networking opportunities with other ASHA-Approved Sponsors, a Sponsor newsletter that is published six times yearly, access to technical assistance for program planning, marketing, implementation, and evaluation, and ASHA's computerized record keeping system (Fagan 1990c).

ISSUES AND CHALLENGES IN CONTINUING EDUCATION

A number of issues and challenges must be addressed in continuing education in the field of communication sciences and disorders.

How do we determine the needed content of preprofessional curricula versus lifelong professional educational plans?

How do we help professionals stay up to date in the ever-expanding fund of knowledge in audiology and speech-language pathology?

Is there a need to focus CE in specialty areas of training?

Where should the profession head regarding mandatory versus voluntary continuing education?

Are there special populations on which the CE provider should focus?

Role Delineation Study

In 1984, ASHA conducted a role delineation study of the professions of speech-language pathology and audiology (Lingwall 1988). The pur-

pose of the study was to identify skills, tasks, and knowledge necessary to practice, and to determine when, in the educational sequence,
those skills and knowledge were acquired. Of the 412 knowledge and
skill statements identified and subsequently rated according to point of
acquisition, 28% were acquired by professionals *after* attaining the Certificate of Clinical Competence (CCC) (Wilcoxen 1989). Clearly, those
professionals participating in the role delineation study felt that many
skills and knowledge could be and were acquired through continuing
education. These findings have significant implications for planners of
continuing education and serve as a valid needs assessment source.

The skills and knowledge identified as being acquired after attaining the CCC (post-CCC) were grouped into six clusters by Wilcoxen
(1989): administration, low incidence, specific resources, emerging
technologies, intervention milieu, and research.

Expanding Knowledge Base

Knowledge in the field of CSD is evergrowing (Nation and Aram 1984).
The explosion of new information has occurred because of the information age, the increased interest in scientific and clinical research, and
the many new journals that provide more avenues for publication.

Scope of Practice

As the scope of practice for audiologists and speech-language pathologists broadens, additional education for specialty training will be
needed. Whether practitioners specialize in one area or are eclectic in
their practice, they need continuing education to provide optimal patient services.

Mandatory Continuing Education

Another issue that continues to be discussed is mandatory versus voluntary continuing education. Bess (1983) offered the opinion that CE
should be required for ASHA certification. This is an issue that should
become more important.

Re-Entry Professionals

A system is needed to accommodate persons re-entering the professions—those wishing to re-enroll in graduate education programs and
those wishing to re-enter professional practice. Individuals seeking re-
enrollment in graduate programs find very few programs that accept
students on a part-time basis. Location of programs and inconvenient

class scheduling are also obstacles. Individuals attempting to re-enter professional practice following a period of absence may find knowledge and technological advances have left their degrees and past experience outdated and inadequate for today's workplace. They are also faced with the lack of a support system to structure their re-learning efforts.

Colleges and universities that re-evaluate their programs to focus not only on the needs of traditional students but also on the needs of re-entry students can help solve this problem. Flexible class scheduling, evening and weekend courses, accelerated summer and intersession courses, off-site practicum experiences, child care facilities, courses offered at satellite campuses, instructional television courses, closed circuit television instruction, and video- and audioteleconferencing have been used successfully, but adoption of such nontraditional delivery systems has not been widespread. Professional associations, licensing bodies, employers, and universities must work cooperatively to assess the needs of and implement programs for professionals returning to the work force (Lingwall 1988).

With shortages of practitioners in various regions of the country (Shewan 1989), our professions can ill afford to ignore individuals seeking re-entry into educational programs and professional practice.

THE FUTURE IN CONTINUING EDUCATION

Professional associations should provide leadership in continuing education. ASHA, through the activities of the Continuing Education Board, the Scientific and Professional Programs Board, the Publications Board, the Convention Program Committee, the Executive Board, and the National Office staff working with related professional associations and state associations, should develop a long-range plan for lifelong learning in CSD. The recent concepts in self-managed professional development must be explored, and we must teach ourselves how to plan for lifelong learning. As mentioned previously, a current trend in CE choices by ASHA members is a preference for independent study and self-study activities, and continued support for these CE approaches is warranted.

The need for a central database of information on CE activities has become increasingly apparent as more and more CE events are offered. By revising and expanding the ASHA Clearinghouse, ASHA could provide access to information, and could connect Sponsors to participants and vice versa. To facilitate the establishment of informal study groups, such as journal or video study groups, ASHA should develop guidelines for its members to promote and document participation in these events for the granting of CEUs. As our professions become more specialized in practice, CEUs could be the method for determining acquisition of skills and knowledge in specialty areas. ASHA is in a unique position to implement required CEUs for specialty recognition.

Earning CE units and advocating for CE are outward signs that our profession is dynamic. Continuing education strengthens the profession and its members and, in turn, benefits the clients we serve. The future of continuing education is bright. The partnerships formed among providers, consumers (learners) and professional organizations will become stronger as the public increasingly demands competent professionals; as professional ethics require providers to strive for more than minimal competencies; and as individuals take pride in providing optimal levels of professional services.

REFERENCES

Advisory Panel on Research Needs in Lifelong Learning During Adulthood. 1978. In *Lifelong Learning during Adulthood*. New York: Future Directions for Learning Society, College Board.

American Speech-Language-Hearing Association. 1990. Code of ethics. *Asha* 32(3):91–92.

Apps, J. 1985. *Improving Practice in Continuing Education*. San Francisco: Jossey-Bass.

Award for Continuing Education: Information Booklet. 1990. Rockville, MD: American Speech-Language-Hearing Association.

Bess, J. 1983. Issue VIII: What should be the role of CPE in meeting the full range of needs of faculty, clinical service providers, administrators and scientists in human communication and its disorders? In *Proceedings of the 1983 National Conference on Undergraduate, Graduate, and Continuing Education* (Report No. 13), eds. N. Rees and T. Snope. Rockville, MD: American Speech-Language-Hearing Association.

Blackstone, S. W. (ed.). 1990. *Augmentative Communication News*. Monterey, CA: Sunset Enterprises.

Brookfield, S. 1984. *Adult Learners, Adult Education, and the Community*. New York: Teachers' College Press, Columbia University.

Butler, K. G. (ed.). 1990. *Topics in Language Disorders*. Frederick, MD: Aspen Publishers, Inc.

Continuing Education Board, American Speech-Language-Hearing Association. 1988. *Continuing Education Board (CEB) Manual for Continuing Education Programs in Speech-Language Pathology and Audiology*. Rockville, MD: Author.

The Continuing Education Unit. 1970. Washington, D.C.: National Task Force on the Continuing Education Unit.

Curlee, R. F. (ed.). 1990. *Seminars in Speech and Hearing*. New York: Theime Medical Publishers.

Dubin, S. S. 1972. Obsolescence or life-long education: A choice for the professional. *American Psychology* 27:486–98.

Fagan, E. C. 1989a. [Annual counts from the ASHA CE registry]. Unpublished raw data.

Fagan, E. C. 1989b. Conferences and workshops are "voter's choice." *Continuing Education Board News Notes* September: 2–6.

Fagan, E. C. 1990a. [Annual counts from the ASHA CE registry]. Unpublished raw data.

Fagan, E. C. 1990b. [Continuing education registry data]. Unpublished raw data.

Fagan, E. C. 1990c. What are the benefits of becoming an ASHA approved CE sponsor? *Continuing Education Board News Notes* May: 1.

Frandson, P. E. 1980. Continuing education for the professions. In *Serving Personal and Community Needs through Adult Education,* eds. E. J. Boone, R. W. Shearon, and E. E. White. San Francisco: Jossey-Bass.

Gratten, C. H. 1955. *In Quest of Knowledge: A Historical Perspective in Adult Education.* New York: Association Press.

Lingwall, J. 1988. Evaluation of requirements for the certificates of clinical competence in speech-language pathology and audiology. *Asha* 30(9):75–78.

Lynch, C. E. 1990. *Continuing Education: Issues and Status* (Report 5-90). Rockville, MD: American Speech-Language-Hearing Association.

Moll, K. L. 1983. Issue II: What should be the content and objective of graduate education in communication disorders? In *Proceedings of the 1983 National Conference on Undergraduate, Graduate, and Continuing Education* (Report No. 13), eds. N. Rees and T. Snope. Rockville, MD: American Speech-Language-Hearing Association.

Nation, J. E., and Aram, D. M. 1984. *Diagnosis of Speech and Language Disorders* (2nd ed). San Diego, CA: Singular Publishing Group.

Northern, J. L. (ed.). 1990. *Seminars in Hearing.* New York: Thieme Medical Publishers.

Paden, E. P. 1975. ASHA in retrospect—fiftieth anniversary reflections. *Asha* 17:151, 831.

Queeney, D. S. 1984. The role of the university in continuing professional education. *Education Record* 65(3):13–17.

Scanlon, C. L. 1985. Practicing with purpose: Goals of continuing professional education. In *New Directions for Continuing Education: Problems and Prospects in Continuing Professional Education* (no. 27), eds. R. M. Cervero and C. L. Scanlon. San Francisco: Jossey-Bass.

Shelton, H., and Craig, R. 1983. Continuing professional development: The employer perspective. In *Power and Conflict in Continuing Professional Education,* ed. M. Stern. Belmont, CA: Wadsworth.

Shewan, C. M. 1989. ASHA work force study. *Asha* 31(3):63–67.

Shewan, C., and Fagan, E. 1990. Be prepared: Continuing education. *Asha* 32(6/7):83.

Smutz, W., and Queeney, D. S. 1990. Professionals as learners: A strategy for maximizing professional growth. In *Visions for the Future of Continuing Professional Education,* eds. R. Cerzero, J. Azzaretto, and Associates. Athens, GA: University of Georgia.

Stubblefield, H. W., and Keane, P. 1989. The history of the adult and continuing education. In *Handbook of Adult and Continuing Education,* eds. S. B. Merrian and P. M. Cunningham. San Francisco: Jossey-Bass.

Suleiman, A. 1983. Private enterprise: The independent provider. In *Power and Conflict in Continuing Professional Education,* ed. M. R. Stern. Belmont, CA: Wadsworth.

Wilcoxen, A. G. 1989. ASHA role delineation study: Implications for continuing education. *Continuing Education Board News Notes* September: 2–4.

Chapter 16

CONTINUING EDUCATION: PROGRAM PLANNING AND MANAGEMENT

Ellen C. Fagan, Jo Williams, and Gloria D. Kellum

This chapter, devoted solely to discussion of program planning and management, does not address the many teaching methods and presentation formats that are applicable in continuing education. Rather, the reader is referred to other chapters where many of the classroom, laboratory, and clinical approaches described can be adapted for use in continuing education offerings, depending on such factors as group size, equipment availability, and instructional setting.

OVERVIEW

Continuing education (CE) is often viewed as professionals' participation in specific, formal educational activities. It is the ongoing, lifelong process of acquiring and updating knowledge to meet professional responsibilities. Professional growth results from formal and informal individual efforts as well as from continuing education activities.

CE quality is measured by its effectiveness, relevancy, accessibility, and efficiency (Suter et al. 1984). Quality CE requires: organizational support, resources, and direction; a mechanism to identify learners' needs; the development of educational objectives and events to address learners' needs; and ongoing program evaluation. CE program planning and management is a configuration of interacting elements, not a series of linear progressions. Planners sometimes temporarily skip steps, work on several tasks simultaneously, and make decisions that defy planning sequence logic (Sork and Caffarella 1989). Planning models can help CE planners understand the complex decision-making process. In this chapter, we use a four-step model for program planning and management. This model is applicable to planning individual activities as well as the overall CE program.

The model's four steps suggest that planners:

1. determine internal and external organizational influences;
2. identify learner needs and program goals and objectives;
3. develop plans to address goals and objectives, marketing, and program delivery; and
4. evaluate all components of the program.

DETERMINING INTERNAL AND EXTERNAL ORGANIZATIONAL INFLUENCES

CE planners work within the constraints of organizations and are influenced by each organization's history, philosophical framework, and operating procedures. Identifying these and related influences helps planners make decisions consistent with organizational constraints (Sork and Caffarella 1989).

Internal factors influencing provision of CE include the organization's (1) mission, charge, and purpose; (2) history and traditions; (3) financial and personnel resources; (4) current governing structure; (5) operating procedures; and (6) philosophies that affect the types of programs sponsored or the audience served. Additional influences include the organization's long range goals; perceived and assessed needs of its members; need to supplement income via CE activities; promotion of the organization, its image, and its products; changes in professional education requirements; need for established forums to exchange new knowledge and information; need for networking opportunities between professionals and between organizations; and obligation to share information about new knowledge, products, and services with the public and practitioners.

External societal and consumer factors influencing an organization's provision of CE include changes in regulatory, credentialing, and licensing requirements; learners' demands for educational opportunities that address their practice needs; public demand for accountability of service providers; needs assessments conducted by outside sources; and changes in the scope of professional practice. External influences also include relationships with other organizations serving the same consumers; appropriateness of the organization to provide CE; market advantage in responding to needs of the members and consumers it serves; and the target audience.

Program planners must consider factors that influence individuals to participate in CE. The tremendous growth and interest in lifelong learning and CE in the United States can be attributed in part to three factors (Cross 1981): demographic changes, social changes, and advances in technology and knowledge.

Demographic Changes

The demographic make-up of the United States is shifting toward an increasing number of adults. One-third of the United States population is now between 30 and 45 years of age (Beck 1990). By the year 2000, more than half of the country's population will be between 25 and 55 years of age. The demographic trends in speech-language pathology and audiology parallel the general population trends. The majority of ASHA members are between 34 and 45 years of age, the median being 37 years (Keough 1990).

Social Changes

Rising educational levels contribute to the growing interest in CE, and educational level is the best predictor of participation in CE (Cross 1981). The largest number of consumers of adult education are between 25 and 34 years of age, and the second largest consumer group is between 34 and 44 years of age (Rachal 1989). A population bulging with competitive, career-minded adults who are highly educated and highly paid is creating a demand for CE. The majority (73%) of American Speech-Language-Hearing Association (ASHA) CE participants are baby boomers between 30 to 49 years old (Fagan 1991). Over the past ten years, the number of individuals participating in CE has increased (Fagan 1990).

The changing roles of women in our society also continue to have a profound effect on the CE system (Rachal 1989). By 1995, more than 59% of the work force will be women (U.S. Bureau of the Census 1987). Women traditionally are more active CE participants than men, and in 1981, surpassed men in the number of job-related courses taken (Rachal 1989). Ten years of CE data on ASHA members indicate that men and women have participated in formal CE activities at a percentage rate equivalent to the ratio of female/male ASHA members. In 1990, the ASHA membership was 89.4% female to 10.6% male (Keough 1990); 91% of the participants in ASHA-Sponsored CE programs were women compared to 9% men (Fagan 1991). Because women make up a large percentage of the professions, active member participation in CE is expected and evident.

Advances in Technology and Knowledge

The information explosion coupled with new technology is changing the way we learn and exchange information (Dubin 1990). Satellite discs and audioteleconferencing provide new options for distance education. Videotape, audiotape, and computer instructional programs promote individual and self-paced CE. Interactive videodisc technology holds great promise as an educational tool, especially for health care professionals. Learners are presented with simulated clinical experiences and real-life situations so that they can practice making decisions without the pressures of working with actual clients.

Today's technology is affecting the learning preferences of speech-language pathologists and audiologists. In 1980, 92% of ASHA CE participants preferred workshops and seminars. By 1989, although workshops and seminars remained the most popular choices, learners showed increased interest in videotapes, videoconferences, and self-study materials (Fagan 1989).

Additional Factors Influencing Continuing Education Participation

Adults participate in CE activities (Cross 1981) to: (1) network and meet new colleagues; (2) meet external expectations (e.g., supervisors' directives); (3) advance professionally; (4) effect change in their routines; (5) improve the welfare of society (e.g., provide better client service); (6) learn for learning's sake; and (7) use information immediately.

Audiologists and speech-language pathologists are motivated by additional factors including the explosion in knowledge and technology; expanding professional practice; change in concept of accepted practice; altered societal expectations; different requirements as mandated by new laws; requirements and expectations of services; accountability demands; new professions; certification and licensing needs; review of knowledge previously acquired; trends in private practice and the need for additional expertise; and need for multiple skills.

IDENTIFYING LEARNERS' NEEDS AND PROGRAM GOALS AND OBJECTIVES

Needs assessment is the process of identifying existing skills, competencies, and knowledge, and determining whether a gap exists between what is known and what needs to be known. Needs assessments also identify areas in which the learner is meeting standards but desires expanded knowledge (McKinley 1973). The development and use of carefully planned needs assessments have an impact on all phases of program planning, participant support and evaluation. Through informed decision-making, planners can select the kinds and amount of educational intervention likely to bring about changes in learners.

Types of Needs Assessments

Successful CE providers conduct needs assessments at several levels: the strategic level, the program level, and the project level (Levine et al. 1984). Strategic level assessments gather data on (1) current issues in the professions; (2) new knowledge and technology affecting clinical practice; (3) social, cultural, and environmental issues; and (4) national, community, and organizational issues. Results are used for long-term planning, decisions about general topics to cover, audiences to target, and CE resources. Program level assessments focus on specific concerns within general topic areas. This level assists the planner in narrowing the topic areas' focus. Project level assessments identify learners' knowledge, skills, and competencies, and develop the instructional level and content that meet learner's needs.

Conducting Needs Assessments

A needs assessment process is a progression leading to objective measures useful for planning present and future CE activities. This process consists of developing needs assessment procedures, collecting data, analyzing data, and formulating a report for planning recommendations.

Developing a Needs Assessment Procedure. Conducting a needs assessment involves several steps. Planners should address the following questions prior to the assessment:

- What is the purpose of the assessment?
- How will results be used?
- Who is the target audience?
- What areas will be addressed?
- How will the results contribute to program planning?
- Are there adequate resources to conduct the assessment?
- What type of data are needed—individual characteristics, individual performance levels, work setting characteristics and demands?
- What are the data sources—professional standards, participants' perceptions of needs, normative sources (studies indicating practice differences), scientific research, new knowledge, client opinion and attitudes?
- What data gathering techniques will be used?
- How will the data be analyzed? How will the planner determine that needs exist?
- What are the causes of the identified needs? Can the needs be addressed through CE?

- What are the priorities of the identified needs?
- How will the planner report these findings?

Gathering Data. It is rare that a single method of collecting data can answer all the planner's questions about learner needs; therefore, most planners find it preferable to use a combination of methods. Planners must consider the cost and time involved in each method and the usefulness of the data collected.

Observing the performance of professionals in the work setting is one way to gather information about desired proficiencies. To acquire valid data, observers must have standards of performance against which to judge observed performance. The disadvantages of this kind of data gathering are the expense of training and paying observers, observers' personal biases and preconceived standards, and the fact that performance is likely to be different because an observer is present.

Interviews with potential participants encourage free expression of opinions and provide insight into learner attitudes. The interviewer has the opportunity to probe for in-depth information. Questions should be field-tested and validated, and all persons being interviewed should be asked the same group of questions. The drawbacks are that interviewing is time-consuming, usually limited to a small group of people, and is difficult to quantify (Levine et al. 1984).

Surveys and questionnaires are used widely to gather information about learners' interests, needs, preferences, and learning styles. This form of data collection is cost effective, easily standardized and analyzed, and allows the learner time to think and reflect on answers. The disadvantages are that low response rates influence data analysis, respondents may not understand the questions, and follow-up is difficult because responses may be anonymous.

Conversations with experts are helpful in identifying needs. Information is obtained easily via phone or face-to-face conversation, is inexpensive, and is likely to spark experts' interest in becoming involved in teaching or attending CE activities. Unfortunately, information obtained via this approach does not necessarily represent the views of potential participants and may be misleading.

Searches of documents, recent texts, articles, and state and federal regulatory interpretations can provide information about emerging topics and learner needs as well as insight into existing problems.

Inspection of records and charts can reflect adequacy of practitioner performance and proficiency. CE planners can audit client records to determine level and appropriateness of care, as well as deficiencies to be addressed later through CE for staff and supervisor development. Planners can use national reports (e.g., child-find data, caseload composition reports) to determine underserved populations. Record inspection is difficult in many settings where confidentiality is stringently enforced, however, and descriptions recorded in charts may not accurately reflect provider/client interaction.

Testing current knowledge, skills, and attitudes helps to identify deficiencies. Planners use written or oral examinations, interest checklists, performance checklists, or simulation exercises to judge learner proficiencies. Collecting data in this manner results in standardized responses that are easily analyzed. Instruments can be re-administered following the activity to determine if needs were addressed and learning occurred. Disadvantages include the expense and time involved in administrating, scoring, and reporting information. Also, taking formal tests to demonstrate knowledge may not reflect adults' typical work performance (Levine et al. 1984).

Group problem analysis asks professionals to identify their problems, needs, and educational deficiencies, and to suggest solutions in terms of topics to be addressed, CE activities, and educational intervention approaches. Various formats for group problem analysis are available.

The nominal group process uses silent problem identification by each individual, followed by group activities for round-robin recording and discussion of ideas, determining priority areas, and ordering of identified priorities.

Additional methods of group problem analysis include *brainstorming sessions, speak-up sessions,* appointment of a *task force* or *advisory group,* and *critical incident techniques.* The critical incident technique requires potential learners to write a paragraph on a practice problem. This process allows anonymous sharing of real concerns and feelings, and provides insight into effective and ineffective learner response to those situations. The disadvantages of this technique are that it is time-consuming and costly to administer, and the data are difficult to analyze.

Analyzing Data. Although data from formal assessments may appear sufficient for planning purposes, adult CE needs are never absolute. Needs are influenced by the learner's behavior and the environment and are constantly changing, even during the CE activity. Ongoing needs assessments are imperative.

To conduct data analysis, several steps should occur, including classifying the data into need areas, establishing the nature and extent of needs, and validating needs by considering learner perspectives. Data from interviews, questionnaires, formal assessments, and group problem analysis procedures are summarized in quantitative and narrative forms. Results are compiled into a needs list or problem area inventory, then used to identify priority areas, plan objectives, and suggest CE formats.

Formulating Recommendations. Planners should document data gathering and analysis in a written report that serves several purposes: to justify allocation of CE funds; to advertise validated reasons for CE offerings; and to formulate specific CE objectives and outcomes. The final report should include the purpose and areas of the needs assessment; the population sampled and the sampling and analysis procedures; and a summary of findings and recommendations.

No needs assessment provides all information necessary to make correct CE planning decisions; however, assessing CE activity effectiveness is accomplished only through knowing the needs, wants, and behaviors of the learners. A well planned and executed needs assessment is important for planning, marketing, and delivering CE, and is a powerful tool in building successful CE programs.

DEVELOPING PLANS TO ADDRESS GOALS
AND OBJECTIVES, MARKETING, AND PROGRAM DELIVERY

The concepts in this section are applicable to a variety of CE activity formats; however, emphasis is on group learning because of its dominance in CE.

Activity Planning: Content, Design, Faculty

Content. Content decisions are based on needs assessment analyses and CE program goals. CE planners should identify and rank objectives for desired learner outcomes (Draves 1984). Content decisions are made by a planning committee, the instructors, and/or the CE planner. A committee of target audience members is very effective (Fischer 1989), but time limitations and group dynamics can pose problems. If the course involves only one instructor, objectives are typically developed by the instructor. If the activity involves multiple presenters, the CE planner usually plays a major role in establishing course objectives and agenda.

Design. Designing the CE program involves matching the learners' energy levels, attention span, and interests to program content, faculty, and meeting-site characteristics. Content is organized in a number of ways: introductory to advanced, concrete to abstract, general to specific, and chronological to historical (Draves 1984).

Depending upon the activity's objectives, a variety of learning formats is available: formal instruction, group discussion, demonstration and hands-on laboratory experiences, and participant presentations (e.g., case exchange). Modular programming, multiple simultaneous tracks, and activity menus offer additional variety. Meals, refreshment breaks, exhibit activities, and social functions accommodate learners' bio-rhythms and vary course pace.

Faculty. Faculty selection decisions focus on four areas: (1) credentials, training, and work experience; (2) expertise in the topic area; (3) speaking ability and delivery style; and (4) appropriateness to program tone and audience ("Working with speakers" 1985). Personal observation is the best way to assess a potential speaker's suitability; however, information can also be obtained through word-of-mouth reports, planning committee advice, previous audiences' perceptions and evaluations, and topic publications.

Once a potential speaker is identified, the planner should discuss general information about program goals, possible topic areas to be covered, reimbursement policy, and the individual's interest and availability. During the discussion, the planner learns more about the prospective speaker's background and experience and also has the opportunity to gain an impression about the person's communication ability. Planners should indicate that the discussion is a preliminary step, not a commitment. Final speaker agreements are written as contract letters.

Planners should have realistic expectations about speakers. Not all presenters are "super-speakers." Programs with multiple speakers and topics should position speakers to balance the program. The faculty should understand the program goals and the needs of the audience (Szczypkowski 1980). Conference calls or meetings involving all the faculty provide opportunities to discuss goals, answer questions, coordinate overall objectives and activities, and balance the content across topic areas.

Program Planning Time Lines

A time line identifying the sequence and tasks of program management is provided in the Appendix at the end of this chapter. This time line was developed for large meetings; but, it can be adapted to smaller meetings.

Marketing

A successful CE program is one in which desired services benefit a targeted audience, and organizational objectives are met. Marketing plays a strategic role in achieving this success. Three basic marketing models (Simerly 1989a) applicable to CE activities are: the traditional model, the exchange model, and the adaptive model. CE providers typically use some combination of the three. The traditional model focuses on organizational needs, persuading the consumer to buy the services. The exchange and adaptive models are more consumer-oriented. Both consumer and organization interests are considered in the exchange model with emphasis on the needs assessment. The adaptive model stresses the consumer's wants, excluding the values, norms, or needs of the CE provider.

Guidelines for Effective Marketing. Basic guidelines for developing effective marketing plans (Simerly 1989a) include:

1. differentiating among marketing, publicity, and advertising,
2. linking marketing directly to the CE organization's mission and goals,
3. using environmental scanning (techniques to collect information about environmental factors having an impact on the organization and the consumers it serves),
4. determining the consumer's role and developing a customer service orientation,
5. collecting, analyzing, and using consumer demographic and psychographic data,
6. segmenting the market into different consumer populations,
7. tracking marketing activity results to determine effectiveness,
8. developing an ongoing marketing plan.

Identifying a Continuing Education Market. There is no single central CE market. The marketing-plan goal is to create a niche in the CE market by providing activities professionals want and need. Data from the needs assessment analysis offer valuable information about the market and about reaching the CE audience. Planners should focus on differentiating their activity from other activities and on creating a unique product, making use of timing, activity format, site and geographic location, faculty, and promotion of the program. Creating a unique program is important in establishing a market niche.

Determining the Marketing Mix. The success of a CE program depends upon the marketing mix (the combination of program planning, promotion, and pricing) and external market forces affecting the marketing mix (consumer purchasing behavior and competition). There are four components of the marketing mix: product, pricing, location, and promotion/advertising (Riggs 1989).

Product is the key element; it is the total package of benefits that consumers obtain when they make a purchase (Riggs 1989). Planners should ask, "What is the consumer buying?" A key decision made by CE providers is that of determining the program's style, features, quality, "packaging," and "branding." The style should reflect organizational image. Features are program components that are added or deleted without affecting quality or style. Quality is the perceived level of effectiveness; "packaging" is the "wrapping" (e.g., the physical appearance of a course manual); and "branding" is a symbol, name, or design distinguishing one organization's CE programs from other offerings (Riggs 1989).

It is also important to consider the program's life-cycle. Products in any marketplace go through a natural cycle from introductory stage to maturity and then decline. CE providers should decide when to introduce and when to remove programs from the CE market.

Pricing strategies fall into three categories. Cost-oriented pricing is based on estimating the total costs associated with the activity plus the profit desired. Demand pricing is used for high demand activities where cost is not an important consideration. Competition-oriented pricing, the most common strategy, bases fees on average market levels. CE planners select pricing strategies based on the organization's marketing objectives, the consumer's market options, and whether the purchaser can pass on costs (Riggs 1989).

Selecting a CE *location* involves choosing a city and a facility site. Selection decisions are based on program goals, course design, programming needs, target audience, and resources (Carson 1989). CE locations can increase the participants' impressions of the activity's overall benefits. Participants perceive CE quality to be higher when activities are held on or near university campuses, in expensive hotels, and in locations that relate to program content (Riggs 1989).

Activity timing is as important as location. The majority of CE activities for speech-language pathologists and audiologists are held in fall (October and November) and spring (March, April, and May). Planners must decide whether to market CE events during these high competition months or during alternate months. Employment settings and funding sources are also important factors in CE timing and scheduling. Private practitioners favor weekend events and are more likely to want meeting/vacation options at resorts. State and federal employees typically do not earn compensatory time for weekend meetings, are on per diem expense allowances, and are expected to use hotel accommodations that offer government discounts. Often, school personnel do not participate in CE offerings during the summer due to lack of employer funding.

Non-paid *promotion* of CE activities includes calendar items, announcements, and articles in professional publications, national and state association newsletters, and journals. CE press releases should be one-page, double-spaced statements of fewer than 300 words, issued on official stationery and stating who, what, where, when, and how, including the name, telephone number, and address of a contact person. The first paragraph should cover essential elements followed by paragraphs that expand on details and generate reader interest (Patterson 1989). Most professional publications also accept paid announcements of upcoming activities.

The most effective direct-mail approaches use (1) selective mailing lists of professionals most likely to need the program and respond, (2) past users of the CE organization's programs, and (3) multiple mailings to target audiences (Elliott 1989). Mailing lists and labels are available from most professional associations and special interest groups.

CE organizations should develop in-house mailing lists that remove non-users from the list and update mailing addresses. In-house lists can be updated using the United States Postal Service's National Change of Address System (NCOA) that tracks address changes within an 18 month period. The NCOA lists are updated biweekly and are available on disk or magnetic tape (Kershner Report 1990).

Planners using direct-mail marketing should also consider lead time on brochure mailings, options and incentives to register. Brochures should be received 12 to 14 weeks prior to the activity; for larger meetings a longer lead time is recommended. Bulk mailings can take from 2 to 6 weeks to reach their destinations after delivery to the post office. Fifty percent of total responses to a brochure mailing generally occur within 3 to 4 weeks following the initial response (Elliott 1989).

Incentives in direct-mail promotion include offering multiple sites and dates; options to attend portions of the program; a variety of payment arrangements; registration options; discounts to organizations with more than one registrant; a free promotional item; and announcement of specifically-desired content areas in advance. Other considerations might include penalties for cancellations, registration by mail only, early registration fees, and acknowledging by mail receipt of registration material (Elliott 1989).

Brochure

Because a brochure is the primary marketing vehicle for most CE activities, content should be planned carefully. Brochure copy should enhance the CE organization's overall image and program, convey comprehensive and accurate program information, and enroll the number of participants needed to meet financial obligations (Simerly 1989b). Brochure copy should also:

- attract the readers' attention within 4–5 seconds;
- use action words and powerful messages;
- display program titles in large print;
- display the CE organization's name prominently;
- use header and headings to re-emphasize program title and dates;

- be written from a participant's point of view;
- emphasize benefits; and
- make sure that information accurately depicts the program.

Brochure Elements. Brochure elements must include the title of the activity, the activity sponsor, program description, intended audience, special features, faculty, general information, and a registration form. The *program title* should emphasize action, excellence, importance, and results (Simerly 1989b), using a catchy or simple title that is not too lengthy or complex (Draves 1984).

The overview and *program description* focuses on content and learner benefits, starting with one or two sentences to attract the interest of a reader. The activity's scope and content should be written in a clear and readable manner. *Course objectives* should be specific and written using action words, describing the specific benefits participants will derive from the CE activity. Testimonials by previous participants can add credibility to the program's "claims" (Markoe 1989).

ASHA uses three general categories to designate *activity content:* basic communication areas, related areas, and professional areas. Using content classifications assists participants in meeting and monitoring CE requirements for licensure renewal, re-certification, and earning the ASHA Award for Continuing Education (ACE). Highlighting the *instructional level* (e.g., Introductory, Intermediate, Advanced, Unspecified) assists learners in determining whether the activity is appropriate for their skill levels. Courses with a variety of instructional levels are designated as "unspecified." Brochure recipients also want to know if the program is suited to their needs and levels of expertise; therefore, the *target audience* should be as specific as possible. *Faculty information* should include each individual's title, degrees, position, and affiliations. A brief description of his/her experience and background as it relates to the topic area may be included. All activities have *special features* to highlight and use as marketing strategies (e.g., a well-known guest speaker, resort atmosphere, unusual program format, and take-home materials). Planners also include background information about and credentials of the *sponsoring organization.* Logos and identifiers of CE accrediting bodies should be displayed as well as ASHA CEUs or certificates of completion to be awarded.

The *agenda* is the time order for activity events. It is not the same as the description of activity or course objectives. For long programs, a detailed agenda with specific days, activities, times, locations, and speakers should be included on the brochure (Markoe 1989).

General information items include the fees (meals, CEUs, social functions), policies and procedures, a contact person, and phone number. If the activity location is a marketing tool, display it prominently. If not, place site and hotel information in the brochure's general information section (Markoe 1989).

Hotel/facility information should include address, telephone number, room rates and tax, accommodation information, special needs, and parking information. A map and directions to the facility from major highways and airports, as well as information on transportation, are helpful.

The *registration form* should include: registrant information (name, day-time telephone number, address, affiliation); special dietary needs or accommodations for persons with disabilities; fee information (what the registration fee includes); how to register (e.g., telephone, address, FAX); and payment options.

Brochure Layout and Design. Effective brochure layout and design can be critical to attracting and securing registrants (Markoe 1989). An effective brochure is one that catches and maintains the reader's attention, most likely accomplished through graphics, color, type, and space. The front cover should attract the reader's attention and generate interest in reading the program information. Information on the front should include program title (prominently displayed in bold print), name of the CE organization, co-sponsors, and dates (Simerly 1989b). An 8½" × 11" format is generally advisable. People are likely to think the activity is unimportant if smaller sizes are used (Simerly 1989b). A frequently overlooked layout consideration is the importance of the back panel. People see the back panel first since that is the location of the mailing label. The back panel can strengthen a brochure's marketing impact if it is visually appealing, includes the program logo, and is used to advertise the activity (Simerly 1989b).

Tracking Effectiveness. The promotion's effectiveness is tracked by looking at the response. Asking participants how they heard about the activity is one way to accomplish this. Measuring mailing lists' effectiveness can be done by tracking responses to various lists. Analyzing the effectiveness of promotional activities helps to refine marketing efforts for future CE activities.

Conducting the Meeting Activity

The program planner should arrive early, meet with facility staff to review the program, and make any necessary adjustments. The planner should become familiar with location and use of audiovisual equipment, lighting and temperature controls, and facility layout. A program that follows the time agenda is greatly appreciated by participants, hotel staff, and faculty. If adhering to the timetable does become a problem, getting back on schedule can be achieved by shortening breaks, meal times, or discussion periods.

EVALUATION OF THE CONTINUING EDUCATION PROGRAM

Evaluation is typically perceived as the final activity of CE programming; however, an effective evaluation system is a dynamic, ongoing process integrated into the entire program. Designing an evaluation plan for all the program's components, although complex, is necessary.

Types of Evaluations

Evaluations can assess program design and implementation, marketing activities, participant satisfaction, knowledge/skills gained, and short- and long-term effects on performance.

There are two types of program evaluations: formative and summative. Formative evaluations focus on improving the educational program; summative evaluations focus on measuring program results and outcomes. Kirkpatrick (1967) recommends using a combination of both to assess the participants' reaction to the program, new knowledge and behavioral change. The ASHA Continuing Education Board (1988) recommends both formative evaluations (focused on course content, instructor effectiveness, teaching aids, and general implementation of the activity) and summative evaluations (focused on learner outcomes).

Participants are typical sources of evaluation information; however, speakers, activity planners, outside consultants, and planning team members are also important sources. Using several sources results in the most useful and comprehensive information.

Evaluation Design

Organizing an evaluation by asking a series of who, what, when, and how questions helps planners to focus on evaluation tasks (Levine, Moore, and Pennington 1984). Evaluation should focus on what is important to know about the activity and the learners. Evaluators' perceptions about room/physical arrangements, cost, location, content, speakers' styles and effectiveness, usefulness of the handout materials and audiovisual aids, and satisfaction with the learning objectives can be assessed.

Most CE providers evaluate participant satisfaction; few evaluate the program based on learner outcomes (Sork and Caffarella 1989). Although measuring learner outcome is not appropriate for all CE activities, a general lack of commitment exists on the part of health care educators to assess outcomes and the impact of CE participation on client services (Green and Walsh 1979). Few studies have been undertaken to assess the relationship of CE and quality of care in health care professions, and no impact studies specific to audiology and speech-language pathology are available.

Determining what participants learn and use as a result of CE should be assessed over a period of time. Immediate learning outcomes usually differ from outcomes measured three or six months later. Outcome measures should evaluate the impact of CE on service delivery as well as on participant perceptions and, in some cases, employer perceptions of change in participant performance. Assessing CE impact on clinical service delivery may take longer to assess but is an important part of the evaluation process.

Traditional methods of outcome assessment use paper and pencil tasks to determine cognitive and attitude changes; questionnaires, surveys, and interviews help determine changes in process and behavior. Newer methods include videotaping, role playing, and comparing test performances. Performance tests can assess acquisition of theoretical as well as practical knowledge (Tecker 1981). Evaluating skill outcome is accomplished by videotaping participants, conducting role-play situations, or conducting participant and employer interviews. Using a combination of traditional and contemporary methods strengthens assessment of the relation between CE and learning outcomes (Green and Walsh 1979). Participants' perceptions are typically assessed through questionnaires and group information discussions. Using a questionnaire is the most common method because it is inexpensive, quick, and easy to standardize. The paper and pencil evaluation can include both open- and closed-set questions. Other frequently used methods are brief, informal group discussions at the end of the event, interviews with participants on site, or postevent contacts via telephone (Tecker 1981).

Technology can facilitate data collection and analysis. An optical scanner can automate data entry of closed-set measures (e.g., rating scales). Having participants enter assessment information directly onto a computer terminal is another way to reduce resource demands.

Reporting Results

The evaluation report's content and format depends on its intended audience. A summary of participants' perceptions or a narrative report of the strengths and weaknesses of the event is one approach. Most summaries report percentages. To facilitate comparison, the report format should be consistent from one CE activity to another. Deciding how an evaluation will be used is a critical consideration made early in the program planning stages.

Vital to the evaluation process is analysis of data, review of the final report by planners, and use of information to effect change in future events. A consistent evaluation will yield positive results for CE providers as well as for participants. Well planned and well executed evaluations are investments in the future. They cause the CE provider to re-evaluate learner needs and planning for future activities.

APPENDIX: ACTIVITY PLANNING TIME LINE

18–24 Months Ahead

1.   Conduct needs assessment
2.   Define program purpose and content
3.   Select dates
4.   Select site
5.   Develop preliminary budget
6.   Identify and contact key faculty

12–18 Months Ahead

1.   Develop program
2.   Contact faculty
3.   Develop marketing plan
4.   Contact exhibitors
5.   Sign contract with facility

9–12 Months Ahead

1.   Refine program
2.   Send out contract letters to faculty
3.   Send out meeting announcements and press releases

6–9 Months Ahead

1.   Make arrangements with travel agency
2.   Revise specifications with facility
3.   Refine budget
4.   Book special events
5.   Develop marketing brochure
6.   Decide goals of program evaluation
7.   Decide format of evaluation questions

3–6 Months Ahead

1. Mail brochures to target audience
2. Confirm special events
3. Develop pre-registration materials
4. Finalize special events
5. Pre-test evaluation instrument
6. Decide how to analyze data from evaluation
7. Decide who will receive results of evaluation

6 Weeks Ahead

1. Complete agenda
2. Complete selection of food and beverage needs
3. Prepare educational handout materials
4. Determine audiovisual needs

4 Weeks Ahead

1. Send specification sheets to facility
2. Send rooming lists to facility
3. Review meals and other function selections and advise facility of any change(s)
4. Review final program with faculty
5. Prepare list of participants
6. Prepare materials to be shipped to site
7. Prepare on-site registration materials

2 Weeks Ahead

1. Ship materials to facility
2. Review audiovisual needs with facility
3. Review program with facility

Day Before Meeting

1. Walk through program and facility
2. Review program and room set-up needs
3. Review master billing and facility agreement
4. Meet with responsible facility staff and contacts

REFERENCES

Beck, M. 1990, Winter/Spring. The geezer boom. *Newsweek*, pp. 62–68.
Carson, C. 1989. Choosing the best locations for continuing education pro-

grams. In *Handbook of Marketing of Continuing Education,* eds. R. Simerly and Associates. San Francisco: Jossey-Bass.

Continuing Education Board, American Speech-Language-Hearing Association. 1988. *Continuing Education Board (CEB) Manual.* Rockville, MD: Author.

Cross, K. 1981. *Adults as Learners.* San Francisco: Jossey-Bass.

Draves, W. 1984. *How to Teach Adults.* Manhattan, KS: Learning Resources Network.

Dubin, S. 1990. Maintaining competence through updating. In *Maintaining Professional Competence,* eds. S. Willis and S. Dubin. San Francisco: Jossey-Bass.

Elliot, R. 1989. Increasing the success of direct-mail marketing. In *Handbook of Marketing of Continuing Education,* eds. R. Simerly and Associates. San Francisco: Jossey-Bass.

Fagan, E. 1989. Conferences and workshops are "voter's choice." *Continuing Education Board News Notes* September: 6.

Fagan, E. 1990. ASHA's CE registry continues to add participants. *Continuing Education Board News Notes* May: 5.

Fagan, E. 1991. Facts and figures: Who's your CE audience? *Continuing Education Board News Notes* April: 4.

Fischer, R. 1989. Involving clients in the development and marketing of programs. In *Handbook of Marketing of Continuing Education,* eds. R. Simerly and Associates. San Francisco: Jossey-Bass.

Green, J., and Walsh, P. 1979. Impact evaluation in continuing medical education—the missing link. In *New Directions for Continuing Education: Assessing the Impact of Continuing Education* (no. 3), ed. A. Knox. San Francisco: Jossey-Bass.

Keough, K. 1990. ASHA demographic profile. Rockville, MD: Research Division, American Speech-Language-Hearing Association.

Kershner Report. 1990, April. Alexandria, VA: Kershner & Company, Inc.

Kirkpatrick, D. 1967. Evaluation of training. In *Training and Development Handbook,* eds. R. Craig and L. Bittel. New York: McGraw Hill Book Company.

Levine, H., Cordes, D., Moore, D., Jr., and Pennington, F. 1984. Identifying and assessing needs to relate continuing education to patient care. In *Continuing Education for the Health Professions,* eds. J. Green, S. Grosswald, E. Suter, and D. Walthall, III. San Francisco: Jossey-Bass.

Levine, H., Moore, D., Jr., and Pennington, F. 1984. Evaluating continuing education activities and outcomes. In *Continuing Education for the Health Professions,* eds. J. Green, S. Grosswald, E. Suter, and D. Walthall, III. San Francisco: Jossey-Bass.

Markoe, J. 1989. How to design and lay out successful brochures and catalogues. In *Handbook of Marketing of Continuing Education,* eds. R. Simerly and Associates. San Francisco: Jossey-Bass.

McKinley, J. 1973. Perspectives on diagnostics in adult education. *Viewpoint* 49:69–83.

Patterson, D. 1989. Developing an overall public relations plan and budget. In *Handbook of Marketing of Continuing Education,* eds. R. Simerly and Associates. San Francisco: Jossey-Bass.

Rachal, J. 1989. The social context of adult and continuing education. In *Handbook of Adult and Continuing Education,* eds. S. Merriam and P. Cunningham. San Francisco: Jossey-Bass.

Riggs, J. 1989. Determining an effective marketing mix. In *Handbook of Marketing of Continuing Education,* eds. R. Simerly and Associates. San Francisco: Jossey-Bass.

Simerly, R. 1989a. The strategic role of marketing for organizational success. In

Handbook of Marketing of Continuing Education, eds. R. Simerly and Associates. San Francisco: Jossey-Bass.

Simerly, R. 1989b. Writing effective brochure copy. In *Handbook of Marketing of Continuing Education*, eds. R. Simerly and Associates. San Francisco: Jossey-Bass.

Sork, T., and Caffarella, R. 1989. Planning programs for adults. In *Handbook of Adult and Continuing Education*, eds. S. Merriam and P. Cunningham. San Francisco: Jossey-Bass.

Suter, E. Green, J., Grosswald, F., Lawrence, K. Walthall, D., and Zeleznik, C. 1984. Introduction: Defining quality for continuing education. In *Continuing Education for the Health Professions*, eds. J. Green, S. Grosswald, E. Suter, and D. Walthall, III. San Francisco: Jossey-Bass.

Szczypkowski, R. 1980. Objectives and activities. In *Developing, Administering, and Evaluating Adult Education*, eds. W. Griffith and H. McClusky. San Francisco: Jossey-Bass.

Tecker, G. 1981. Speaker selection and orientation—Learning methodology from A.S.A.E. Education Directors Certificate Program Course #5. Trenton, NJ: Tecker Consultants.

U.S. Bureau of the Census. 1987. *Statistical Abstract of the United States* (107th ed.). Washington, DC: Author.

Working with speakers: An information central executive briefing. 1985. In *Fundamentals of Association Management*, ed. S. Blackwell. Washington, DC: American Society of Association Executives.

Chapter 17

Epilogue:
Integration of Person and Process

Judith A. Rassi and Margaret D. McElroy

The notion of learning as a lifelong process, of involving oneself in some form of continuing education to stay current in a field and/or to upgrade skills has been acknowledged and accepted by many professionals. Certification, licensure, and attendant continuing education requirements notwithstanding, these individuals recognize their own learning needs and seek to have them met. Through journals and books, conventions and teleconferences, workshops and study groups, professionals have unprecedented access to information.

There is little question about input. But what of output? Does received information translate into applied information? Not necessarily. In some cases, it may be applied in a timely fashion; in others, not until years after it was obtained; and, in still others, it may never be applied. Application may not be within a professional's control, depending on work setting, budget, or decision-making constraints. More often, however, there simply may be a reluctance on the part of professionals to institute change. Cloaked in such excuses as being content with current techniques and materials or not having enough time or space, an underlying combination of fear, apathy, and/or inertia may be the real reason for lack of change.

Professionals, by definition, aspire to the highest standards of their profession. High standards presume state-of-the-art practice in administration, clinical service (in CSD), research, and teaching. Each professional is responsible for his/her own continued learning *and* application in each relevant area. This responsibility is critical to advancement of knowledge, to growth of a profession, and to ongoing devel-

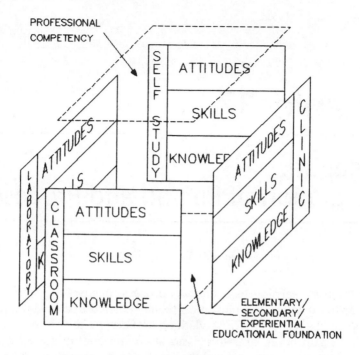

CONCEPTUAL MODEL:
BUILDING AN
INTEGRATED CURRICULUM

Figure 1. Conceptual model: Building an integrated curriculum.

opment of every professional. Relative to the context of this book, continued learning and its applications underscore the importance of these two postulates:

Those who teach at undergraduate, graduate, or continuing education levels in this field are responsible not only for imparting current information but also for using state-of-the-art instructional and supervisory approaches.

Those who teach at undergraduate, graduate, or continuing education levels in this field are responsible for exemplifying and fostering in their students the joy of learning (and of teaching!); the challenge of problem solving; the excitement of experimentation; the gratification of scholarly discourse and exchange of ideas with colleagues; and the rewards of creativity, discovery, and innovation.

Experience, whether administrative, clinical, research, or instructional, has its place in professional growth, but only when supplemented by expert guidance through continuing education efforts, including self-study and other intellectual stimulation. Although trial-and-error approaches sometimes have their place, the practice of subjecting students, or anyone else, to classroom and laboratory instructors with no preparation for teaching or to supervisors with no preparation for supervision is ill-advised.

We wish to end by returning to the concept of an integrated curriculum. As depicted in figure 1, our conceptual visualization of a lifelong-learning curriculum is made up of a foundation with elementary, secondary, and experiential educational bases, upon which rests acquisition of attitudes, skills, and knowledge via four interdependent learning modes—classroom, laboratory, clinic, and self-study. Together, they provide the framework for and give support to professional competency. Two conceptual points are especially noteworthy: (1) curricular balance does not end with higher education, but is necessary for maintaining competency beyond the graduate degree; and (2) self-study must be cultivated throughout the span of lifelong learning, not deferred until the postgraduate continuing education period.

For both teacher and learner—and, eventually, they are one and the same—the integration of person and process should endure a lifetime.

And gladly wolde he lerne, and gladly teche.[1]

---

[1] From Chaucer, Geoffrey. *Canterbury Tales*. 1948. In *Chaucer's Canterbury Tales. An Interlinear Translation*, V. F. Hopper. p. 20, line 308. Woodbury, NY: Barron's Educational Series, Inc.

SECTION V

APPENDICES

Appendix A

Standards for the Certificates of Clinical Competence*

Adopted October 23, 1988
Effective for Applications for Certification Postmarked on
January 1, 1993 and thereafter

The American Speech-Language-Hearing Association issues Certificates of Clinical Competence to individuals who present evidence of their ability to provide independent clinical services to persons who have disorders of communication. Individuals who meet the standards specified by the Association's Council on Professional Standards may be awarded a Certificate of Clinical Competence in Speech-Language Pathology (CCC-SLP) or a Certificate of Clinical Competence in Audiology (CCC-A). Individuals who meet the standards in both professional areas may be awarded both Certificates.

STANDARD I: DEGREE

Applicants for either certificate must have a master's or doctoral degree. Effective January 1, 1994, all graduate coursework and graduate clinical practicum required in the professional area for which the certificate is sought must have been initiated and completed at an institution whose program was accredited by the Educational Standards Board of the American Speech-Language-Hearing Association in the area for which the certificate is sought.

---

*For implementation procedures, see ASHA (1991a).

STANDARD II: ACADEMIC COURSEWORK
(75 SEMESTER CREDIT HOURS)

Applicants for either certificate must have earned at least 75 semester[1] credit hours that reflect a well-integrated program of study dealing with (1) the biological/physical sciences and mathematics, (2) the behavioral and/or social sciences, including normal aspects of human behavior and communication, and (3) the nature, prevention, evaluation, and treatment of speech, language, hearing, and related disorders. The coursework should address, where appropriate, issues pertaining to normal and abnormal human development and behavior across the life span and to culturally diverse populations.
—At least 27 of the 75 semester credit hours must be in Basic Science Coursework (See Standard II-A).
—At least 36 of the 75 semester credit hours must be in Professional Coursework (See Standard II-B).

STANDARD II-A: BASIC SCIENCE COURSEWORK
(27 OF 75 SEMESTER CREDIT HOURS)

Applicants for either certificate must earn at least 27 semester credit hours in the basic sciences.
—At least 6 semester credit hours must be in the biological/physical sciences and mathematics.
—At least 6 semester credit hours must be in the behavioral and/or social sciences.
—At least 15 semester credit hours must be in the basic human communication processes, to include coursework in each of the following three areas of speech, language, and hearing: the anatomic and physiologic bases; the physical and psychophysical bases; the linguistic and psycholinguistic aspects.

STANDARD II-B: PROFESSIONAL COURSEWORK
(36 OF 75 SEMESTER CREDIT HOURS)

Applicants for either certificate must earn at least 36 semester credit hours in courses that concern the nature, prevention, evaluation, and treatment of speech, language, and hearing disorders. Those 36 semester credit hours must encompass courses in speech, language, and hearing that concern disorders primarily affecting children as well as disorders primarily affecting adults. At least 30 of the 36 semester credit hours must be in courses for which graduate credit was received, and at least 21 of those 30 must be in the professional area for which the certificate is sought.

---

[1]One quarter credit hour is equivalent to two-thirds of a semester credit hour.

Certificate of Clinical Competence
in Speech-Language Pathology(CCC-SLP)

—At least 30 of the 36 semester credit hours of professional coursework must be in speech-language pathology. At least 6 of the 30 must be in speech disorders and at least 6 must be in language disorders.

—At least 6 of the 36 semester credit hours of professional coursework must be in audiology. At least 3 of the 6 must be in hearing disorders and hearing evaluation, and at least 3 must be in habilitative/rehabilitative procedures with individuals who have hearing impairment.

—A maximum of 6 academic semester credit hours associated with clinical practicum may be counted toward the minimum of 36 semester credit hours of professional coursework, but those hours may not be used to satisfy the minimum of 6 semester credit hours in speech disorders, 6 hours in language disorders, 6 hours in audiology, or in the 21 graduate credits in the professional area for which the certificate is sought.

Certificate of Clinical Competence in Audiology (CCC-A)

—At least 30 of the 36 semester credit hours of professional coursework must be in audiology. At least 6 of the 30 must be in hearing disorders and hearing evaluation and at least 6 must be in habilitative/rehabilitative procedures with individuals who have hearing impairment. Credits in courses that concern the nature, prevention, evaluation, and treatment of speech and language disorders associated with hearing impairment may be counted.

—At least 6 of the 36 semester credit hours of professional coursework must be in speech-language pathology. At least 3 of the 6 must be in speech disorders and at least 3 must be in language disorders. This coursework in speech-language pathology must concern the nature, prevention, evaluation, and treatment of speech and language disorders not associated with hearing impairment.

—A maximum of 6 academic semester credit hours associated with clinical practicum may be counted toward the minimum of 36 semester credit hours of professional coursework, but those hours may not be used to satisfy the minimum of 6 semester credit hours in hearing disorders/evaluation, 6 hours in habilitative/rehabilitative procedures, 6 hours in speech-language pathology, or in the 21 graduate credits in the professional area for which the certificate is sought.

STANDARD III: SUPERVISED CLINICAL OBSERVATION AND PRACTICUM
(375 CLOCK HOURS)

Applicants for either certificate must complete the requisite number of clock hours of supervised clinical observation and supervised clinical practicum that are provided by the educational institution or by one of its cooperating programs. The supervision must be provided by an individual who holds the Certificate of Clinical Competence in the appropriate area of practice.

STANDARD III-A: CLINICAL OBSERVATION
(25 CLOCK HOURS)

Applicants for either certificate must complete at least 25 clock hours of supervised observation prior to beginning the initial clinical practicum. Those 25 clock hours must concern the evaluation and treatment of children and adults with disorders of speech, language, or hearing.

STANDARD III-B: CLINICAL PRACTICUM
(350 CLOCK HOURS)

Applicants for either certificate must complete at least 350 hours of supervised clinical practicum that concern the evaluation and treatment of children and adults with disorders of speech, language, and hearing. No more than 25 of the clock hours may be obtained from participation in staffings in which evaluation, treatment, and/or recommendations are discussed or formulated, with or without the client present.
—At least 250 of the 350 clock hours must be completed in the professional area for which the certificate is sought while the applicant is engaged in graduate study.
—At least 50 supervised clock hours must be completed in each of three types of clinical settings.

Certificate of Clinical Competence
in Speech-Language Pathology (CCC-SLP)

The applicant must have experience in the evaluation and treatment of children and adults, and with a variety of types and severities of disorders of speech[2], language, and hearing.
—At least 250 of the 350 supervised clock hours must be in speech-language pathology. At least 20 of those 250 hours must be completed in each of the eight categories listed below:
1. Evaluation: Speech disorders in children
2. Evaluation: Speech disorders in adults
3. Evaluation: Language disorders in children
4. Evaluation: Language disorders in adults
5. Treatment: Speech disorders in children
6. Treatment: Speech disorders in adults
7. Treatment: Language disorders in children
8. Treatment: Language disorders in adults
—Up to 20 clock hours in the major professional area may be in related disorders.
—At least 35 of the 350 clock hours must be in audiology. At least 15 of those 35 clock hours must involve the evaluation or screening of indi-

[2]"Speech" disorders include disorders of articulation, voice, and fluency.

viduals for hearing disorders, and at least 15 must involve habilitation/ rehabilitation of individuals who have hearing impairment.

Certificate of Clinical Competence in Audiology (CCC-A)

The applicant must have experience with the evaluation and treatment[3] of children and adults, with a variety of types and severities of disorders of hearing, speech, and language, and with the selection and use of amplification and assistive devices.

—At least 250 of the 350 supervised clock hours must be in audiology. At least 40 of those 250 clock hours must be completed in each of the first four categories listed below,[4] and at least 20 of those 250 clock hours must be completed in the fifth category:
1. Evaluation: Hearing in children
2. Evaluation: Hearing in adults
3. Selection and use: Amplification and assistive devices for children
4. Selection and use: Amplification and assistive devices for adults
5. Treatment: Hearing disorders in children and adults
—Up to 20 clock hours in the major professional area may be in related disorders.
—At least 35 of the 350 clock hours must be in speech-language pathology. At least 15 of those 35 clock hours must involve the evaluation or screening of individuals for speech and language disorders unrelated to hearing impairment, and at least 15 must involve the treatment of individuals with speech and language disorders unrelated to hearing impairment.

STANDARD IV: NATIONAL EXAMINATIONS IN SPEECH-LANGUAGE PATHOLOGY AND AUDIOLOGY

Applicants must pass the national examination in the area for which the certificate is sought.

STANDARD V: THE CLINICAL FELLOWSHIP

After completion of the academic coursework (Standard II) and clinical observation and clinical practicum (Standard III), the applicant then must successfully complete a clinical fellowship. The fellowship shall consist of at least

---

[3]"Treatment" for hearing disorders refers to clinical management and counseling, including auditory training, speech reading, and speech and language services for those with hearing impairment.

[4]This section of Standard III B has been revised so that: "At least 80 hours must be completed in categories 3 and 4 with a minimum of 10 hours in each of these categories." See ASHA (1990, 1991b).

36 weeks of full-time professional experience or its part-time equivalent. The fellowship must be completed under the supervision of an individual who holds the Certificate of Clinical Competence in the area for which the certificate is sought.

— The professional experience shall primarily involve clinical activities.

— The supervisor shall periodically conduct a formal evaluation of the applicant's progress in development of professional skills.

REFERENCES

American Speech-Language-Hearing Association. 1990. Council on Professional Standards. Revision of certification standards and clarification of ESB standards. *Asha* 32(12):81.

American Speech-Language-Hearing Association. 1991a. Clinical Certification Board. Implementation procedures for the standards for the certificates of clinical competence. *Asha* 33(5):47–53.

American Speech-Language-Hearing Association. 1991b. Council on Professional Standards. Revision of certification standard IIIB, clinical practicum, CCC-A. *Asha* 33(6/7):65.

American Speech-Language-Hearing Association. 1991c. Standards for the certificates of clinical competence. *Asha* 33(3):121–22.

Appendix B

Standards for Accreditation of Educational Programs

Final Revised Standards
Effective January 1, 1993

(The effective date applies to all programs regardless of their accreditation status on that date.)

The American Speech-Language-Hearing Association (ASHA) is committed to ensuring that quality speech-language pathology and audiology services are provided to the public. The ASHA believes that the quality of educational preparation for delivery of clinical services is highly correlated with the quality of services provided by certified professional practitioners. Consequently, the ASHA maintains a system of accreditation for college and university educational programs that offer a master's degree[1] with a major emphasis in speech-language pathology and/or audiology. Although quality education can be achieved in a variety of ways, the Association's Council on Professional Standards in Speech-Language Pathology and Audiology (Standards Council) believes that certain components are essential to effect quality education in the profession. Five areas have been delineated for the establishment of standards for accreditation of master's-level educational programs:

— administration
— instructional staff
— curriculum
— clinical education
— program self-analysis

The Standards Council has adopted the following standards as necessary conditions for accreditation of educational programs at the master's level.[1] **Pro-**

---

[1]Wording changes have been proposed to expand the scope of ESB accreditation "to include professional preparation components of doctoral degree programs, as well as master's programs. . . . " See ASHA (1991a).

grams must satisfy all standards to be awarded accreditation. The Educational Standards Board (ESB) of the ASHA has the responsibility to evaluate the adequacy of the program's efforts in satisfying each requirement. The ESB recognizes that a variety of means may be available to satisfy each of the Standards.

Compliance with the following standards represents the minimum requirements for accreditation. The Standards Council and the ESB encourage programs to exceed these Standards to achieve educational excellence.

STANDARD 1.0: ADMINISTRATION

The program must have an administrative structure that provides reasonable autonomy for the academic and clinical program within the institution, reasonable access to the higher levels of administration, and appropriate and sufficient resources with which to carry out its mission.

1.1   The applicant institution must have regional accreditation.

1.2   The applicant institution must comply with the laws, regulations, and executive orders with respect to equitable treatment of students, staff, and clients without regard to gender, sexual orientation, age, race, creed, national origin, or handicapping condition.

1.3   The program must have physical facilities (classrooms, offices, clinic rooms, research laboratories), instructional materials, equipment, library holdings, and support services that are appropriate and sufficient to meet its present needs and its projected needs during the accreditation period.

1.4   The program must have an appropriate curriculum that leads to a master's degree[1] with a major emphasis in speech-language pathology and/or audiology.

1.5   The program must have criteria for accepting students for graduate study in speech-language pathology and/or audiology that are consistent with the institutional policy for admission to graduate study.

1.6   The person responsible for the program of professional education must hold a graduate degree with a major emphasis in speech-language pathology, audiology, or in speech, language, or hearing science and must hold a full-time appointment in the institution.

1.7   The applicant institution must make regular budgetary allocations for personnel, space, equipment, and materials that are appropriate and sufficient for the continued operation of the program.

1.8   The program must maintain documentation on each of its students that verifies how the student has satisfactorily completed each requirement for the graduate degree and for the ASHA CCC. That documentation must be made available to the student upon request.

1.9   The program must maintain adequate records to assist students in meeting state certification and licensure requirements.

1.10   The program must demonstrate how information concerning its accreditation status, resources, admission policies and standards, academic offerings, policies with regard to satisfactory academic progress, fees and other charges and graduation rates and requirements does not mislead students, prospective students or the public.

STANDARD 2.0:   INSTRUCTIONAL STAFF

The program must have an instructional staff who competently teach the academic and clinical components of the speech-language pathology and audiology program for which they are responsible.

2.1   The instructional staff must be sufficient in number to meet the instructional, clinical, research, and advising responsibilities without carrying a greater load than is traditional for instructional staff in the applicant institution.

2.2   There must be at least three full-time instructional staff members in the program who hold earned doctorates from regionally accredited institutions. There must be at least one full-time doctoral-level member of the instructional staff whose major emphasis in doctoral study was in the area(s) for which accreditation is sought. Further, at least three full-time equivalent members of the instructional staff must have earned doctorates with a major emphasis in [communication sciences and/or disorders][2].

2.3   There must be at least two full-time members of the instructional staff who hold the ASHA CCC in each area for which accreditation is sought, each of whom contribute full-time in that area. If the program seeks accreditation in only one area, there must be at least one additional full-time equivalent member of the instructional staff holding the ASHA CCC in the other area.

2.4   A reasonable portion of a student's academic contacts must be with members of the instructional staff holding full-time appointments in the program.

2.5   Programs that have undergraduate, doctoral, or other educational offerings[1] must demonstrate that sufficient personnel are available to ensure the quality of the master's education in speech-language pathology and audiology.

2.6   The program must ensure that the instructional staff/student ratio at the master's level[1] is at least one full-time equivalent member of the instructional staff to each six full-time equivalent master's level students in the program.

2.7   There must be a demonstrated commitment by the applicant institution with regard to full-time instructional staff that will ensure the continuity of the program.

2.8   The program must provide opportunities for and ensure that its instructional staff members do continue their own professional education.

STANDARD 3.0:   CURRICULUM

The program must have appropriate and sufficient curricular offerings to support the mission, goals, and objectives established by its instructional staff.

3.1   The instructional staff must have responsibility for making decisions regarding the substance of academic and clinical education (i.e., supervised clinical practicum experiences) in speech-language pathology and audiology.

---

[2]This part of the Standard 2.2 statement has been clarified to read: " . . . in speech-language pathology, audiology or in speech, language, or hearing science." See ASHA (1991b).

3.2   The curriculum must reflect a commitment to the scientific and research bases of the profession.

3.3   The curriculum must be updated on an ongoing basis to reflect current knowledge, technology, and scope of practice.

3.4   The program's curriculum must be sufficient to permit students to fulfill Standard II of the ASHA *Standards for the Certificates of Clinical Competence* in the area(s) in which accreditation is sought, or it must demonstrate how its students meet those requirements. If appropriate coursework to meet those requirements is taken in other departments of the program's institution or at other colleges and universities, the program must show how the course content and quality of instruction meet the requirements of Standard II of the ASHA *Standards for the Certificates of Clinical Competence.*

3.5   The program must establish and maintain an appropriate sequence of academic and clinical education that adheres to the principle that the basic sciences of communication should *precede* the study of communication disorders and their treatment.

3.6   The program must establish and maintain an appropriate sequence of academic and clinical education that adheres to the principle that appropriate professional coursework in communication should precede, or be concurrent with, clinical education in those disorders.

3.7   The program must include instruction in the current ASHA Code of Ethics, the current ASHA *Standards for the Certificates of Clinical Competence* when appropriate, current state certification and licensure requirements.

STANDARD 4.0:   CLINICAL EDUCATION

Clinical education that reflects current knowledge, technology, and scope of practice and that meets the standards and ethics of the ASHA is vital to the development of competent speech-language pathologists and audiologists.

4.1   The program must demonstrate that it has access to a client base sufficiently large and diverse to permit students to fulfill the ASHA *Standards for the Certificates of Clinical Competence* in the area(s) in which accreditation is sought.

4.2   The program must ensure that each student's clinical observations that are used to meet Standard III-A of the ASHA *Standards for the Certificates of Clinical Competence* are in compliance with that standard.

4.3   The program must be able to provide students with all clinical education necessary to fulfill the ASHA *Standards for the Certificates of Clinical Competence* in the area(s) in which accreditation is sought.

4.4   The program must ensure that students earn clinical clock hours only for time during which they are involved in providing services for the client or the client's family as specified by Standard III-B of the ASHA *Standards for the Certificates of Clinical Competence.*

4.5   The program must ensure that all clinical education in speech-language pathology and audiology, both on and off the campus, is supervised by persons holding the ASHA CCC in the appropriate area.

4.6   Clinical education obtained outside the jurisdiction of the program must be coordinated and monitored by a member of the program's instructional staff holding the ASHA CCC.

4.7 The program must ensure that supervised clinical education is obtained as specified by Standard III-B of the ASHA *Standards for the Certificates of Clinical Competence.*

4.8 The program must ensure that the first 25 hours of each student's supervised clinical education provided by that program are supervised directly by a member of the program's instructional staff.

4.9 The program must ensure that the nature and amount of clinical supervision is adjusted to the experience and ability of the student and that appropriate guidance and feedback are provided to the student.

— At least 50% of *each diagnostic evaluation,* including screening and identification, in speech-language pathology and audiology must be observed directly by the supervisor.

— At least 25% of *each student's total contact time in clinical treatment with each client* must be observed directly by the supervisor. Observation of clinical treatment must be scheduled appropriately throughout the treatment period.

4.10 The program must ensure that all major decisions by students regarding evaluation and treatment of a client are implemented or communicated only after approval by the supervisor.

4.11 The program must ensure that the welfare of each client served by its students is protected. A person holding the appropriate ASHA CCC must be available on site for consultation at all times when a student is providing clinical services as part of the student's clinical education, both on and off the campus.

STANDARD 5.0: PROGRAM SELF ANALYSIS

The program's administration and instructional staff must have a mechanism for ongoing, systematic appraisal of program strengths and limitations in order to accommodate and plan for those changes that are necessary to provide the highest quality education possible.

5.1 The program must have clearly specified goals and objectives that are consistent with its academic and clinical mission and with the mission of the applicant institution. The instructional staff must be aware of those goals and objectives and must critically evaluate the ways in which they are achieved.

5.2 The program must have ongoing plans for evaluating the currency and effectiveness of both academic and clinical education and must demonstrate how it uses the results of those evaluations to achieve its goals and objectives and to improve its quality.

5.3 The program must make verifiable and ongoing evaluations of the academic and clinical preparation of its students and must document specific outcome measures that are used in those evaluations, including, for example, data on the percentage of students who successfully complete the master's program[1] in the area for which accreditation is sought, and the percentage of students who pass the NESPA examination in the area for which accreditation is sought. The program further must demonstrate how those evaluations are used to improve educational preparation of its students.

5.4   The program must have verifiable and consistent mechanisms that are ongoing and that are utilized for the periodic assessment of the quality and effectiveness of the professional performance of its graduates for at least a five-year period. The program also must demonstrate the ways in which those assessment data are used to improve preparation of students.

5.5   The program must engage in a continuing process of self-analysis and appropriate modification in order to establish and maintain a high quality academic and clinical education in speech-language pathology and audiology.

REFERENCES

American Speech-Language-Hearing Association. 1990. Standards for accreditation of educational programs. *Asha* 32(6/7):93-94, 100.

American Speech-Language-Hearing Association. 1991a. Council on Professional Standards. Proposed change in scope of ESB accreditation. *Asha* 33(3):97.

American Speech-Language-Hearing Association. 1991b. Council on Professional Standards. Revision of certification standards and clarification of ESB standards. *Asha* 32(12):81.

Appendix C

Clinical Supervision in Speech-Language Pathology and Audiology

TASKS OF SUPERVISION

A central premise of supervision is that effective clinical teaching involves, in a fundamental way, the development of self-analysis, self-evaluation, and problem-solving skills on the part of the individual being supervised. The success of clinical teaching rests largely on the achievement of this goal. Further, the demonstration of quality clinical skills in supervisors is generally accepted as a prerequisite to supervision of students, as well as those in the Clinical Fellowship Year or employed as certified speech-language pathologists or audiologists.

Outlined in this paper are 13 tasks basic to effective clinical teaching and constituting the distinct area of practice which comprises clinical supervision in communication disorders. The committee stresses that the level of preparation and experience of the supervisee, the particular work setting of the supervisor and supervisee, and client variables will influence the relative emphasis of each task in actual practice.

The tasks and their supporting competencies which follow are judged to have face validity as established by experts in the area of supervision, and by both select and widespread peer review. The committee recognizes the need for further validation and strongly encourages ongoing investigation. Until such time as more rigorous measures of validity are established, it will be particularly important for the tasks and competencies to be reviewed periodically through quality assurance procedures. Mechanisms such as Patient Care Audit and Child Services Review System appear to offer useful means for quality assurance in the supervisory tasks and competencies. Other procedures appropriate to specific work settings may also be selected.

The tasks of supervision discussed above follow:

1. establishing and maintaining an effective working relationship with the supervisee;

2. assisting the supervisee in developing clinical goals and objectives;
3. assisting the supervisee in developing and refining assessment skills;
4. assisting the supervisee in developing and refining clinical management skills;
5. demonstrating for and participating with the supervisee in the clinical process;
6. assisting the supervisee in observing and analyzing assessment and treatment sessions;
7. assisting the supervisee in the development and maintenance of clinical and supervisory records;
8. interacting with the supervisee in planning, executing, and analyzing supervisory conferences;
9. assisting the supervisee in evaluation of clinical performance;
10. assisting the supervisee in developing skills of verbal reporting, writing, and editing;
11. sharing information regarding ethical, legal, regulatory, and reimbursement aspects of professional practice;
12. modeling and facilitating professional conduct; and
13. demonstrating research skills in the clinical or supervisory processes.

COMPETENCIES FOR EFFECTIVE CLINICAL SUPERVISION

Although the competencies are listed separately according to task, each competency may be needed to perform a number of supervisor tasks.

1.0 Task: Establishing and maintaining an effective working relationship with the supervisee.

Competencies required:

1.1 Ability to facilitate an understanding of the clinical and supervisory processes.

1.2 Ability to organize and provide information regarding the logical sequences of supervisory interaction, that is, joint setting of goals and objectives, data collection and analysis, evaluation.

1.3 Ability to interact from a contemporary perspective with the supervisee in both the clinical and supervisory process.

1.4 Ability to apply learning principles in the supervisory process.

1.5 Ability to apply skills of interpersonal communication in the supervisory process.

1.6 Ability to facilitate independent thinking and problem solving by the supervisee.

1.7 Ability to maintain a professional and supportive relationship that allows supervisor and supervisee growth.

1.8 Ability to interact with the supervisee objectively.

1.9 Ability to establish joint communications regarding expectations and responsibilities in the clinical and supervisory processes.

1.10 Ability to evaluate, with the supervisee, the effectiveness of the ongoing supervisory relationship.

2.0 Task: Assisting the supervisee in developing clinical goals and objectives.
Competencies required:
    2.1 Ability to assist the supervisee in planning effective client goals and objectives.
    2.2 Ability to plan, with the supervisee, effective goals and objectives for clinical and professional growth.
    2.3 Ability to assist the supervisee in using observation and assessment in preparation of client goals and objectives.
    2.4 Ability to assist the supervisee in using self-analysis and previous evaluation in preparation of goals and objectives for professional growth.
    2.5 Ability to assist the supervisee in assigning priorities to clinical goals and objectives.
    2.6 Ability to assist the supervisee in assigning priorities to goals and objectives for professional growth.
3.0 Task: Assisting the supervisee in developing and refining assessment skills.
Competencies required:
    3.1 Ability to share current research findings and evaluation procedures in communication disorders.
    3.2 Ability to facilitate an integration of research findings in client assessment.
    3.3 Ability to assist the supervisee in providing rationale for assessment procedures.
    3.4 Ability to assist supervisee in communicating assessment procedures and rationales.
    3.5 Ability to assist the supervisee in integrating findings and observations to make appropriate recommendations.
    3.6 Ability to facilitate the supervisee's independent planning of assessment.
4.0 Task: Assisting the supervisee in developing and refining management skills.
Competencies required:
    4.1 Ability to share current research findings and management procedures in communication disorders.
    4.2 Ability to facilitate an integration of research findings in client management.
    4.3 Ability to assist the supervisee in providing rationale for treatment procedures.
    4.4 Ability to assist the supervisee in identifying appropriate sequences for client change.
    4.5 Ability to assist the supervisee in adjusting steps in the progression toward a goal.
    4.6 Ability to assist the supervisee in the description and measurement of client and clinician change.
    4.7 Ability to assist the supervisee in documenting client and clinician change.

4.8 Ability to assist the supervisee in integrating documented client and clinician change to evaluate progress and specify future recommendations.

5.0 Task: Demonstrating for and participating with the supervisee in the clinical process.

Competencies required:

5.1 Ability to determine jointly when demonstration is appropriate.

5.2 Ability to demonstrate or participate in an effective client-clinician relationship.

5.3 Ability to demonstrate a variety of clinical techniques and participate with the supervisee in clinical management.

5.4 Ability to demonstrate or use jointly the specific materials and equipment of the profession.

5.5 Ability to demonstrate or participate jointly in counseling of clients or family/guardians of clients.

6.0 Task: Assisting the supervisee in observing and analyzing assessment and treatment sessions.

Competencies required:

6.1 Ability to assist the supervisee in learning a variety of data collection procedures.

6.2 Ability to assist the supervisee in selecting and executing data collection procedures.

6.3 Ability to assist the supervisee in accurately recording data.

6.4 Ability to assist the supervisee in analyzing and interpreting data objectively.

6.5 Ability to assist the supervisee in revising plans for client management based on data obtained.

7.0 Task: Assisting the supervisee in development and maintenance of clinical and supervisory records.

Competencies required:

7.1 Ability to assist the supervisee in applying record-keeping systems to supervisory and clinical processes.

7.2 Ability to assist the supervisee in effectively documenting supervisory and clinically related interactions.

7.3 Ability to assist the supervisee in organizing records to facilitate easy retrieval of information concerning clinical and supervisory interactions.

7.4 Ability to assist the supervisee in establishing and following policies and procedures to protect the confidentiality of clinical and supervisory records.

7.5 Ability to share information regarding documentation requirements of various accrediting and regulatory agencies and third-party funding sources.

8.0 Task: Interacting with the supervisee in planning, executing, and analyzing supervisory conferences.

Competencies required:

8.1 Ability to determine with the supervisee when a conference should be scheduled.

8.2 Ability to assist the supervisee in planning a supervisory conference agenda.

8.3 Ability to involve the supervisee in jointly establishing a conference agenda.

8.4 Ability to involve the supervisee in joint discussion of previously identified clinical or supervisory data or issues.

8.5 Ability to interact with the supervisee in a manner that facilitates the supervisee's self exploration and problem solving.

8.6 Ability to adjust conference content based on the supervisee's level of training and experience.

8.7 Ability to encourage and maintain supervisee motivation for continuing self-growth.

8.8 Ability to assist the supervisee in making commitments for changes in clinical behavior.

8.9 Ability to involve the supervisee in ongoing analysis of supervisory interactions.

9.0 Task: Assisting the supervisee in evaluation of clinical performance.
Competencies required:

9.1 Ability to assist the supervisee in the use of clinical evaluation tools.

9.2 Ability to assist the supervisee in the description and measurement of his/her progress and achievement.

9.3 Ability to assist the supervisee in developing skills of self-evaluation.

9.4 Ability to evaluate clinical skills with the supervisee for purposes of grade assignment, completion of Clinical Fellowship Year, professional advancement, and so on.

10.0 Task: Assisting the supervisee in developing skills of verbal reporting, writing, and editing.
Competencies required:

10.1 Ability to assist the supervisee in identifying appropriate information to be included in a verbal or written report.

10.2 Ability to assist the supervisee in presenting information in a logical, concise, and sequential manner.

10.3 Ability to assist the supervisee in using appropriate professional terminology and style in verbal and written reporting.

10.4 Ability to assist the supervisee in adapting verbal and written reports to the work environment and communication situation.

10.5 Ability to alter and edit a report as appropriate while preserving the supervisee's writing style.

11.0 Task: Sharing information regarding ethical, legal, regulatory, and reimbursement aspects of the profession.
Competencies required:

11.1 Ability to communicate to the supervisee a knowledge of professional codes of ethics (e.g., ASHA, state licensing boards, and so on).

11.2 Ability to communicate to the supervisee an understanding of legal and regulatory documents and their impact on the practice of the profession (licensure, PL 94-142, Medicare, Medicaid, and so on).

11.3 Ability to communicate to the supervisee an understanding of reimbursement policies and procedures of the work setting.

11.4 Ability to communicate to the supervisee rights and appeal procedures specific to the work setting.

12.0 Task: Modeling and facilitating professional conduct.
Competencies required:

12.1 Ability to assume responsibility.

12.2 Ability to analyze, evaluate, and modify own behavior.

12.3 Ability to demonstrate ethical and legal conduct.

12.4 Ability to meet and respect deadlines.

12.5 Ability to maintain professional protocols (respect for confidentiality, etc.).

12.6 Ability to provide current information regarding professional standards (PSB, ESB, licensure, teacher certification, etc.).

12.7 Ability to communicate information regarding fees, billing procedures, and third-party reimbursement.

12.8 Ability to demonstrate familiarity with professional issues.

12.9 Ability to demonstrate continued professional growth.

13.0 Task: Demonstrating research skills in the clinical or supervisory processes.
Competencies required:

13.1 Ability to read, interpret, and apply clinical and supervisory research.

13.2 Ability to formulate clinical or supervisory research questions.

13.3 Ability to investigate clinical or supervisory research questions.

13.4 Ability to support and refute clinical or supervisory research findings.

13.5 Ability to report results of clinical or supervisory research and disseminate as appropriate (e.g., in-service, conferences, publications).

REFERENCE

American Speech-Language-Hearing Association. 1985. Committee on Supervision in Speech-Language Pathology and Audiology. Position Statement. *Asha* 27(6):57–60.

Appendix D

Questions to Consider in Evaluating a College Course

Consider each of the following questions and check those that are appropriate for the specific course you are evaluating.

I.   Course Rationale
    _____ A. What population of students is the course intended to serve?
    _____ B. What student needs is the course intended to service?
    _____ C. What institutional, community or societal needs is the course intended to serve?
    _____ D. What other defensible reasons exist for offering this course?
    _____ E. What other courses serve these same needs?
    _____ F. To what extent does this course overlap with or duplicate these other courses?
    _____ G. On what grounds is the continued existence of this course justified and warranted?

II.   Development and Current Status of the Course
    _____ A. When and under what circumstances was the course developed?
    _____ B. How frequently and how regularly has the course been offered?
    _____ C. To what extent has the enrollment increased, decreased or stabilized from year to year?
    _____ D. What problems have been associated with the course and how have they been resolved?
    _____ E. To what extent is the course intended to be replicable from instructor to instructor or from term to term?
    _____ F. To what degree do the plans or design for the course exist in a written or documented form? In what documents (course approval forms, course outlines or syllabi, memos, etc.) do these plans exist?

_____ G. How does the current version of the course differ from earlier versions? Why?

III.   Credit and Curricular Implications

_____ A. What credit is awarded for successful completion of the course? On what basis is this credit allocation justifiable?

_____ B. In what ways can credit for this course be applied towards fulfillment of graduate and degree requirements?

_____ C. At what level (lower division, upper division or graduate) is the course classified? Why? On what basis is this classification justified?

_____ D. How does the course fit into the overall curriculum of the sponsoring department and college?

_____ E. In which departments is the course cross-listed? Why? How does it fit into the curriculum of these departments or colleges?

_____ F. What prerequisite skills or experiences are needed in order to succeed in this course?

_____ G. What problems are experienced by students who do not have these prerequisites?

IV.   Course Objectives

_____ A. What are the formal, stated objectives of the course?

_____ B. How feasible and realistic are these objectives in terms of the abilities of the target population and the available time and resources?

_____ C. How are the stated objectives related to the adult life-role competencies students will need in everyday life outside of school?

_____ D. How are the objectives related to the competencies students will need in their subsequent academic careers?

_____ E. If the course is designed to prepare students for a specific professional or vocational field, how are the objectives related to the competencies they are likely to need in their future careers?

_____ F. What values are affirmed by the choice of these objectives as goals for this course?

_____ G. What other purposes, intents, or goals do the faculty, administrators, and other interested audiences have for the course?

_____ H. What goals and expectations do students have for the course?

_____ I. To what extent are these additional goals and expectations compatible with the stated course objectives?

V.   The Content of the Course

_____ A. What (1) information, (2) processes, and (3) attitudes and values constitute the subject-matter or content of the course?

_____ B. How are the various content elements related to the course's objectives?

     _____ 1. Which objectives receive the most coverage or emphasis? Why?

_____ 2. Which objectives receive only minor coverage? Why?

_____ C. How is the content sequenced or arranged? Why is this sequence appropriate/inappropriate?

_____ D. What means are used to integrate and unify the various elements into a coherent pattern or structure? To what extent does fragmentation or lack of coherence appear to be a problem?

_____ E. What values and assumptions are implicit in the decisions which have been made regarding content selection and emphasis?

VI.   Instructional Strategies

_____ A. What kinds of learning activities are utilized?

      _____ 1. What activities are the students expected to engage in during class sessions?

      _____ 2. What assignments or projects are students expected to complete outside of class?

      _____ 3. In what ways are these activities appropriate or inappropriate in light of the course objectives?

      _____ 4. How could these activities be made more effective?

_____ B. What instructional materials are utilized?

      _____ 1. How and for what purpose are the materials used?

      _____ 2. How accurate and up-to-date are the materials?

      _____ 3. In what ways do the materials need to be improved?

      _____ 4. How could the materials be utilized more effectively?

_____ C. What instructional roles or functions are performed by the teacher(s)?

      _____ 1. How could these roles be performed more effectively?

      _____ 2. What important instructional roles are not provided or are performed inadequately? Why?

_____ D. What premises and assumptions about learning and the nature of the learner underly the selection of instructional strategies? How and to what extent are these assumptions warranted?

VII.   Procedures and Criteria for Evaluating Students' Achievements

_____ A. What instruments and procedures are employed as a means of collecting evidence of the students' progress and achievement?

_____ B. What criteria are used to assess the adequacy of the students' work and/or achievement? On what basis were these criteria selected?

_____ C. How well do the assessment procedures correspond with the course content and objectives? Which objectives or content areas are not assessed? Why?

———— D.   To what extent do the assessment procedures appear to be fair and objective?

———— E.   What evidence is there that the assessment instruments and procedures yield valid and reliable results?

———— F.   How are the assessment results used? Are the results shared with the students within a reasonable amount of time?

———— G.   How consistently are the assessment criteria applied from instructor to instructor and from term to term?

———— H.   What indications are there that the amount of assessment is excessive, about right or insufficient?

VIII.   Organization of the Course

———— A.   How is the course organized in terms of lectures, labs, studios, discussion sections, field trips and other types of scheduled class sessions?

———— B.   How frequently and for how long are the various types of class meetings scheduled? Is the total allocation of time sufficient/insufficient? Why?

———— C.   If there is more than one instructor, what are the duties and responsibilities of each? What problems result from this division of responsibilities?

———— D.   What outside-of-class instruction, tutoring or counseling is provided? By whom? On what basis?

———— E.   How well is the student workload distributed throughout the course?

———— F.   To what extent are the necessary facilities, equipment, and materials readily available and in good working condition when needed?

IX.   Course Outcomes

———— A.   What proportion of the enrollees completed the course with credit during the regular term? How does the completion rate vary from instructor to instructor or from term to term?

———— B.   What proportion of the enrollees withdrew from or discontinued attending the course? Why?

    ———— 1.   To what degree does their discontinuance appear to be related to factors associated with the course?

    ———— 2.   How does the attrition rate vary from instructor to instructor or from term to term?

———— C.   At the end of the course, what evidence is there that students have achieved the stated objectives?

    ———— 1.   For which objectives was the course most/least successful?

    ———— 2.   For what kinds of students was the course most/least successful?

———— D.   What effects does the course appear to have had upon students' interest in the subject-matter and their desire to continue studying and learning about this subject?

_____ E. What other effects did the course have upon the students?
     _____ 1. How were their values, attitudes, priorities, interests or aspirations changed?
     _____ 2. How were their study habits or other behavioral patterns modified?
     _____ 3. How pervasive and/or significant do these effects appear to be?
_____ F. What evidence is there that students who have completed this course were adequately/inadequately prepared for subsequent courses for which this course is intended to prepare them?
_____ G. To what extent do students rate their experience in the course as producing a meaningful and worthwhile contribution to their self-development?
     _____ 1. In what ways were the students satisfied or dissatisfied with the course?
     _____ 2. What suggestions do they have for improving the course?
_____ H. What evidence is there, if any, that the experience of teaching the course has a positive or negative effect upon faculty members?

X.   Institutional Costs & Benefits
_____ A. What are the time, space, equipment and facilities requirements of the course?
_____ B. What are the requirements of the course in terms of faculty and staff?
_____ C. What other support services are required by the course?
_____ D. What direct instructional costs are associated with this course?
_____ E. What benefits derive to the department, the college and the institution for having offered this course?

REFERENCE

Sudweeks, R. R., and Diamond, R. M. 1989. Questions to consider in evaluating a college course. In *Designing and Improving Courses and Curricula in Higher Education. A Systematic Approach,* ed. R. M. Diamond. San Francisco: Jossey-Bass. Reproduced with permission of publisher.

Index

(Page numbers in italics indicate material in tables or figures)